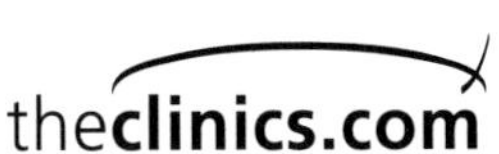

A. Simon Turner, BVSc, MS
CONSULTING EDITOR

VETERINARY CLINICS OF NORTH AMERICA

Equine Practice

Wound Management

GUEST EDITOR
Christine L. Theoret, DMV, PhD

April 2005 • Volume 21 • Number 1

SAUNDERS

An Imprint of Elsevier, Inc.
PHILADELPHIA LONDON TORONTO MONTREAL SYDNEY TOKYO

W.B. SAUNDERS COMPANY
A Division of Elsevier Inc.

The Curtis Center • Independence Square West • Philadelphia, Pennsylvania 19106

http://www.vetequine.theclinics.com

THE VETERINARY CLINICS OF NORTH AMERICA: EQUINE PRACTICE
April 2005
Editor: John Vassallo

Volume 21, Number 1
ISSN 0749-0739
ISBN 1-4160-2836-6

The Veterinary Clinics of North America: Equine Practice (ISSN 0749-0739) is published in April, August, and December by W.B. Saunders Company. Corporate and editorial offices: The Curtis Center, Independence Square West, Philadelphia, PA 19106-3399. Accounting and circulation offices: 6277 Sea Harbor Drive, Orlando, FL 32887-4800. Subscription prices are $145.00 per year for US individuals, $230.00 per year for US institutions, $73.00 per year for US students and residents, $169.00 per year for Canadian individuals, $285.00 per year for Canadian institutions, $185.00 per year for international individuals, $285.00 per year for international institutions and $93.00 per year for Canadian and foreign students/residents. To receive student/resident rate, orders must be accompanied by name of affiliated institution, date of term, and the *signature* of program/residency coordinator on institution letterhead. Orders will be billed at individual rate until proof of status is received. Foreign air speed delivery is included in all *Clinics* subscription prices. All prices are subject to change without notice. POSTMASTER: Send address changes to *The Veterinary Clinics of North America: Equine Practice*, Elsevier, Customer Service Department, 6277 Sea Harbor Drive, Orlando, FL 32887-4800, USA; phone: (+1) (877) 8397126 [toll free number for US customers], or (+1) (407) 3454020 [customers outside US]; fax: (+1) (407) 3631354; e-mail: usjcs@elsevier.com

Reprints. For copies of 100 or more, of articles in this publication, please contact the Commercial Reprints Department, Elsevier Inc., 360 Park Avenue South, New York, New York 10010-1710. Tel. (212) 633-3813 Fax: (212) 462-1935 email: reprints@elsevier.com

The Veterinary Clinics of North America: Equine Practice is covered in *Index Medicus, Excerpta Medica, Current Contents/Agriculture, Biology and Environmental Sciences, and ISI.*

Printed in the United States of America.

CONSULTING EDITOR

A. SIMON TURNER, BVSc, MS, Diplomate, American College of Veterinary Surgeons; Professor, Department of Clinical Sciences, College of Veterinary Medicine and Biomedical Sciences, Colorado State University, Fort Collins, Colorado

GUEST EDITOR

CHRISTINE L. THEORET, DMV, PhD, Diplomate, American College of Veterinary Surgeons; Associate Professor, Département de biomédecine vétérinaire, Faculté de médecine vétérinaire, Université de Montréal, St-Hyacinthe, Québec, Canada

CONTRIBUTORS

SPENCER M. BARBER, DVM, Diplomate, American College of Veterinary Surgeons; Professor of Surgery, Large Animal Clinical Sciences, Western College of Veterinary Medicine, University of Saskatchewan, Saskatoon, Saskatchewan, Canada

GARY M. BAXTER, VMD, Diplomate, American College of Veterinary Surgeons; Professor of Equine Surgery and Lameness, Department of Clinical Sciences, College of Veterinary Medicine and Biomedical Sciences, Veterinary Medical Center, Colorado State University, Fort Collins, Colorado

DAVID G. BRISTOL, DVM, Diplomate, American Board of Veterinary Practitioners (Equine Practice); Diplomate, American College of Veterinary Surgeons; Associate Dean and Director of Academic Affairs, College of Veterinary Medicine, North Carolina State University, Raleigh, North Carolina

GORDON W. BRUMBAUGH, DVM, PhD, Diplomate, American College of Veterinary Internal Medicine; Diplomate, American College of Veterinary Clinical Pharmacology, Wellborn, Texas

CHRISTOPHE J. CÉLESTE, DMV, IPSAV, DES, Clinical Instructor in Equine Surgery and Emergency, Faculté de Médecine Vétérinaire, Centre Hospitalier Universitaire Vétérinaire, Université de Montréal, Montréal, Québec, Canada

ANDREW J. DART, BVSc, Diplomate, American College of Veterinary Surgeons; Diplomate, European College of Veterinary Surgeons; Associate Professor and Hospital Director, University Veterinary Centre Camden, Faculty of Veterinary Science, University of Sydney, New South Wales, Australia

BRAD A. DOWLING, BVSc, FACVSc, Senior Registrar and Head of the Equine Unit, University Veterinary Centre Camden, Faculty of Veterinary Science, University of Sydney, New South Wales, Australia

JORGE H. GOMEZ, MVZ, MS, Diplomate, American College of Veterinary Surgeons; Instructor in Equine Surgery, Department of Clinical Sciences, College of Veterinary Medicine, Auburn University, Auburn, Alabama

R. REID HANSON, DVM, Diplomate, American College of Veterinary Surgeons; Diplomate, American College of Veterinary Emergency and Critical Care; Associate Professor, Department of Clinical Sciences, College of Veterinary Medicine, Auburn University, Auburn, Alabama

DEAN HENDRICKSON, DVM, MS, Diplomate, American College of Veterinary Surgeons; Associate Professor, Equine Surgery, Clinical Sciences, James L. Voss Veterinary Teaching Hospital, Colorado State University, Fort Collins, Colorado

SAM M. HENDRIX, DVM, Resident, Equine Surgery and Lameness, Department of Clinical Sciences, College of Veterinary Medicine and Biomedical Sciences, Veterinary Medical Center, Colorado State University, Fort Collins, Colorado

HENRY JANN, DVM, MS, Diplomate, American College of Veterinary Surgeons; Oklahoma State University, College of Veterinary Medicine, Stillwater, Oklahoma

CHRIS PASQUINI, DVM, MS, Associate Professor, St. George's University, St. George, Grenada, West Indies

CHRISTINE L. SMITH, DVM, Diplomate, American College of Veterinary Surgeons; Senior Registrar, University Veterinary Centre Camden, Faculty of Veterinary Science, University of Sydney, New South Wales, Australia

MIHÀLY O. SZÖKE, DMV, DES, MSc, Diplomate, American College of Veterinary Surgeons; Diplomate, European College of Veterinary Surgeons; Hôpital Vétérinaire Lachute, Lachute, Québec, Canada

CHRISTINE L. THEORET, DMV, PhD, Diplomate, American College of Veterinary Surgeons; Associate Professor, Département de biomédecine vétérinaire, Faculté de médecine vétérinaire, Université de Montréal, St-Hyacinthe, Québec, Canada

P. RENÉ VAN WEEREN, DVM, PhD, Diplomate, European College of Veterinary Surgeons; Department of Equine Sciences, Faculty of Veterinary Medicine, University of Utrecht, Utrecht, The Netherlands

JOANNA VIRGIN, James L. Voss Veterinary Teaching Hospital, Colorado State University, Fort Collins, Colorado

JACINTHA M. WILMINK, DVM, PhD, Woumarec, Wageningen, The Netherlands

DAVID A. WILSON, DVM, MS, Diplomate, American College of Veterinary Surgeons; Associate Professor of Equine Surgery, Section Head, Equine Medicine and Surgery, Associate Chair for Clinical Affairs, Department of Veterinary Medicine and Surgery, University of Missouri, Columbia, Missouri

CONTENTS

GOAL STATEMENT

The goal of the *Veterinary Clinics of North America: Equine Practice* is to keep practicing veterinarians up to date with current clinical practice in equine medicine by providing timely articles reviewing the state of the art in equine care.

ACCREDITATION

The *Veterinary Clinics of North America: Equine Practice* will be offering continuing education credits, to be awarded by a school of veterinary medicine, contract pending.

The aforementioned school of veterinary medicine is a designated provider of continuing veterinary education. Veterinarians participating in this learning activity may earn up to 6 credits per issue up to a maximum of 18 credits per year. Credits awarded may not apply toward license renewal in all states. It is the responsibility of each participant to verify the requirements of their state licensing board.

Credit can be earned by reading the text material, taking the examination online at ***http://www.theclinics.com/home/cme,*** and completing the program evaluation. Each test question must be answered correctly; you will have the opportunity to retake any questions answered incorrectly. Following successful completion of the test and the program evaluation, you may print your certificate.

TO ENROLL

To enroll in the *Veterinary Clinics of North America: Equine Practice* Continuing Education program, call customer service at 1-800-654-2452 or sign up online at ***http://www.theclinics.com/home/cme***. The CME program is available to subscribers for an additional annual fee of $49.95.

FORTHCOMING ISSUES

August 2005

Neonatal Medicine and Surgery
L. Chris Sanchez, DVM, PhD, *Guest Editor*

December 2005

New Therapies in Joint Disease
Troy N. Trumble, DVM, PhD, *Guest Editor*

RECENT ISSUES

December 2004

Infection Control
Fairfield T. Bain, DVM,
J. Scott Weese, DVM, DVSc, *Guest Editors*

August 2004

Updates in Ophthalmology
Tim J. Cutler, MVB, MS, *Guest Editor*

April 2004

Critical Care for All Ages
Pamela A. Wilkins, DVM, PhD, *Guest Editor*

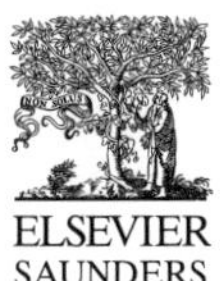

ELSEVIER
SAUNDERS

Vet Clin Equine 21 (2005) xi–xii

VETERINARY
CLINICS
Equine Practice

Preface

Wound Management

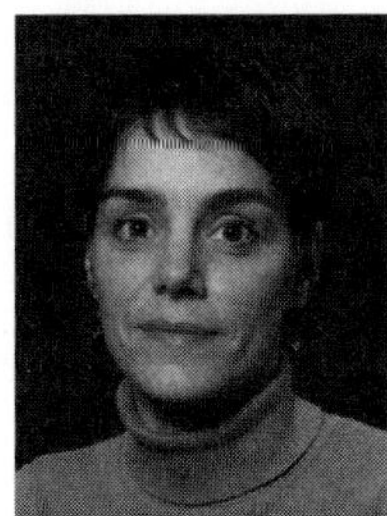

Christine L. Theoret, DMV, PhD
Guest Editor

Sixteen years have passed since the last issue on wound management was published in the *Veterinary Clinics of North America: Equine Practice*. Although many general principles guiding the clinical approach to a traumatic wound remain applicable, several innovative treatments have been developed, often based on the progressive investigations of our peers in human and veterinary medicine. Because many aspects of the horse's healing response are unique, it is the species-specific research that is likely to yield the most valuable information. Fortunately, several basic science and clinical studies have been performed in the horse and pony in recent years and have generated useful data to clarify these important distinctions. Since then, a handful of novel therapies have been tested, with mixed success. Such varied success underscores the critical need for continued research, particularly in view of the zeal of the pharmaceutical industry to synthesize many molecules associated with wound repair. Indeed, it is estimated that in the United States alone, more than a billion dollars is spent annually on the management of wounds in human beings. As such, the ability to influence the repair process directly is a powerful impetus for research and development by drug companies. In this perspective, it can be said that the underlying theme of this issue is "innovation."

The first article summarizes the important concepts pertaining to the host's response to wounding, whereas the second article further explores this issue as it specifically pertains to the equine species. The third article then addresses the various factors that can exert a negative impact on the physiologic mechanisms involved in repair. This first section thus serves as an introduction to the theme.

0749-0739/05/$ - see front matter
doi:10.1016/j.cveq.2004.11.013 *vetequine.theclinics.com*

The fourth article emphasizes the importance of a thorough assessment of the wound and the patient. Various actions include hemostasis, cleansing, debriding, and disinfecting the wound as well as closure, when indicated, in the first few hours after injury. The author of the fifth article shares his expertise relating to the use of antimicrobials in wound management, whereas the sixth and seventh articles review topical treatments and then dressings and bandages, respectively, used in the management of equine wounds. These latter articles focus on the manipulation of the cytokine profile and the wound environment through the use of therapeutic agents in an effort to accelerate the rate and improve the quality of repair but highlight the inability of one single agent in achieving these objectives as a result of the complex processes involved.

The remaining articles are devoted to the management of specific entities, including burn injuries (eighth article); skin grafting techniques used in the management of extensive or complicated wounds that cannot heal by primary intention (ninth article); wounds involving deep structures on the limb (tenth article); hoof injuries (eleventh article); neck and head injuries (twelfth article); and complicated wounds, such as degloving injuries, nerve and vessel trauma, osseous sequestration and foreign bodies, and wounds involving body cavities (thirteenth article).

It is my hope that this compilation of articles serves as a means for equine veterinarians to manage a wide variety of wounds successfully. Furthermore, this issue provides practitioners with the knowledge required to understand some of the current research-based publications and to formulate a critical opinion of the numerous new treatments proposed by pharmaceutical companies.

Christine L. Theoret, DMV, PhD
Département de biomédecine vétérinaire
Faculté de médecine vétérinaire
Université de Montréal
CP 5000
3200 rue Sicotte
St-Hyacinthe
Québec, Canada J2S 7C6

E-mail address: Christine.theoret@umontreal.ca

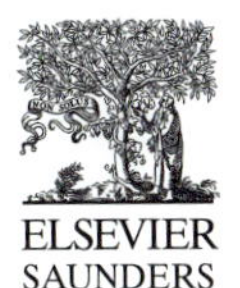
ELSEVIER
SAUNDERS

Vet Clin Equine 21 (2005) 1–13

VETERINARY
CLINICS
Equine Practice

The Pathophysiology of Wound Repair

Christine L. Theoret, DMV, PhD

Département de biomédecine vétérinaire, Faculté de médecine vétérinaire, Université de Montréal, CP 5000, St-Hyacinthe, Québec J2S 7C6, Canada

Veterinarians in equine practice are frequently called on to manage traumatic wounds, which can be labor-intensive and expensive. To minimize cost and time spent on treatment, practitioners must be meticulous in their selection of techniques, dressings, and medications, which should be based on a clear understanding of the mechanisms involved in wound repair. One objective of this article is thus to review the physiologic, cellular, and biochemical responses to wounding.

Since the last issue on equine wound management was published in this journal, much research aimed at elucidating and possibly augmenting the reparative mechanisms of the body has been performed and has yielded advances in the field of cytokines and the ability to readily synthesize most molecules associated with wound repair [1]. Because you are likely to come across some of these novelties in your quest for continuing education, another objective of this article is to familiarize you with these influential and ubiquitous proteins and then to place them in the context of wound repair. Indeed, many new therapies are cytokine based not only in soft tissue repair but in the realm of orthopedics.

Cytokines in wound repair

Wound repair begins as soon as a cellular barrier is broken and follows a predictable pattern in re-establishing an epithelial shield and recovering tissue integrity, strength, and function. Although oversimplified, a conceptual distinction between phases of the healing response helps us to understand the individual events occurring during repair. These can be divided into synchronized and overlapping phases that include acute inflammation, cellular proliferation, and, finally, extracellular matrix (ECM) synthesis and remodeling with scar formation. It is increasingly

E-mail address: christine.theoret@umontreal.ca

0749-0739/05/$ - see front matter
doi:10.1016/j.cveq.2004.11.001 **vetequine.theclinics.com**

apparent that each phase relies on complex interactions between many cell types, their mediators (particularly cytokines), and the ECM.

Cytokines are proteins whose secretion is induced within platelets and inflammatory cells at the wound border and that act on the same cell, an adjacent cell, or a distant cell to initiate and amplify the host response to trauma. The most common activities stimulated by cytokines are cellular migration, proliferation, and protein synthesis, all of which are essential to the repair process. The term *cytokine* loosely encompasses colony-stimulating factors (CSFs), interferons (IFNs), interleukins (ILs), tumor necrosis factors (TNFs), and various growth factors. The following discussion briefly reviews the key features of cytokines that have been attributed a role in dermal wound repair, with an emphasis placed on those studied in the horse.

Colony-stimulating factors

CSFs promote the differentiation and maturation of hematopoietic stem cells into granulocytes, monocytes, macrophages, and lymphocytes. These mature inflammatory cells then invade the wound during the acute inflammatory phase of repair and secrete or produce other cytokines with ensuing effects on inflammation, angiogenesis, epithelialization, and fibroplasia [2,3]. Equine granulocyte-macrophage CSF has recently been cloned [4].

Interferons

IFNs are mostly known for their antiviral properties but can modulate wound repair via their influence on immunity. For example, they activate macrophage functions that may stimulate the inflammatory response to trauma and lead to the release of additional cytokines with secondary effects on the repair process. IFNγ may prevent excessive fibrosis from occurring in the later phases of repair by inhibiting fibroblast proliferation as well as by suppressing collagen synthesis and increasing its degradation [5]. IFNγ seems to enhance epithelialization by facilitating the migration of epithelial cells, whereas IFNα inhibits their proliferation [6] as well as wound contraction [7]. Cloning and sequencing of equine IFNγ cDNA have been achieved [8].

Interleukins

The majority of cells are a source of and a target for ILs. IL-1 is the most studied of the ILs and is an essential mediator of inflammation, although it also modulates the later phases of repair. In particular, it favors epithelialization by stimulating migration of epithelial cells and also influences ECM synthesis and remodeling via enhancement of fibroblast proliferation and collagen degradation [9].

Equine IL-1α and IL-1β [10] as well as their natural inhibitor, IL-1 receptor antagonist [11], cDNAs have been cloned, sequenced, and expressed.

Tumor necrosis factor-α

Although TNFα is probably less important for wound repair than for systemic inflammation, it does seem to encourage epithelialization [12], angiogenesis, and ECM remodeling. The gene encoding equine TNFα has been cloned [13].

Connective tissue growth factor

Unlike other cytokines, the effects of connective tissue growth factor (CTGF) are not widespread. Rather, this growth factor acts mostly on the fibroblast, in which it mediates TGFβ activity and indirectly stimulates the production of fibrous tissue [14].

Although equine CTGF has not been cloned, equine and human CTGF appear similar [15]. Interestingly, CTGF is present in equine tear fluid, which might explain why corneal ulceration often leads to profound stromal fibrosis and scarring.

Epidermal growth factor and transforming growth factor-α

Epidermal growth factor (EGF) and transforming growth factor (TGF)-α exhibit similar biologic activities and are thus considered together. Aggregating platelets release EGF in the immediate period after wounding, and this growth factor is also abundant in saliva, which may represent the physiologic basis for wound licking. TGFα, conversely, is synthesized by activated macrophages and epithelial cells [16]. Both growth factors enhance epithelial cell migration and proliferation, thus accelerating epithelialization. Although EGF also influences remodeling by activating protein and matrix metalloproteinase (MMP) synthesis [17], TGFα is considered a more potent inducer of angiogenesis [18]. The coding sequence for equine EGF shows 60% to 70% identity with EGF of other species [19].

Fibroblast growth factor

Basic fibroblast growth factor (bFGF) is the most extensively studied member of the fibroblast growth factor family and was one of the first angiogenic growth factors characterized [20]. Trauma triggers release of bFGF by inflammatory cells, dermal fibroblasts, and microvascular endothelial cells, to name a few. Within the hypoxic wound environment, bFGF stimulates migration and growth of endothelial cells into the newly deposited granulation tissue [21]. Furthermore, bFGF boosts epithelialization and may stimulate wound contraction via the enhancement of TGF-β1 activity [22]. Finally, bFGF affects remodeling by halting collagen synthesis while encouraging its degradation [23].

Insulin-like growth factor

Insulin-like growth factor (IGF) has insulin-like activity and is released by platelets during clotting to exert potent effects on microvascular endothelial cells, encouraging their migration and growth into the wound bed [24]. IGF also enhances epithelial cell proliferation [25] and stimulates collagen synthesis by fibroblasts. Equine IGF-1 cDNA has been cloned and sequenced [26].

Keratinocyte growth factor

Keratinocyte growth factor (KGF) is a member of the FGF family; indeed, KGF is sometimes referred to as FGF-7. Whereas most FGFs influence proliferation or differentiation of various cell types, KGF acts specifically on epithelial cells to exert effects similar to those of EGF and TGFα [27].

Platelet-derived growth factor

Although platelets are the largest source of platelet-derived growth factor (PDGF), a number of other cell types are also triggered by trauma to express it [16], such that wound tissues are bathed in PDGF throughout the repair process. PDGF acts initially to enhance inflammatory cell and fibroblast migration and then stimulates growth of mesenchymal cells through the release of other growth factors, namely, TGFβ, from activated macrophages [28]. By a similar indirect mechanism, PDGF may participate in angiogenesis [28], stimulating the production of granulation tissue, and increase the enzymatic activity of the wound fibroblast required for remodeling.

Transforming growth factor-β

This growth factor has the broadest range of activities in repair because of the wide variety of cell types that produce or respond to it and the spectrum of those responses [29]. A unique feature of this peptide is that it can regulate its own production by monocytes and activated macrophages, which sustains its expression at the wound site and extends the effectiveness of the initial burst of TGFβ released on injury as well as TGFβ that might be applied to a wound [30].

TGFβ's most notable effects are to enhance migration and growth of fibroblasts and to modulate the accumulation of ECM, central to increasing the strength of wounds. It does this by encouraging the synthesis of a great number of proteins while concurrently inhibiting matrix turnover by reducing overall enzymatic activity. For this reason, TGFβ is often referred to as "profibrotic." Indeed, a cause-and-effect relation has been established between TGFβ and fibrosis in various tissues [31,32]. TGFβ also promotes angiogenesis by stimulating endothelial cell migration, differentiation, and tubule formation. Some of these effects may be indirect, via the release of bFGF and vascular endothelial growth factor (VEGF) from TGFβ-activated macrophages [33]. TGFβ seems to favor epithelial cell migration and enhance wound contraction [34]. The cDNA for equine TGF-β1 has been cloned and found to be 99% identical to human TGF-β1 [35].

Vascular endothelial growth factor

VEGF, predominantly produced by macrophages, is a potent angiogenic factor through stimulation of proliferation, migration, and tube formation by microvascular endothelial cells [36]. Cloning of equine VEGF cDNA has recently been completed.

Phases of wound repair

Acute inflammation

The severity of trauma usually determines the degree of the resultant vascular and cellular responses, referred to as inflammation. The first reaction of the damaged blood vessel is to constrict for 5 to 10 minutes. Dilation then follows and promotes the passage of cells, fluid, and protein across the vessel wall into the wound space. At this point, blood coagulation and platelet aggregation form a clot that ensures hemostasis and serves as a scaffold for future cell migration.

Platelets, once activated, also release potent mediators that initiate and amplify the subsequent phases of repair. Over time, the clot desiccates to form a scab, which is eventually sloughed. During the inflammatory phase, most of the wound strength is provided by fibrin within the blood clot. This provisional ECM consisting of products released by platelets and inflammatory cells is replaced by granulation tissue in the next phase of repair.

Inflammatory leukocytes are rapidly recruited from circulating blood and directed to the site of injury by the numerous chemoattractants supplied by the coagulation and activated complement pathways as well as by injured or activated wound cells [37]. For example, the activated platelet releases cytokines (IL-1β and TNFα) and growth factors (PDGF, TGFα, TGFβ, EGF, and IGFs) which stimulate leukocyte migration. The combination of wound fluid, tissue debris, and neutrophils is referred to as pus. The primary role of the neutrophil is to destroy debris and bacteria through phagocytosis and subsequent degradation, mechanisms that are enhanced by IL-1 and TNFα [38]. Once contaminating particles are cleared from the site of injury, neutrophil migration and phagocytosis cease and most cells become entrapped within the clot. The neutrophils remaining within viable tissue die in a few days and are phagocytosed by the macrophage. Although the neutrophil is important in creating a propitious wound environment and serves as a source of proinflammatory cytokines, it is mostly useful in infected wounds [39].

Macrophages carry out debridement, microbial killing, and coordination of the later phases of repair. In particular, activated macrophages have the ability to synthesize and secrete cytokines necessary to the recruitment and activation of cells involved in fibroplasia, angiogenesis, and epithelialization. Monocyte recruitment from the circulating blood pool is mediated by numerous chemoattractants released by platelets and neutrophils, together with matrix degradation products and inflammatory proteins. Once adhered to the wound bed, macrophages express CSF-1, which is necessary to their survival; IL-1 and TNFα, which are proinflammatory cytokines; or PDGF and TGFβ, which are potent chemoattractants and growth factors for fibroblasts [37]. Macrophages participate in bacterial killing and clearance of damaged ECM components via mechanisms similar to those described for the neutrophil. In normally healing wounds, macrophages remain for days to weeks.

Acute inflammation is generally considered essential to the normal outcome of wound repair. Conversely, should inflammation not resolve within a certain interval, this may contribute to the pathogenesis of diseases characterized by excessive fibrosis or scarring. For inflammation to terminate, inciting stimuli must be inactivated and normal microvascular permeability must be restored to prevent continued passage of blood cells into the wound space. Likewise, the secretory activities of inflammatory cells must be halted, mediator receptors must be downregulated or inhibitory factors must be produced, and, ultimately, neutrophils and macrophages must die and be cleared from the wound bed [40].

Cellular proliferation

Fibroplasia

The proliferative phase, which begins before complete resolution of inflammation, includes the formation of granulation tissue, also referred to as fibroplasia, as well as epithelialization. Granulation tissue is formed by three elements that move into the wound space simultaneously: macrophages produce mediators stimulating angiogenesis and fibroplasia, fibroblasts proliferate and synthesize ECM components, and new blood vessels carry oxygen and nutrients necessary for cell growth. This characteristic red granular stroma begins to invade the defect approximately 5 days after injury to protect against infection and to provide a surface on which epithelial cells can migrate. Although there is no apparent gain in wound strength at this time, replacement of the clot by granulation tissue ensures the orderly progression of repair.

The signals for fibroblasts to proliferate and migrate probably include a number of chemoattractants and cytokines or growth factors emanating from inflammatory cells, particularly IL-1, TNFα, IGF-1, PDGF, EGF, FGF, and especially TGFβ. Cellular migration into the blood clot is facilitated by a variety of fibroblast-derived degradative enzymes, the production and secretion of which are stimulated by PDGF and TGFβ. Initially, fibroblasts proliferate; they then switch their major function to protein synthesis and commence the replacement of provisional matrix (fibrin, fibronectin, and hyaluronan) by glycoproteins, proteoglycans, and immature (type III) and, eventually, mature (type I) collagen to bind the wound edges together. Profibrotic TGFβ indirectly regulates fibroblast proliferation and directly stimulates matrix production and inhibits its degradation [29]. Soon after the matrix is deposited, protein synthesis ceases and fibroblasts subsequently undergo apoptosis [41] or acquire smooth muscle characteristics and transform into myofibroblasts, which initiate wound contraction.

Angiogenesis

Angiogenesis involves the formation of new blood vessels from preexisting ones and relies on an orderly sequence that includes augmented microvascular permeability, degradation of basement membrane, migration into the local stroma, cellular proliferation and formation of new blood vessels, stabilization, and, eventually, regression and involution of the newly formed vasculature [42]. Wounding causes tissue hypoxia, followed by the release of mediators by activated cells, such as the platelet, monocyte, and wound macrophage. Some of these soluble mediators are specific angiogenic factors, such as bFGF and VEGF [42]. Other cytokines found to exhibit angiogenic activity (TGF-β1, TNFα, EGF, and PDGF) seem to act by enhancing the production of bFGF and VEGF by macrophages and endothelial cells [42]. bFGF is especially active during the first few days of repair, when it promotes endothelial cell migration by facilitating capillary basement membrane digestion. Likewise, bFGF and VEGF favor the binding of endothelial cells to ECM, and hence their migration [43]. Thus, endothelial cells at the tip of existing capillaries begin their migration into the wound space on the second day after wounding in response to angiogenic stimuli. Microvascular endothelial cells remaining in the parent vessel begin to proliferate, providing a continuous source of cells for angiogenesis to proceed [37]. Proliferative stimuli are believed to resemble the migratory stimuli and include bFGF, VEGF, EGF, TGFβ, and PDGF [43]. Proliferating endothelial cells form a lumen through which blood flows and whose diameter depends on a balance between bFGF-induced proteolysis and TGFβ-induced antiproteolysis [44]. New capillaries oriented perpendicular to the wound surface are then stabilized within 24 hours as TGFβ encourages the interaction of endothelial cells with the new basement membrane [44]. As the need for a rich vascular supply fades, most of the recently formed microvessels quickly vanish through apoptosis of endothelial cells. The wound color fades as the capillary bed disappears from the granulation tissue.

Epithelialization

Within hours of wounding, basal epidermal cells at the wound margin undergo marked alterations that favor mobility and phagocytic activity. EGF and TGFα are considered essential to epithelial migration and proliferation [17,45] because they encourage lysis and ingestion of debris found along the migratory path by epithelial cells attempting to advance beneath the clot. IL-1 and TNFα released from inflammatory cells also seem to facilitate epithelial migration by increasing their secretion of degradative enzymes [12] and KGF [46]. TGFβ is thought to enhance the synthesis of epithelial cell-surface receptors for various ECM components and thus to favor migration. Although epithelial migration is evident at a cellular level before the acute inflammatory response has resolved, the characteristic pink rim of new epithelium becomes visible at the edge of a full-thickness wound, healing by second intention only 5 to 7 days after trauma. Epithelialization continues until the wound is covered and migration ceases because of contact inhibition.

Epithelial proliferation begins at the wound edge 1 to 2 days after wounding to replenish the migratory front. Proliferation is maximal within 48 to 72 hours and is evident histologically as epithelial hyperplasia. Several growth factors enhance proliferation, particularly KGF and TGFα [47], whereas others are thought to halt the proliferative potential of epithelial cells, specifically TGFβ [48]. The newly established monolayer of cells becomes attached to the new basement membrane and differentiates into a stratified epidermis, which may take weeks to months, such that in some large wounds, complete epithelialization may never be achieved, whereas in others, the new epidermis at the center may be thin and fragile [49].

Epithelialization is more rapid in superficial (partial thickness) wounds, because migrating cells arise not only from the residual epithelium at the wound periphery but from remaining dermal appendages (hair follicles and sweat glands). The rate of wound closure depends on the animal species as well as on the wound site, substrate, and size.

Matrix synthesis and remodeling

Contraction

During the second week after injury, wound edges are progressively brought together by a physical phenomenon termed *contraction*. Wound contraction is attributed to cells combining the characteristics of fibroblasts and smooth muscle cells, referred to as myofibroblasts [50]. Their most striking feature is a well-developed α-smooth muscle actin (α-SMA) microfilamentous system arranged parallel to the cell's long axis, which itself lies parallel to the lines of contraction within the wound in contrast to capillaries and macrophages. Bundles of these microfilaments are referred to as "stress fibers" and are in continuity with the ECM on which they exert tension [50]. Factors producing and regulating contraction in vivo are presently unknown but seem to include TGFβ [51] and, possibly, PDGF [52,53].

Wound contraction is greater in regions of the body with loose skin than in regions in which skin is under tension, such as the distal part of the limb in the horse. It seems that wound shape does not influence the process of contraction [54]. Wound contraction can be divided clinically into three phases: a lag phase lasting 5 to 10 days in which wound size increases because of swelling as well as centrifugal tension forces in the surrounding skin; a phase of rapid contraction; and, finally, a phase of slow contraction as the wound becomes fully epithelialized. As contraction ceases, myofibroblasts revert to a resting fibroblast or disappear by means of apoptosis [41]. Should myofibroblast numbers be inadequate, contraction may be deficient. In contrast, when myofibroblasts persist beyond the time required for wound closure, they may favor ECM accumulation and pathologic contracture, a condition leading to significant morbidity, particularly when it involves joints or body orifices. TGFβ promotes myofibroblast survival through prevention of apoptosis [55], adding to this cytokine's profibrotic effects, whereas IFNγ decreases α-SMA expression [56].

Matrix remodeling

Simultaneous with wound contraction, the ECM is being formed and remodeled as granulation tissue evolves toward mature scar tissue. Proteoglycans replace hyaluronan in the ECM during the second week of repair to improve the resilience of the matrix. Collagen type I gradually provides the wound with tensile strength as deposition peaks between 7 and 14 days. Although this corresponds to the period of most rapid gain in strength, only 20% of the final strength of the wound is achieved in the first 3 weeks of repair. After this time, collagen synthesis is balanced by degradation and collagen contents level off. Collagen remodeling, however, continues beyond the synthetic phase of repair and depends on continued synthesis and catabolism of collagen at a low rate. Proteolytic enzymes, many from the MMP class, are released from wound cells. MMPs are not normally expressed in intact skin but are induced in response to exogenous signals like cytokines and growth factors whenever proteolysis is required, such as during cell migration and matrix remodeling [57]. To date, a dozen different MMPs have been characterized [58], of which the best-known subgroup are the interstitial collagenases. Other subgroups of MMPs are the stromelysins, which possess broad substrate specificity; the metallogelatinases, which efficiently degrade denatured collagens (gelatins) and also attack basement membranes; and matrilysin, which is a strong proteoglycanase.

The balance between collagen synthesis and degradation during the remodeling phase depends on the simultaneous presence of MMPs and their natural specific inhibitors, the tissue inhibitors of metalloproteinases (TIMPs). Any disparity between MMPs and TIMPs may lead to abnormal resolution and delayed repair.

Tensile strength of the repair tissue continues to increase slowly over some months as a result of collagen remodeling, with the formation of larger collagen bundles that are oriented along the lines of tension as well as an increase in the number of intermolecular cross-links in the maturing scar. Full-thickness skin wounds acquire only 75% to 80% of the strength of normal surrounding tissue, because the final end point of normal repair is a nonfunctional scar [59].

Summary

The equine practitioner who is presented with a wounded horse should fully understand the physiologic mechanisms involved in repair so as to design an appropriate treatment plan. In the following articles of this issue, experienced authors share their thoughts on the management of specific injuries, and the reader should benefit from acquisition of knowledge about the different phases of healing as well as the cytokines that regulate them, because these data dictate the approach to follow, particularly in complicated wounds, such as those afflicted by chronic inflammation and/or an excessive proliferative response.

References

[1] Kirsner RS, Eaglstein WH. The wound healing process. Dermatol Clin 1993;11:629–40.
[2] Metcalf D. The granulocyte-macrophage colony stimulating factors. Science 1985;229: 16–22.
[3] Mann A, Breuhahn K, Schirmacher P, et al. Keratinocyte-derived granulocyte-macrophage colony stimulating factor accelerates wound healing: stimulation of keratinocyte proliferation, granulation tissue formation, and vascularization. J Invest Dermatol 2001;117: 1382–90.
[4] Steinbach F, Mauel S, Beier I. Recombinant equine interferons: expression cloning and biological activity. Vet Immunol Immunopathol 2002;84:83–95.
[5] Laato M, Heino J, Gerdin B, et al. Interferon-gamma-induced inhibition of wound healing *in vivo* and *in vitro*. Ann Chir Gynaecol 2001;90(Suppl 215):19–23.
[6] Gyulai R, Hunyadi J, Kenderessy-Szabo A, et al. Chemotaxis of freshly separated and cultured human keratinocytes. Clin Exp Dermatol 1994;19:309–11.
[7] Nedelec B, Shen YJ, Ghahary A, et al. The effect of interferon alpha 2b on the expression of cytoskeletal proteins in an *in vitro* model of wound contraction. J Lab Clin Med 1995;126: 474–84.
[8] Curran JA, Argyle DJ, Cox P, et al. Nucleotide sequence of the equine interferon gamma cDNA. DNA Seq 1994;4:405–7.
[9] Unemori EN, Ehsani N, Wang M, et al. Interleukin-1 and transforming growth factor-α: synergistic stimulation of metalloproteinases, PGE_2, and proliferation in human fibroblasts. Exp Cell Res 1994;210:166–71.

[10] Howard RD, McIlwraith CW, Trotter GW, et al. Cloning of equine interleukin 1 alpha and equine interleukin 1 beta and determination of their full-length cDNA sequences. Am J Vet Res 1998;59:704–11.

[11] Howard RD, McIlwraith CW, Trotter GW, et al. Cloning of equine interleukin 1 receptor antagonist and determination of its full-length cDNA sequence. Am J Vet Res 1998;59: 712–6.

[12] Bechtel MJ, Reinartz J, Rox JM, et al. Upregulation of cell-surface-associated plasminogen activation in cultured keratinocytes by interleukin-1 beta and tumor necrosis factor-alpha. Exp Cell Res 1996;223:395–404.

[13] Su X, Deem Morris D, McGraw RA. Cloning and characterization of gene TNFα encoding equine tumor necrosis factor alpha. Gene 1991;107:319–21.

[14] Grotendorst GR. Connective tissue growth factor: a mediator of TGF-β action on fibroblasts. Cytokine Growth Factor Rev 1997;8:171–9.

[15] Ollivier FJ, Brooks DE, Schultz GS, et al. Connective tissue growth factor in tear film of the horse: detection, identification and origin. Graefes Arch Clin Exp Ophthalmol 2004;242(2): 165–71.

[16] Martin P, Hopkinson-Woolley J, McCluskey J. Growth factors and cutaneous wound repair. Prog Growth Factor Res 1992;4:25–44.

[17] Nanney LB, King LE. Epidermal growth factor and transforming growth factor-α. In: Clark RAF, editor. The molecular and cellular biology of wound repair. 2nd edition. New York: Plenum Press; 1996. p. 171–94.

[18] Ono M, Okamuro K, Nakayama Y, et al. Induction of human microvascular endothelial tubular morphogenesis by human keratinocytes: involvement of transforming growth factor-alpha. Biochem Biophys Res Commun 1992;189:601–9.

[19] Stewart F, Power CA, Lennard SN, et al. Identification of the horse epidermal growth factor (EGF) coding sequence and its use in monitoring EGF gene expression in the endometrium of the pregnant mare. J Mol Endocrinol 1994;12:341–50.

[20] Burgess W, Maciag T. The heparin-binding (fibroblast) growth factor family of proteins. Annu Rev Biochem 1989;58:575–606.

[21] Kuwabara K, Ogawa S, Matsumoto M, et al. Hypoxia-mediated induction of acidic/basic fibroblast growth factor and platelet-derived growth factor in mononuclear phagocytes stimulates growth of hypoxic endothelial cells. Proc Natl Acad Sci USA 1995;92:4606–10.

[22] Finesmith TH, Broadley DN, Davidson JM. Fibroblasts from wounds of different stages of repair vary in their ability to contract a collagen gel in response to growth factors. J Cell Physiol 1990;144:99–107.

[23] Abraham JA, Klagsbrun M. Modulation of wound repair by members of the fibroblast growth factor family. In: Clark RAF, editor. The molecular and cellular biology of wound repair. 2nd edition. New York: Plenum Press; 1996. p. 195–248.

[24] Taylor WR, Alexander RW. Autocrine control of wound repair by insulin-like growth factor 1 in cultured endothelial cells. Am J Physiol 1993;265:C801–5.

[25] Ando H, Jensen PJ. EGF and IGF-1 enhance keratinocyte migration. J Invest Dermatol 1993;100:633–9.

[26] Otte K, Rozell B, Gessbo A, et al. Cloning and sequencing of an equine insulin-like growth factor I cDNA and its expression in fetal and adult tissues. Gen Comp Endocrinol 1996;102: 11–5.

[27] Werner S. Keratinocyte growth factor: a unique player in epithelial repair processes. Cytokine Growth Factor Rev 1998;9:153–65.

[28] Heldin CH, Westermark B. Role of platelet-derived growth factor *in vivo*. In: Clark RAF, editor. The molecular and cellular biology of wound repair. 2nd edition. New York: Plenum Press; 1996. p. 249–73.

[29] Roberts AB, Sporn MB. Transforming growth factor-β. In: Clark RAF, editor. The molecular and cellular biology of wound repair. 2nd edition. New York: Plenum Press; 1996. p. 275–308.

[30] O'Kane S, Ferguson MWJ. Transforming growth factor βs and wound healing. Int J Biochem Cell Biol 1997;29:63–78.
[31] Shah M, Foreman DM, Ferguson MWJ. Neutralization of TGF-β1 and TGF-β2 or exogenous addition of TGF-β3 to cutaneous rat wounds reduces scarring. J Cell Sci 1995; 108:985–1002.
[32] Huang JS, Wang YH, Ling TY, et al. Synthetic TGF-beta antagonist accelerates wound healing and reduces scarring. FASEB J 2002;16:1269–70.
[33] Kim KY, Jeong SY, Won J, et al. Induction of angiogenesis by expression of soluble type II transforming growth factor-beta receptor in mouse hepatoma. J Biol Chem 2001;276: 38781–6.
[34] Desmoulière A, Geinoz A, Gabbiani F, et al. Transforming growth factor β1 induces α-smooth muscle actin expression in granulation tissue myofibroblasts in quiescent and growing cultured fibroblasts. J Cell Biol 1993;122:103–11.
[35] Penha-Goncalves MN, Onions DE, Nicolson L. Cloning and sequencing of equine transforming growth factor-beta 1 (TGF beta-1) cDNA. DNA Seq 1997;7:375–8.
[36] Dvorak HF, Brown LF, Betmar M, et al. Vascular permeability factor/vascular endothelial growth factor, microvascular hyperpermeability, and angiogenesis. Am J Pathol 1995;146: 1029–39.
[37] Singer AJ, Clark RAF. Cutaneous wound healing. N Engl J Med 1999;341:738–46.
[38] Dinarello CA. Interleukin-1: a proinflammatory cytokine. In: Gallin JI, Snyderman R, editors. Inflammation: basic principles and clinical correlates. 3rd edition. New York: Lippincott, Williams & Wilkins; 1999. p. 443–61.
[39] Leibovitch SJ, Ross R. The role of the macrophage in wound repair: a study with hydrocortisone and antimacrophage serum. Am J Pathol 1975;78:71–100.
[40] Haslett C, Henson P. Resolution of inflammation. In: Clark RAF, editor. The molecular and cellular biology of wound repair. 2nd edition. New York: Plenum Press; 1996. p. 143–68.
[41] Desmoulière A, Redard M, Darby I, et al. Apoptosis mediates the decrease in cellularity during the transition between granulation tissue and scar. Am J Pathol 1995;146:56–66.
[42] Li J, Zhang Y-P, Kirsner RS. Angiogenesis in wound repair: angiogenic growth factors and the extracellular matrix. Microsc Res Tech 2003;60:107–14.
[43] Liekens S, De Clerq E, Neyts J. Angiogenesis: regulators and clinical applications. Biochem Pharmacol 2001;61:253–70.
[44] Pepper MS, Montesano R. Proteolytic balance and capillary morphogenesis. Cell Differ Dev 1990;32:319–28.
[45] Kim I, Mogford JE, Chao JD, et al. Wound epithelialization deficits in the transforming growth factor-alpha knockout mouse. Wound Repair Regen 2001;9:386–90.
[46] Brauchle M, Angermeyer K, Hubner G, et al. Large induction of keratinocyte growth factor expression by serum growth factors and pro-inflammatory cytokines in cultured fibroblasts. Oncogene 1994;9:3199–204.
[47] Dlugosz AA, Cheng C, Denning MF, et al. Keratinocyte growth factor receptor ligands induce transforming growth factor alpha expression and activate the epidermal growth factor receptor signaling pathway in cultured epidermal keratinocytes. Cell Growth Differ 1994;5:1283–92.
[48] Sarret Y, Woodley DT, Grigsby K, et al. Human keratinocyte locomotion: the effect of selected cytokines. J Invest Dermatol 1992;98:12–6.
[49] Hosgood G. Wound repair and specific tissue response to injury. In: Slatter D, editor. Textbook of small animal surgery. 3rd edition. Philadelphia: WB Saunders; 2003. p. 66–86.
[50] Desmoulière A, Gabbiani G. The role of the myofibroblast in wound healing and fibrocontractive diseases. In: Clark RAF, editor. The molecular and cellular biology of wound repair. 2nd edition. New York: Plenum Press; 1996. p. 391–423.
[51] Desmoulière A. Factors influencing myofibroblast differentiation during wound healing and fibrosis. Cell Biol Int 1995;19:471–6.

[52] Clark RAF, Folkvord JM, Hart CE, et al. Platelet isoforms of platelet-derived growth factor stimulate fibroblasts to contract collagen matrices. J Clin Invest 1989;84:1036–40.

[53] Ehrlich HP, Freedman BM. Topical platelet-derived growth factor in patients enhances wound closure in the absence of wound contraction. Cytokines Cell Mol Ther 2002;7:85–90.

[54] Madison JB, Gronwall RR. Influence of wound shape on wound contraction in horses. Am J Vet Res 1992;53:1575–8.

[55] Zhang H-Y, Phan SH. Inhibition of myofibroblasts apoptosis by TGF-β1. Am J Respir Cell Mol Biol 1999;21:658–65.

[56] Desmoulière A, Rubbia-Brandt L, Abdiu A, et al. α-Smooth muscle actin is expressed in a subpopulation of cultured and cloned fibroblasts and is modulated by γ-interferon. Exp Cell Res 1992;201:64–73.

[57] Kahari VM, Saariallio KU. Matrix metalloproteinases in skin. Exp Dermatol 1997;6:199–213.

[58] Mignatti P, Rifkin DB, Welgus HG, et al. Proteinases and tissue remodeling. In: Clark RAF, editor. The molecular and cellular biology of wound repair. 2nd edition. New York: Plenum Press; 1996. p. 427–74.

[59] Levenson SM, Geever EF, Crowley LV, et al. The healing of rat skin wounds. Ann Surg 1965;161:293–308.

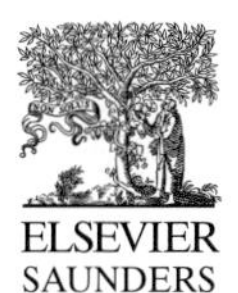

ELSEVIER
SAUNDERS

Vet Clin Equine 21 (2005) 15–32

VETERINARY
CLINICS
Equine Practice

Second-Intention Repair in the Horse and Pony and Management of Exuberant Granulation Tissue

Jacintha M. Wilmink, DVM, PhD[a,*],
P. René van Weeren, DVM, PhD[b]

[a] *Woumarec, Hamsterlaan 4, 6705 CT Wageningen, The Netherlands*
[b] *Department of Equine Sciences, Faculty of Veterinary Medicine, University of Utrecht, Yalelaan 12, 3584 CM Utrecht, The Netherlands*

Horses frequently suffer traumatic wounds. Healing of these wounds is often delayed and complicated compared with that occurring in other species, which leads to significant wastage, because a considerable number of animals are not able to continue their athletic career as a result of persisting lameness, swollen limbs, and extensive scars. Although primary or delayed closure is the preferred way of treatment, this can be followed by partial or total dehiscence of the wound, necessitating second-intention healing. Also, in cases of unmanageable contamination, excessive tissue loss, or severe compromise of the tissue, wound healing by second intention is often the only option [1].

Second-intention healing is lengthy, and complications, such as wound infection and the formation of exuberant granulation tissue or hypertrophic scars, are frequent. These difficulties particularly afflict limb wounds, whereas extensive body wounds heal relatively well [2,3]. Furthermore, wound healing in ponies is significantly faster and of superior quality to that occurring in horses [4,5]. This can be largely attributed to differences in the inflammatory response as well as to more pronounced and faster wound contraction in body wounds compared with limb wounds and in ponies compared with horses.

This article reviews those major differences. It also addresses the various options available for managing the exuberant granulation tissue that often develops subsequent to second-intention healing.

* Corresponding author.
E-mail address: j.m.wilmink@tiscalimail.nl (J.M. Wilmink).

0749-0739/05/$ - see front matter
doi:10.1016/j.cveq.2004.11.014

Phases during the second-intention wound healing process

Wound healing can be divided into four macroscopically apparent events: inflammation, formation of granulation tissue, wound contraction, and epithelialization. Remarkable differences in these phases between horses and ponies and body and limb wounds determine the speed and efficiency of healing [4,5].

Inflammation

During this phase polymorphonuclear (PMN) cells and macrophages migrate to the wound site to clear it of contaminating bacteria and nonviable tissue. Macrophages additionally release a plethora of biologically active substances that are essential for the recruitment of more inflammatory and mesenchymal cells and initiate the healing process [6].

Formation of granulation tissue

Fibroblasts, endothelial cells, and macrophages move into the wound space as a unit and are dependent on each other [7]. Macrophages provide a continuing source of cytokines and growth factors necessary for the stimulation of fibroplasia and angiogenesis, fibroblasts construct the new extracellular matrix (ECM) needed to support cell ingrowth, and blood vessels transport oxygen and nutrients necessary to cell metabolism [8]. Fibroblasts use the fibrin clot as a provisional matrix and rapidly replace it with a new loose ECM consisting of glycoproteins (fibronectin and laminin), proteoglycans (hyaluronic acid), and collagens (initially mainly type III, later type I) [9]. Granulation tissue fills the gap and is the basis for wound contraction and epithelial migration.

Wound contraction

Wound contraction is caused by the action of differentiated fibroblasts (myofibroblasts) in the granulation tissue, which contain filaments of smooth muscle actin. Contraction of these fibroblasts makes the wound margins move centripetally [8,10], reducing the wound area by means of original full thickness skin. Wound contraction largely determines the speed of second-intention wound healing and the final cosmetic appearance of the scar.

Epithelialization

Epithelialization occurs during the final phase of wound closure and is a slow process (1 mm per 10 days at the most in limb wounds of horses) [11]. Although epithelialization starts a few hours after trauma with the migration of epithelial cells, macroscopically, it can only be observed starting approximately 2 weeks after wounding. Proliferation occurs after approximately 2 days, evoked by the secretion of many cytokines and growth factors by fibroblasts, inflammatory cells, and the keratinocytes themselves [9,12]. Epithelialization is impaired by fibrin remnants of the clot and chronic inflammation [13]. Newly formed epithelium lacks skin adnexa and is thin and fragile because it has few epidermal projections [2], and this part of the wound remains visible as a superficial scar.

Differences in second-intention healing between horses and ponies

Standardized deep excisional wounds on the metatarsi and hindquarters of horses and ponies show a different healing pattern [4,5]. During the first week, all wounds increase in size. Thereafter, the body wounds of horses and ponies and the limb wounds of ponies decrease rapidly in size. In contrast, the limb wounds of horses increase further to almost twice their original size after 2 weeks, with a subsequent slow decrease, regaining their original size only after 6 weeks. All pony wounds healed in 7 to 9 weeks, whereas only two body wounds of horses healed within the 12-week observation period and healing of the other horse wounds took longer. This experiment revealed that wounds heal significantly faster in ponies than in horses and confirmed that wounds heal significantly faster on the body than on the limbs [2,4]. Because such disparity may provide information about the basic biology of second-intention healing within the equine species, other studies were undertaken to investigate the differences further.

Inflammatory phase

A healthy granulation bed develops more rapidly in ponies, whereas it remains irregular and purulent in horses for longer, with persistent fibrin deposits [4]. Histologically, the initial influx of leukocytes into the wound is faster in ponies than in horses, resulting in a higher number of PMNs during the first 3 weeks of healing in ponies. The PMNs subsequently disappear rapidly in these wounds. In horses, the influx is slower, and the initial number of PMNs is lower but thereafter remains persistently elevated [5].

Further research showed that leukocytes of ponies produce more reactive oxygen species (ROS), which are necessary for bacterial killing [14]. They also produced higher initial levels of several inflammatory mediators (tumor necrosis factor-α [TNFα], interleukin [IL]-1, chemoattractants, and transforming growth factor-β [TGFβ]) [14,15], which are essential for the reinforcement of the inflammatory response, for the induction of granulation tissue, and for wound contraction. The greater production of these mediators can thus explain the higher initial influx of leukocytes into wounds of ponies. The migrated leukocytes, in turn, release more biologically active substances, thus creating a positive feedback loop that further enhances the inflammatory response [6,16]. This loop can explain the faster cellular debridement of nonviable tissue and fibrin deposits in ponies and the more efficient local defense against contaminating bacteria, resulting in better prevention of wound infection [17]. A stronger acute inflammatory response thus prevents the development of chronic inflammation and leads to faster preparation of the wound for repair. Indeed, chronic inflammation perpetuates the release of tissue-damaging lysosomal enzymes as well as mediators, such as TGFβ, which overstimulate fibroplasia, leading to the formation of exuberant granulation tissue [6,18–20] and inhibiting contraction. In summary, the inflammatory response in ponies is a more efficient initiator of wound healing, whereas the lower initial production of TNFα, IL-1, chemoattractants, TGFβ, and ROS in horses can explain the weak onset of the inflammatory response and the ensuing persistence of inflammation.

Formation of granulation tissue

Granulation tissue is formed faster in horses than in ponies [7]. This new and abundant tissue seems to push the wound edges apart, which may explain why limb wounds in horses enlarge so dramatically after 2 weeks (Fig. 1). Additionally, the granulation tissue is traversed by grooves and clefts for a much longer period and presents a purulent surface up to week 5 after wound creation [4], which may relate to the weak and delayed onset of the inflammatory phase. In contrast, the granulation tissue of pony wounds is smooth, regular, and of a healthy pink color significantly sooner than that of horse wounds (see Fig. 1).

It is apparent microscopically that fibroblasts continue to proliferate in horse wounds even after granulation tissue has filled the wound bed contrary to pony fibroblasts, which cease proliferation at this time. Additionally, granulation tissue seems to be chaotic and subject to persistent inflammation in horses, whereas it is regularly organized in pony wounds [5]. As mentioned previously, there may exist a causal relation between persistent inflammation and the continuous proliferation of fibroblasts and synthesis of granulation tissue via the activity of mediators like TNFα, IL-1, IL-6, platelet derived growth factor (PDGF), TGFβ, and basic fibroblast growth factor (bFGF), which are know to induce fibrosis [19,21].

The formation of granulation tissue was less extensive in ponies despite initially higher levels of TNFα, IL-1, and TGFβ [4,14], which mediate the migration and proliferation of fibroblasts and endothelial cells [19]. Furthermore, fibroblasts of ponies are known to proliferate faster in vitro than those of horses [22,23]. Apparently, the balance of mediators in vivo is more important than actual levels in determining cellular proliferative rate, stressing once again the importance of the overall course of the inflammatory response.

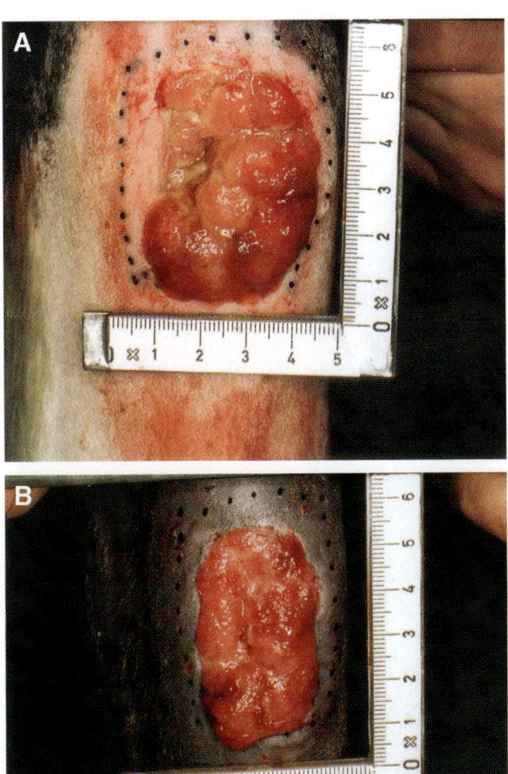

Fig. 1. Experimental metatarsal (*A*) and hindquarter (*C*) wounds of a horse and metatarsal (*B*) and hindquarter (*D*) wounds of a pony 14 days after creation. Tattoos are located 5 mm from the original wound margins. (*A*) The limb wound of the horse has enlarged to almost twice the original size. The formation of granulation tissue has been fast, and exuberant granulation tissue has developed. The tissue shows grooves and clefts and has a purulent aspect. (*B*) In contrast, the limb wound of the pony is decreasing in size after having maximally enlarged during the first week after creation. The formation of granulation tissue has been less extensive. The tissue has become regular significantly sooner, and it has developed a pink, glistening, and healthy surface significantly earlier. The body wounds of the horse (*C*) and pony (*D*) have decreased in size. The surface of the granulation tissue is more regular and healthy in body wounds compared with limb wounds. Protrusion of the granulation tissue over the wound margins is present in limb wounds (*A*, *B*) and body wounds (*C*, *D*).

The formation of granulation tissue in horses is thus excessively fast, not only compared with other species, as was found in the past [24], but compared with ponies [4]. The fast formation and persistent proliferation, no doubt related to an unrelenting inflammatory response, probably result in the formation of exuberant granulation tissue [4,5].

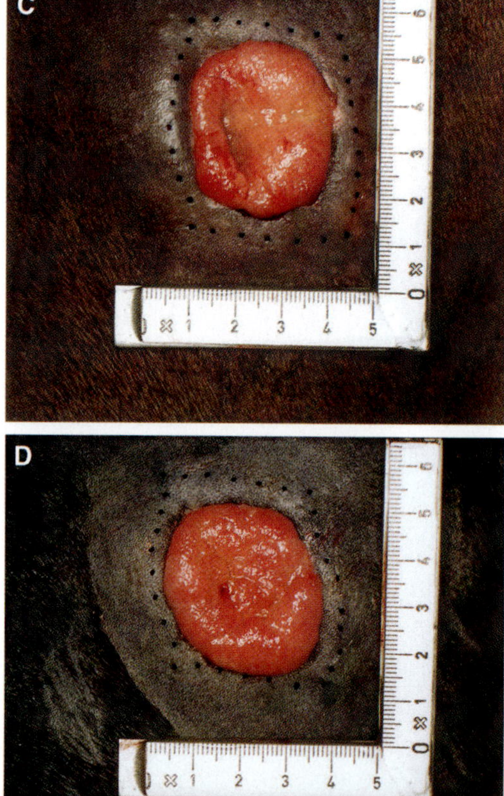

Fig. 1 (*continued*)

Wound contraction

Contraction is important to wound healing in the equine species because it results in fast closure of the wound by full-thickness skin. Consequently, wound contraction is a critical determinant of the speed of second-intention wound healing as well as the final cosmetic appearance of the scar.

Wound contraction is faster and more pronounced in ponies than in horses (Figs. 2, 3) [4]. Wound contraction occurs when the forces exerted by the myofibroblast exceed the centrifugal forces and the local resistance to movement from the environment. Centrifugal forces present in horse and pony skin are similar, as evidenced by the identical enlargement immediately after creation of experimental wounds. Moreover, there is no reason to assume that the local resistance to contraction in horses and ponies differs.

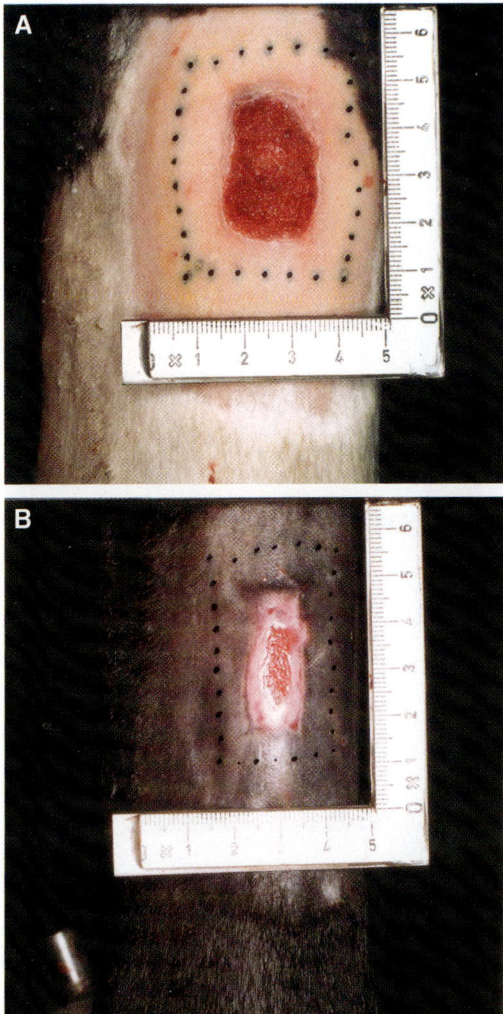

Fig. 2. Experimental metatarsal (*A*) and hindquarter (*C*) wounds of a horse and metatarsal (*B*) and hindquarter (*D*) wounds of a pony 42 days after creation. (*A*) The limb wound of the horse has almost not contracted, as is visualized by the tattoos. The wound area has decreased in size, mainly by epithelialization. The granulation tissue has finally become regular and healthy. (*B*) In contrast, the limb wound of the pony shows wound contraction and epithelialization. The body wounds of the horse (*C*) and pony (*D*) have decreased in size, mainly by wound contraction, which is more evident in the pony (*D*) than in the horse (*C*), as demonstrated by the tattoos.

Therefore, the differences in wound contraction are most likely related to differences in the contractile forces generated by myofibroblasts in the granulation tissue. Although myofibroblasts are better organized in the wounds of ponies [5], the inherent contraction capacity of fibroblasts from

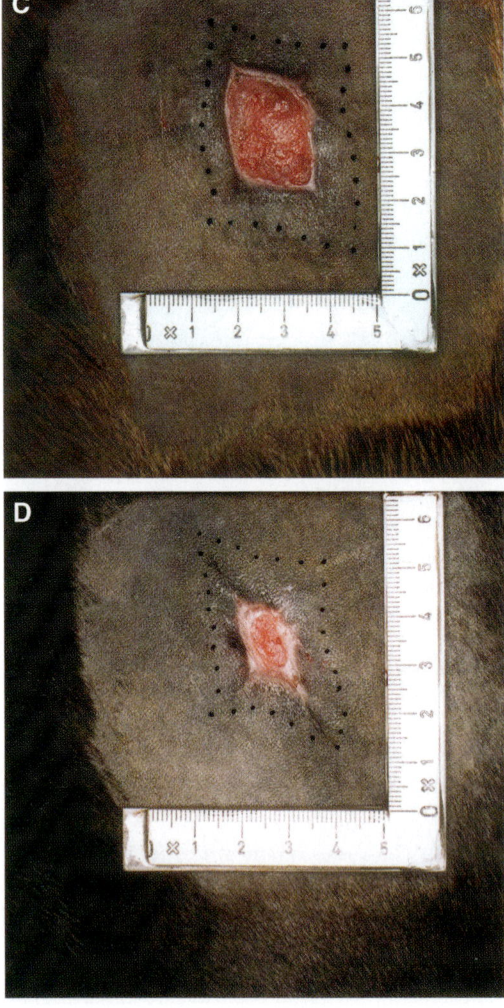

Fig. 2 (*continued*)

ponies and horses is similar, at least in vitro [22]. This suggests that environmental factors, such as the presence of inflammatory mediators, determine the contractile forces exerted by myofibroblasts, and hence the extent of wound contraction. Indeed, inflammatory mediators, particularly TGFβ, exert major effects on wound contraction. Interestingly, it has been shown that TGFβ levels are significantly higher in the early granulation tissue of pony wounds [15]. This may explain the faster organization of myofibroblasts and the more extensive wound contraction in ponies, because TGFβ stimulates the differentiation of fibroblasts into myofibroblasts [25], creates other conditions necessary for contraction [26], and

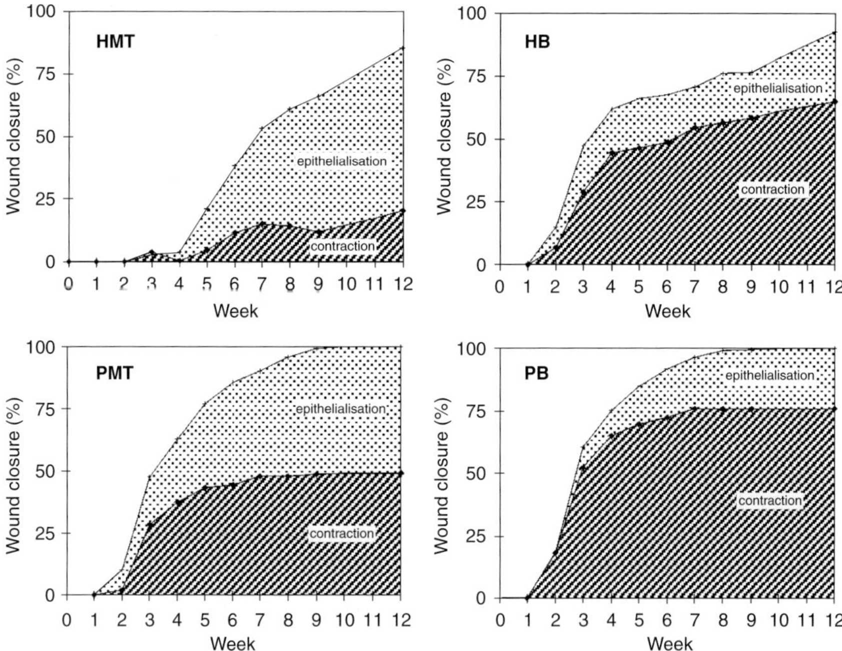

Fig. 3. Relative contribution of contraction and epithelialization to wound closure. HB, horse body wounds; HMT, horse metatarsal wounds; PB, pony body wounds; PMT, pony metatarsal wounds. (*From* Wilmink JM, Stolk PWT, van Weeren PR, et al. Differences in second-intention wound healing between horses and ponies: macroscopical aspects. Equine Vet J 1999;31:53–60; with permission.)

enhances contractile forces [27]. Furthermore, because other inflammatory mediators, such as prostaglandin (PG) E_1, PGE_2, TNFα, IL-1, IL-6, and interferon-γ (IFNγ) inhibit contractility [28], the chronic inflammatory response characteristic of horse wounds might exacerbate the deficient contraction noted in these wounds.

In summary, the greater contribution of contraction to wound closure in ponies compared with horses results in a faster second-intention wound healing process in the former (see Figs. 2, 3). Differences in wound contraction are not caused by disparity in the contractile capacity of the fibroblasts but by mediators present in the granulation tissue.

Epithelialization

Epithelialization is the slowest phase of the wound healing process and concludes wound closure. The mitotic activity of epithelial cells is similar for horses and ponies during the first weeks of healing. After the third week, however, an inverse relation between the epithelialized area and wound contraction develops: wounds demonstrating more contraction show less epithelialization (see Figs. 2, 3) [4]. This is likely related to a decrease in the length of the wound margins furnishing migrating and proliferating epithelial cells. Thus, more epithelialization is seen when limited wound contraction occurs, such as in limb wounds of horses (see Fig. 2) [4], which leads to a larger area of newly formed inferior-quality epithelium and the most pronounced scars [2,4].

Epithelialization is also affected by persistent inflammation, which promotes leukocyte release of toxic products and lysosomal enzymes. These not only induce tissue damage but inhibit epithelial mitosis by altering the critical balance of cytokines and growth factors on which epithelial cells depend [13].

Differences in second-intention healing between body and limb wounds

Clinical experience suggests that the healing of limb wounds is often delayed and complicated, whereas extensive body wounds usually heal remarkably well. These impressions have been experimentally confirmed [2,4] and further investigated.

Inflammatory phase

The influx of leukocytes is faster in body wounds than in limb wounds, resulting in higher numbers during the first 3 weeks of healing in body wounds. Thereafter, the number of PMNs decreases more rapidly in body wounds than in limb wounds [5].

Further research on the local inflammatory response has shown that the number of macrophages before and during local inflammation is significantly higher in tissue cages implanted in the neck than in the limb [14], although the levels of proinflammatory cytokines TNFα, IL-1, and IL-6, produced mainly by macrophages, do not differ. Contrary to the slower influx of leukocytes, the production of chemoattractants is significantly higher in limb cages, apparently as a result of greater susceptibility to repeat bleeding of the granulation tissue in the limb cages [14]. Interestingly, temporal expression of TGFβ, originating from leukocytes and fibroblasts, differs between the two sites [15,29]. Total TGFβ, active TGFβ, and TGF-β_1 reach a peak in body wounds during the first few days after wounding, after which levels return to baseline. Levels also peak early in limb wounds but remain persistently elevated thereafter [15,29].

The stronger and shorter inflammatory response in body wounds compared with limb wounds cannot be explained by differences in production of inflammatory mediators by leukocytes. Indeed, systemic leukocytes are genetically identical and can thus be expected to exhibit similar functions, independent of their environment, although subtle differences may exist in the way they are activated at various body sites. Variations in the inflammatory response may thus relate to differences in the anatomic environment, such as local temperature, local perfusion, and resident leukocyte population. Slightly higher temperature in body wounds compared with limb wounds may speed up biologic processes in general. The deepest layers of limb wounds often consist of cortical bone or tendon, whereas they almost invariably correspond to muscle in body wounds, which offers better perfusion, resulting in a faster supply of nutrients, oxygen, mediators, and leukocytes. Furthermore, the resident leukocyte population may differ between various sites on the body, as demonstrated in tissue cages [14]. It is also possible that local differences exist in vascular beds, the presence of receptors, and the reaction to cytokines, which can influence the migration of leukocytes. Greater numbers of immigrant or resident leukocytes intensify the inflammatory response through a positive feedback mechanism and can explain the faster initiation of the inflammatory response in body wounds compared with limb wounds. This results in more rapid cellular debridement and an earlier transition to repair in body wounds.

Formation of granulation tissue

Granulation tissue is formed more slowly and its surface takes a shorter time to become regular, pink, and healthy in body wounds compared with limb wounds [2,4] (see Fig. 1). This corresponds microscopically to a faster disappearance of clefts containing fibrin deposits and debris in body wounds [2,4], no doubt in relation to the stronger inflammatory response of the latter. Furthermore, fibroblast proliferation ceases sooner in body wounds, perhaps in response to decreasing levels of TGFβ [5,15,29], and the cells and ECM achieve a regular orientation earlier [2,5]. Conversely, persisting levels of TGFβ in limb wounds encourage the development of exuberant granulation tissue, because TGFβ not only stimulates inflammation and contraction but mediates migration and proliferation of fibroblasts and endothelial cells [19]. Although in apparent contradiction, the faster in vitro proliferation of fibroblasts from the rump compared with those from the limb [22,23] simply reflects the influence of the local environment on cellular function.

Wound contraction

Research has confirmed that wound contraction starts sooner and is more pronounced in body wounds than in limb wounds [4] (see Fig. 2). Restricted wound contraction may result from weaker centripetal forces, stronger centrifugal forces, or greater local resistance in limb wounds compared with body wounds. Centripetal forces exerted by the myofibroblast should be equivalent at various body sites, because the inherent contraction capacity of fibroblasts from the limb and the body is similar [22]. Additionally, peak levels of TGFβ, an important instigator of wound contraction, are not lower in limb wounds than in body wounds [15,29].

Centrifugal forces exerted by the environment seem to be smaller in limbs, which is evidenced by experimental wounds that enlarge significantly less in this location than on the body immediately after creation. Therefore, differences in wound contraction between body and limb wounds no doubt relate to a disparity in local resistance, which is probably higher in limbs, because the skin is more rigidly fixed to the skeleton in this area [2,4]. It is known that resistance to contraction can induce the expression of more TGFβ, which may subsequently downregulate TGFβ receptors and limit the response of the fibroblast (M.W.J. Ferguson, DDS, PhD, personal communication, 2000). This supports the finding that TGFβ levels persist and that fibroblasts are less differentiated and organized in limb wounds [5,15,29], which seems to be unfavorable for wound contraction. Moreover, limited contraction results in delayed reduction in wound size and contributes to the prolonged inflammation and persisting TGFβ levels, because the area exposed to environmental stimuli remains larger [30]. Prolonged inflammation inhibits contraction, is self-perpetuating, and contributes to the formation of exuberant granulation tissue, which, in turn, physically impedes wound contraction.

Epithelialization

The inverse relation between epithelialization and wound contraction probably results from the decrease in length of the wound margins by means of contraction, from which epithelialization occurs. Limited epithelialization and pronounced wound contraction result in stellate scars in body wounds (see Fig. 2) [2,4]. Limb wounds showing comparatively more epithelialization develop a larger area of inferior-quality neoepithelium and the most pronounced scars, which tend toward a circular shape [2,4]. The effect of faster epithelialization on the speed of healing is limited, because the process is inherently slow.

Development and treatment of exuberant granulation tissue

The formation of exuberant granulation tissue is a frequent complication in limb wounds of horses healing by second intention. Exuberant granulation tissue is typically unhealthy in appearance, its surface is riddled with many grooves and clefts, and it protrudes above the wound margins. The clefts contain fibrin deposits that have not been cleared by the acute inflammatory response; chronic inflammation ensues and proliferation is active. On histologic examination, the tissue has a chaotic, unorganized, cellular appearance [5]. Physiologically, the tissue may produce more TGFβ [31], and a greater population of fibroblasts translates into increased numbers of TGFβ receptors [32], stimulating the formation of surplus ECM. A recent study suggests that the excessive accumulation of ECM within the limb wounds of horses may also be caused by microvascular occlusion and deficient apoptosis (Professor C.L. Theoret, DMV, PhD, personal communication, 2004). Microvascular occlusion resulting in hypoxia would then stimulate excessive production of ECM components by fibroblasts by way of up-regulation of angiogenic and fibrogenic factors such as TGF-β. Furthermore, impaired apoptosis leads to persistence of an excess number of fibroblasts, compounding the imbalance between collagen synthesis and degradation, ultimately leading to excessive tissue formation. Thus, it seems that granulation tissue becomes exuberant as a result of dysregulated fibroplasia, whereas, in fact, normal regression of the acute inflammatory response should occur as well as a decrease in synthesis of ECM components and differentiation of proliferative and synthetic fibroblasts into contractile myofibroblasts.

Origins

Two important reasons for the high incidence of exuberant granulation tissue in limb wounds of horses are the development of chronic inflammation [33] and the common use of bandages in the management of such wounds. Chronic inflammation can develop as a result of other factors, such as bony sequestration, foreign bodies, disruption of the wound by motion, or the use of irritating or caustic agents in the wound, but it can also inherently develop in horses because of a less effective acute inflammatory response. The weak acute inflammatory response and the ensuing chronic inflammatory response contribute to the formation of exuberant granulation tissue and the lesser degree of wound contraction. The former, with lower TGFβ levels, retards differentiation of proliferating and synthesizing fibroblasts into myofibroblasts, which promotes tissue formation and restricts contraction. During the latter, several mediators (TNFα, IL-1, IL-6, PDGF, TGFβ, and bFGF additionally stimulate exuberant granulation tissue formation and others (PGE_1, PGE_2, TNFα, IL-1, IL-6, and IFNγ) inhibit contraction. The mutual influence of chronic inflammation, development of exuberant granulation tissue, and lack of wound contraction results in a self-perpetuating process.

It has been shown that the application of bandages and casts to full-thickness wounds promotes the formation of exuberant granulation tissue [34,35] not only in limb wounds but in body wounds [4]. Bandages and casts increase the oxygen gradient between tissue and the wound surface, which stimulates angiogenesis [36], and they can reduce oxygen tension in tissue, stimulating fibroblast proliferation [37]. Additionally, they create a moist and warm environment with a low pH, and some dressings can irritate the wound and trap exudate at the wound surface. All these factors tend to favor the development of exuberant granulation tissue [38]. In this respect, the use of pressure bandages in an attempt to impair granulation tissue formation is counterproductive. These bandages may effectively suppress the swelling of young edematous granulation tissue but generally do not impair its formation. Nevertheless, bandages also have many positive influences on wound healing. They keep the wound clean and prevent contamination and irritation by environmental factors, such as dirt and straw, which induce inflammation. They also allow topical treatments to be administered. Additionally, casts restrict movement in highly mobile regions, thus reducing disruption to the healing process and reducing the chance of exuberant granulation tissue formation.

Prevention and treatment

The prevention and treatment of exuberant granulation tissue focus on resolution of chronic inflammation. The wound should be carefully examined for possible irritants, such as bone sequestra, necrotic parts of tendons, foreign bodies, and motion resulting in disruption of the granulation tissue. Elimination of these factors, the use of casts in highly mobile areas, and the reduction of deleterious environmental influences contribute to the prevention and treatment of exuberant granulation tissue.

The formation of exuberant granulation tissue can be prevented largely by leaving the wound unbandaged [38]. This can be a reasonable choice when less intensive treatment is desired, for example, when costs must be limited. The best time to do this is after the wound has filled in with healthy-appearing granulation tissue. Leaving the wound unbandaged is not always the best or even a feasible option, however.

The treatment of exuberant granulation tissue is simple in most cases, and surgical excision seems to be the best choice [33]. It should be done as soon as granulation tissue protrudes above the wound margins [5]. Excision removes not only excess tissue but nonviable parts, contaminants, and the undue number of leukocytes present in the superficial layer of the granulation tissue. Excision thus purges the wound of triggers of chronic inflammation [33]. Furthermore, healing receives a new impulse: wound contraction occurs and epithelialization takes place. Usually, resection must be repeated a few times.

Environmental contaminants as triggers of chronic inflammation can be reduced by aseptic preparation of the wound site, followed by sterile bandaging. A period of topical antibacterial treatment or antiseptic dressings can assist in decreasing bacterial numbers at the wound surface and in clefts. The topical treatment must be chosen carefully, because some products can irritate the wound and delay healing [35].

Corticosteroids inhibit the formation of exuberant granulation tissue [39] by decreasing the overall chronic inflammatory response and levels of inflammatory mediators that induce fibrosis. There is evidence that some corticosteroids may selectively reduce the release of profibrotic TGF-β1 and TGF-β2 from monocytes and macrophages, reducing fibroblast proliferation and ECM formation. This makes corticosteroid use somewhat rational in the treatment of newly formed excessive granulation tissue [40]. If corticosteroids are used, it is suggested that one or two applications at the first signs of excessive fibroplasia are often all that is needed. Continued application is not recommended because it may exert negative effects on angiogenesis, wound contraction, and epithelialization [41].

Skin grafting or delayed (partial) closure of the wound can be used in the prevention or during treatment of exuberant granulation tissue to reduce the wound area. This results in a faster healing process. The wound area that is exposed to environmental stimuli is also reduced, resulting in a decline of inflammation and a reduction in the chance of exuberant granulation tissue formation, which further promotes healing.

The use of caustic agents or cryogenic surgery is not recommended because these seriously delay healing by inducing necrosis of the granulation tissue and the migrating and proliferating epithelium [3,11,38]. Necrosis exacerbates chronic inflammation and the release of mediators that inhibit wound contraction and overstimulate cellular proliferation. When wounds treated in this way eventually heal, they frequently have developed unacceptable scars [3].

Many other treatments have been tested unsuccessfully in the prevention and treatment of exuberant granulation tissue, namely, topical agents to affect collagen metabolism [38,42] and physical methods, such as electromagnetic stimulation [43]. A factor complicating the interpretation of these studies is that the treatment effect is often not correctly evaluated. During some treatments, it is advised to leave the wound unbandaged, which has a preventive influence on exuberant granulation tissue, and the real effect of the treatment can be disputed.

A current investigation is evaluating the efficacy of a silicone gel dressing (CicaCare; Smith & Nephew, Hull, England) in preventing the development of proud flesh in wounds located at the distal aspect of the limb in horses (C.L. Theoret, DVM, PhD, personal communication, 2004). This treatment is successful in reversing hypertrophic scarring in human burn patients, apparently by exerting pressure on the microvasculature of the scar and altering levels of various cytokines. The silicone gel dressing greatly surpassed a conventional nonadherent absorbent dressing in preventing the formation of exuberant granulation tissue in the experimental wounds of horses. Contraction and epithelialization progressed faster, possibly as a result of the healthier granulation tissue.

Finally, treatments focused on reducing the chronic inflammatory response are likely to be effective in preventing and treating exuberant granulation tissue. Therefore, the development of future medications based on a thorough knowledge of inflammatory mediators and cytokines looks promising.

Summary

Second-intention repair is faster in ponies than in horses and faster in body wounds than in limb wounds. To a large extent, the differences between horses and ponies can be explained by differences in the local inflammatory response, which are a result of the functional capacity of leukocytes. In ponies, leukocytes produce more inflammatory mediators, resulting in better local defense, faster cellular debridement, and a faster transition to the repair phases, with more wound contraction. In horses, leukocytes produce fewer mediators, initiating a weak inflammatory response, which becomes chronic. This inhibits wound contraction and gives rise to the formation of exuberant granulation tissue. The anatomic environment that influences the inflammatory response and wound contraction most probably determines the differences between body and limb wounds. In body wounds, better perfusion results in faster initiation of the inflammatory phase. The weaker local resistance results in a greater degree of contraction. In limb wounds, particularly of horses, the initial inflammatory response is weak and wound contraction is restricted. Both factors give rise to chronic inflammation, which further inhibits wound contraction and promotes exuberant granulation tissue. The high incidence of exuberant granulation tissue in limb wounds of horses can thus be explained by the chronicity of the inflammatory response as well as by the common use of bandages during treatment. Chronic inflammation is often not recognized as a cause of exuberant granulation tissue. It must be prevented and treated to promote the healing process. Bandages and casts stimulate the formation of exuberant granulation tissue; however, they are advantageous in many respects and play an important role in support of the overall healing process.

References

[1] Caron JP. Management of superficial wounds. In: Auer JA, Stick JA, editors. Equine surgery, vol. 1. 2nd edition. Philadelphia: WB Saunders; 1999. p. 129–40.

[2] Jacobs KA, Leach DH, Fretz PB, et al. Comparative aspects of the healing of excisional wounds on the leg and body of horses. Vet Surg 1984;13:83–90.

[3] Knottenbelt DC. Equine wound management: are there significant differences in healing at different sites on the body? Vet Dermatol 1997;8:273–90.

[4] Wilmink JM, Stolk PWT, van Weeren PR, et al. Differences in second-intention wound healing between horses and ponies: macroscopical aspects. Equine Vet J 1999;31:53–60.

[5] Wilmink JM, van Weeren PR, Stolk PWT, et al. Differences in second-intention wound healing between horses and ponies: histological aspects. Equine Vet J 1999;31:61–7.

[6] Cotran SC, Kumar V, Robbins SL. Cellular growth and differentiation: normal regulation and adaptations; inflammation and repair. In: Schoen FJ, editor. Robbins pathologic basis of disease, vol. 1. 5th edition. Philadelphia: WB Saunders; 1994. p. 35–92.

[7] Clark RAF. Cutaneous tissue repair: basic biologic considerations I. J Am Acad Dermatol 1985;5:701–25.

[8] Clark RAF. Biology of dermal repair. Dermatol Clin 1993;11:647–66.

[9] Moulin V. Growth factors in skin wound healing. Eur J Cell Biol 1995;68:1–7.

[10] Darby I, Skalli O, Gabbiani G. α-Smooth muscle actin is transiently expressed by myofibroblasts during experimental wound healing. Lab Invest 1990;63:21–9.

[11] Stashak TS. Principles of wound healing. In: Equine wound management. Philadelphia: Lea & Febiger; 1991. p. 1–18.
[12] Clark RAF. Basics of cutaneous wound repair. J Dermatol Surg Oncol 1993;19:693–706.
[13] Stadelmann WK, Digenis AG, Tobin GR. Physiology and healing dynamics of chronic cutaneous wounds. Am J Surg 1998;176:26–38.
[14] Wilmink JM, van den Boom R, Veenman JN, et al. Differences in polymorphonucleocyte function and local inflammatory response as a possible cause for differences in wound healing efficiency between horses and ponies. Equine Vet J 2003;35:561–9.
[15] Van Den Boom R, Wilmink JM, O'Kane S, et al. Transforming growth factor-β levels during second intention healing are related to the different course of wound contraction in horses and ponies. Wound Rep Regen 2002;10:188–94.
[16] Rook G, Balkwil F. Cell-mediated immune reactions. In: Crowe L, editor. Immunology. 5th edition. London: Mosby International; 1998. p. 121–38.
[17] Wilmink JM, van Herten J, van Weeren PR, et al. Study of primary-intention healing and sequester formation in horses compared to ponies. Equine Vet J 2002;34:270–3.
[18] Wahl SM. The role of lymphokines and monokines in fibrosis. Ann NY Acad Sci 1985;460: 224–31.
[19] Turck C, Dohlman JG, Goetzl E. Immunological mediators of wound healing and fibrosis. J Cell Physiol 1987;5:89–93.
[20] Roberts AB, Sporn MB, Assoian RK, et al. Transforming growth factor type β: rapid induction of fibrosis and angiogenesis in vivo and stimulation of collagen formation in vitro. Proc Natl Acad Sci USA 1986;83:4167–71.
[21] Kovacs EJ. Fibrogenic cytokines: the role of immune mediators in the development of scar tissue. Immunol Today 1991;12:17–23.
[22] Wilmink JM, Nederbragt H, van Weeren PR, et al. Differences in wound contraction between horses and ponies: the in vitro contraction capacity of fibroblasts. Equine Vet J 2001;33:499–505.
[23] Miller CB, Wilson DA, Keegan KG, et al. Growth characteristics of fibroblasts isolated from the trunk and distal aspect of the limb of horses and ponies. Vet Surg 2000;29:1–7.
[24] Chvapil M, Pfister T, Escalada S, et al. Dynamics of the healing of skin wounds in the horse as compared with the rat. Exp Mol Pathol 1979;30:349–59.
[25] Desmoulière A, Geinoz A, Gabbiani F, et al. Transforming growth factor-β1 induces α-smooth muscle actin expression in granulation tissue myofibroblasts and in quiescent and growing cultured fibroblasts. J Cell Biol 1993;122:103–11.
[26] Ignotz RA, Heino J, Massagué J. Regulation of cell adhesion receptors by transforming growth factor-β. J Biol Chem 1989;264:389–92.
[27] Montesano R, Orci L. Transforming growth factor β stimulates collagen-matrix contraction by fibroblasts: implications for wound healing. Proc Natl Acad Sci USA 1988;85:4894–7.
[28] Ehrlich HP, Wyler DJ. Fibroblast contraction of collagen lattices in vitro: inhibition by chronic inflammatory cell mediators. J Cell Physiol 1983;116:345–51.
[29] Theoret CL, Barber SM, Moyana TN, et al. Expression of transforming growth factor β_1, β_3, and basic fibroblast factor in full-thickness skin wounds of equine limbs and thorax. Vet Surg 2001;30:269–77.
[30] Greenhalgh DG. The role of apoptosis in wound healing. Int J Biochem Cell B 1998;30: 1019–30.
[31] Theoret CL, Barber SM, Moyana TN, et al. Preliminary observations on expression of transforming growth factors β1 and β3 in equine full-thickness skin wounds healing normally or with exuberant granulation tissue. Vet Surg 2002;31:266–73.
[32] De Martin I, Theoret CL. Spatial and temporal expression of types I and II receptors for transforming growth factor β in normal equine skin and dermal wounds. Vet Surg 2004;33: 70–6.
[33] Wilmink JM, van Weeren PR. The ins and outs of exuberant granulation tissue. North Am Vet Conf 2003;17:270–1.

[34] Fretz PB, Martin GS, Jacobs KA, et al. Treatment of exuberant granulation tissue in the horse: Evaluation of four methods. Vet Surg 1983;12:137–40.

[35] Berry DB, Sullins KE. Effects of topical application of antimicrobials and bandaging on healing and granulation tissue formation in wounds of the distal aspect of the limbs in horses. Am J Vet Res 2003;64:88–92.

[36] Knighton DR, Silver IA, Hunt TK. Regulation of wound-healing angiogenesis. Effect of oxygen gradients and inspired oxygen concentration. Surgery 1981;90:262–70.

[37] Kirsner RS, Eaglstein WH. The wound healing process. Dermatol Clin 1993;11:629–40.

[38] Bertone AL. Management of exuberant granulation tissue. Vet Clin N Am Equine Pract 1989;5:551–62.

[39] Barber SM. Second intention wound healing in the horse: the effect of bandages and topical corticosteroids. Proc Am Assoc Equine Pract 1990;35:107–16.

[40] Beck LS, Deguzman L, Lee WP, et al. TGF-beta 1 accelerates wound healing: reversal of steroid-impaired healing in rats and rabbits. Growth Factors 1991;5:295–304.

[41] Hashimoto I, Nakanishi H, Shono Y, et al. Angiostatic effects of corticosteroid on wound healing of the rabbit ear. J Med Invest 2002;49:61–6.

[42] Blackford J, Shires M, Goble D, et al. The use of N-butyl cyanoacrylate in the treatment of open leg wounds in the horse. Proc Am Assoc Equine Pract 1986;32:349–55.

[43] Steckel RR, Page EH, Geddes LA, et al. Electrical stimulation on skin wound healing in the horse: preliminary studies. Am J Vet Res 1984;45:800–3.

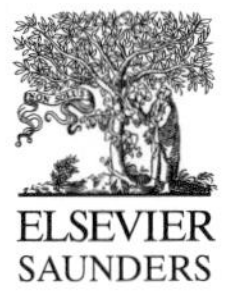

ELSEVIER
SAUNDERS

Vet Clin Equine 21 (2005) 33–44

VETERINARY
CLINICS
Equine Practice

Factors that Affect Equine Wound Repair

Dean Hendrickson, DVM, MS*, Joanna Virgin

Equine Surgery, Clinical Sciences, James L. Voss Veterinary Teaching Hospital, Colorado State University, 300 West Drake Road, Fort Collins, CO 80523–1678, USA

This article provides a general overview of the major factors influencing wound repair. The mechanism and time of onset, the location of a wound, its degree of contamination, and any previous therapy aid in determining the most appropriate management of the wound and the patient.

Wound type

Wounds can be categorized as closed (bruise, hematoma, and contusion) or open (abrasion, erosion, puncture, incision, laceration, and burn). Wound type is an important indicator of the vascular supply, degree of contamination, and viability of surrounding tissue, which reliably determine the best mode of management. For example, relatively uncontaminated incisions and lacerations, such as shearing injuries produced by sharp objects, can heal by primary intention, because tissue devitalization and risk of infection are minimal. Conversely, primary closure of crushing injuries, such as those sustained on limb entrapment, is usually not successful because of the extent of microvascular disruption and tissue trauma that inhibits local defense mechanisms, increasing the risk of infection. Indeed, a lower bacterial load is required to cause infection after blunt trauma compared with other types of wounds. In these cases, second-intention healing is often the best alternative.

Degree of contamination

Wounds are classified into the following categories based on their degree of bacterial contamination: clean, clean-contaminated, contaminated, and infected (Table 1). The degree of bacterial contamination is considered

* Corresponding author.
E-mail address: Dean.Hendrickson@colostate.edu (D. Hendrickson).

doi:10.1016/j.cveq.2004.11.002 **vetequine.theclinics.com**

Table 1
Comparison of wound classifications based on degree of contamination

Wound classification	Description
Clean	Nontraumatic surgical wounds
	Hollow viscus is not entered
	Incision does not pass through infected or nonviable tissue [3,9]
Clean-contaminated	Surgical wounds in which the lumen of the alimentary, urogenital, or respiratory tract may be entered but with minimal invasiveness and contamination [3,9]
Contaminated	Traumatic wounds
	Relatively clean source of wounding
	Commonly accompanied by inflammation
	Include surgical wounds that contain "spill" from another organ and traumatic wounds older than 4 to 6 hours [1,3,9]
Infected	Old traumatic wounds
	Pus and/or abscess is present
	Preoperative entry into viscera may have occurred [3,9]

a reliable predictor of the potential for wound infection. Although the categories are broad and do not evaluate potential confounding risk factors, these basic distinctions serve as the basis for directing wound management.

Clean and clean-contaminated wounds should be sutured when there is adequate surrounding tissue to close the wound with minimal tension and the vascular supply is sufficient. The incidence of infection subsequent to primary closure of clean and clean-contaminated wounds is significantly lower than that in contaminated or infected wounds [1,2].

The accepted protocol for contaminated and infected wounds is thorough lavage and debridement, followed by open wound management and delayed primary closure or second-intention healing as appropriate [3,4]. Other factors, such as vascular supply to the wound, location, and mechanism of onset, also play a role in ascertaining the best management. The time elapsed since injury is not always an accurate factor to rule out primary closure of contaminated wounds. For example, clean-contaminated and "fresh"-contaminated wounds can be converted to clean wounds by thorough lavage and debridement, enabling subsequent primary closure [3,4]. Based on documented lower infection rates, however, most authors advocate open wound management, with or without delayed primary closure, as the preferred repair method [1,2].

Location

The specific limitations and needs of a wound are dependent on its location and severity [5]. By predicting delays and obstacles to the normal reparative processes of wounds in different locations of the body, the veterinarian can adjust management practices to account for these differences.

Particularities of wounds of the distal extremities

Certain anatomic locations on the horse heal more successfully than others because of better physiologic healing characteristics [6]. In human beings, wounds to the head and neck heal more quickly and cosmetically than those in other areas because of a better blood supply, greater number of adnexal structures, and thinner epidermis [6]. In the horse, distal limb wounds exhibit persistent inflammation, greater retraction, and premature cessation of contraction as well as slower rates of epithelialization [7,8]. Healing in this area is also complicated by the formation of exuberant granulation tissue, hypertrophic scarring, and cell transformation.

Some of the challenges presented by wounds on the distal limb can be attributed to the anatomic and physiologic particularities in this area. These include skin with a decreased vascular supply, numerous bony prominences, absence of supporting deep musculature, highly mobile joints, and a generally higher degree of contamination than found in other body sites [5,9–12]. Recent studies have suggested that distal limb wounds exhibit increased collagen synthesis because of prolonged expression of profibrotic growth factors [11], persistent heightened numbers of fibroblasts, and decreased collagen degradation [10]. In comparison to wounds of the distal limb, those on the body exhibit better oriented myofibroblasts, which should lead to more efficient contraction and superior cosmetic results [10]. This no doubt accounts for the clinical observation that body wounds, even extensive ones, usually close successfully even when allowed to heal by second intention.

Because of the elevated tension, relatively poor blood supply, and high degree of contamination common in traumatic wounds of the limb, primary and delayed closures are not always appropriate methods of repair in this location. Conversely, second-intention healing often leads to excessive granulation tissue and cell transformation. Although a moist wound environment is beneficial to most wounds, controlled studies show that occlusive bandages can promote excessive fibroplasias in equine distal limb wounds [13,14]. Occlusive bandages are only beneficial until a healthy bed of granulation tissue fills the defect and is flush with surrounding skin. Thereafter, continued occlusion in the form of bandages stimulates the formation of proud flesh, slowing contraction and epithelialization. Repair and management of this type of wound should be directed toward accelerating healing by restricting movement in the wound bed and promoting wound contraction. This is best achieved by maintaining a fine balance between a moist wound environment and granulation tissue formation.

Primary closure or delayed primary closure can be used on wounds of the distal limb if there is adequate tissue to close the wound with minimal tension. Surgical incisions or noncontaminated lacerations on the limb can be closed primarily and immobilized with a stent, encircling bandage, cast, or other method that minimizes movement, especially that occurring over joints. Suturing limb wounds may necessitate prior undermining or relief incisions or tension-relieving suture techniques.

Contaminated limb wounds require debridement, lavage, and open wound management. The selection of topical medications, bandages, and immobilization techniques should be made according to this location's typical impairments. For example, excessive bandage changes and inappropriate dressings that can traumatize the fragile epithelial cells should be avoided [15]. Compression bandages and rigid limb casting are useful in the management of distal limb wounds because they restrict movement and have also been indicated to reduce the formation of exuberant granulation tissue [5,8]. Care must be taken to avoid applying bandages too tightly because this reduces perfusion of the wound by hindering the local blood supply [5]. Specific dressings and their uses are discussed in further detail elsewhere in this issue. Skin grafting is also an option for repair of lower limb wounds if contraction has ceased and the granulation bed is healthy [8].

Movement

A wound over an area with excessive mobility, such as a joint, is prone to chronic inflammation because of the repetitive disruption of capillary buds, collagen deposits, and fragile new epithelium [5,15]. Conversely, complete immobilization of the wounded area can lead to a disorganized arrangement of new collagen within the wound bed that lessens the resultant tensile strength [5,15]. The predicted amount of movement should dictate dressing and suture choice such that tension is minimized; in some instances, the application of a splint or cast is warranted to provide the best opportunity for strong wound healing.

Structure involvement

The location of a wound determines the potential for deep structure involvement, which is another important consideration of wound management. Repair of wounds that involve or are near synovial structures, such as joints, tendon sheaths, or bursae, necessitates strict aseptic techniques and timely management to prevent contamination and infection. If involvement of a synovial structure is suspected, digital palpation or synovial distention can confirm whether or not the wound communicates with or has entered the structure. If synovial involvement is established, the wound must be thoroughly lavaged and managed with appropriate wound dressing, bandaging, and an antibiotic regimen. Rigid limb casting is recommended to minimize movement in wounds involving tendons and ligaments [5]. Contaminated and infected wounds or those with substantial tissue loss should be managed by delayed primary closure or second-intention healing.

Wounds to the distal limb and head often involve bone exposure, which may lead to sequestrum formation after damage to the periosteum [5]. It is important to note that bony sequestration can take weeks to develop, often beneath a cover of unhealthy granulation tissue, making it difficult to detect [5]. The possibility of a fracture or tendon and ligament involvement should be investigated first by radiography and wound exploration [5]. If either is confirmed, the area should be debrided and immobilized.

Other locations also warrant special attention to rule out involvement of underlying structures. Deep wounds or lacerations to the chest require careful exploration to determine whether the pleural cavity has been penetrated because this can lead to pneumothorax; auscultation, radiography, and an ultrasound examination are warranted. Abdominal wounds require close inspection for herniation of abdominal viscera [5]. Wounds involving body cavities often require surgical repair, are complicated by high rates of infection, and necessitate immediate emergency treatment [5].

Cosmetic locations

Wounds in areas of cosmetic importance, such as the face, head, and neck, should be repaired by techniques that minimize scarring and approximate the original appearance. Although wounds to the head heal well by second intention, grafting and primary closure are options to speed healing and improve the appearance of the wound site [5,15].

Vascularization

Deficient blood flow to a wound bed increases the risk of infection and slows the rate of healing. Although the skin of some areas, such as the distal limb, possesses an inferior blood supply, the latter can also be impaired in other locations secondary to wounding. Indeed, damage to major surrounding vessels, thrombosis, edema, contusion, ischemia, anemia, and local anesthetic agents that promote vasoconstriction lead to delays in capillary formation [5]. It is vital that pressure bandages and anesthetic agents be used fittingly during wound management to avoid such problems. Furthermore, primary closure and skin grafting are unsuitable for repair in areas in which tissue is poorly perfused [3,4,6].

Bony prominences

Wounds over bony prominences heal more slowly than those in other areas because of decreased vascularity and increased tissue tension. This is an important consideration when addressing whether the wound edges can be approximated or if reconstructive and cosmetic approaches are appropriate.

Tension

Tension is a key factor influencing wound repair because it can alter the cosmetic outcome of the wound and impair healing by decreasing blood flow, increasing the inflammatory response, and compromising surrounding tissues [16]. Therefore, tension often determines which management techniques are suitable. For example, suturing is inappropriate in wounds in which the resulting tension leads to ischemia and pressure necrosis of the surrounding tissue [6,17]. In cases in which closure is possible, it is often necessary to implement tension-relieving techniques to avoid these complications. If suturing techniques alone cannot reduce the tension to an optimum level, other tension-relieving techniques, such as undermining, should be used before closure to mobilize the wound edges [17].

Nature of wound

Exudate

Certain types of wounds are characterized by excessive exudate, including burns, wounds with large amounts of skin loss, extensive grazing injuries, and nonhealing wounds with chronic infection [5]. Wound exudate contains nutrients and growth factors produced by key cells in the wound repair process [18,19], and current evidence suggests that allowing wound fluid to stay in contact with the wound is beneficial to healing, at least in the case of acute wounds [18–20].

Indeed, there is evidence supporting the benefits of acute wound fluid on fibroblast migration, growth, and contractile activity [16,19,21,22]. For example, it has been shown that in vitro, human burn blister fluid promotes contraction, whereas acute wound fluid stimulates growth of endothelial cells and dermal fibroblasts [19,21,22]. Conversely, chronic wound fluid induces fibroblast senescence, [23] contains higher levels of protein-degrading enzymes [18,24,25], and dramatically decreases collagen synthesis [23], with an overall effect of retarding healing.

Maintenance of a moist wound environment is considered optimal in many instances [5,6,18,26,27], because such conditions encourage a higher rate of revascularization and epithelialization, increased collagen synthesis and rate of epithelialization, decreased healing time, and decreased pain [26–29]. Nevertheless, although a moist wound environment seems to be conducive to healing in most types of wounds, surplus amounts of exudate may cause tissue maceration; protein, electrolyte, and zinc loss; and anemia [5]. Certain wounds characterized by abundant exudate should be managed by methods favoring its resolution, such as debridement, drains, appropriate dressings, and pressure bandages. Studies in the horse show that occlusive bandages can promote excessive granulation tissue formation if used inappropriately [13,14].

Bacteriology

The degree of bacterial contamination determines the most appropriate method of managing a wound. Thus, quantitative and qualitative wound cultures can be important tools in wound management. The common guideline for predicting the success of healing without infection is based on a bacterial load less than 105 bacteria per gram of tissue [30,31]. Wound infection and healing are affected not only by the dose of bacteria but by the virulence and pathogenicity of the organisms as well as the host's resistance [30,32]. Therefore, it is ill-advised to rely solely on quantitative bacteriology when estimating the risk of infection. Qualitative cultures provide information about the organism's pathogenicity and its interactions with surrounding microflora, which determine the infective dose of the organism [30,31].

There are several ways to culture a wound, including tissue biopsy, swab culture, and fluid aspiration. In addition to identifying the most effective antimicrobial therapy for the wound, the culture and sensitivity testing may pinpoint factors that could impair healing, such as an altered pH caused by certain bacteria [5].

Most wounds are colonized by a normal level of bacteria that does not harm the host or impede healing [30,31]. In fact, colonization by commensal organisms is thought to accelerate wound repair and increase granulation tissue formation by enhancing the immune response in the wound [20,31]. In this case, a moist environment can be maintained; however, wounds that are critically contaminated or infected must first be addressed by reducing the bacterial load through debridement and antibacterial therapy [31].

Necrotic tissue and foreign bodies

Foreign bodies commonly found in equine wounds include wood, metal, surgical implants (eg, plates, screws), suture, and necrotic tissue. The presence of a foreign body within the wound is a source of infection and irritation [5,33]. Before any other treatment, the presence of a foreign body should be ruled out in a wound exhibiting delayed repair. This can be done by manual exploration, ultrasound, plain and contrast radiology, CT, and MRI. If the presence of a foreign body is confirmed within the wound, debridement and lavage are necessary to ensure a clean and moist granular wound bed before the wound can be repaired.

Wound dimensions

The shape, size, and depth of a wound affect the amount and rate of contraction in human patients [34,35]. Linear wounds closed the fastest, followed by rectangular and then circular wounds. This pattern has not been confirmed in the horse, where the shape of a wound does not seem to influence contraction [36].

Wound shape sometimes limits whether skin edges can be successfully approximated or not. Additionally, wound shape and orientation in relation to the tension lines of the skin determine the tautness in the wound, and consequently govern blood flow and closure technique. This must be kept in mind when creating wounds; whenever possible, incisions should be parallel to tension lines to minimize gaping and the amount of suture material required for closure as well as to maximize the ultimate strength of the repair.

Previous treatment

Prior treatment is another important factor to consider during wound management because it conveys information about the condition of the wound and the state of healing. Topical and systemic treatments can negatively influence wound healing by slowing cellular proliferation and hindering the immune response of the host [6,37,38]. Thus, by pondering all previous therapy dispensed by the owner or another veterinarian, the practitioner can estimate the wound's degree of contamination and any impairment in the host's defenses, which may obviate primary closure of the wound.

Hydrogen peroxide and concentrated solutions of povidone-iodine exert cytotoxic effects on human fibroblasts and keratinocytes and delay wound healing in animal models [39,40], such that ultimate wound strength may be reduced. It is therefore critical to lavage the wound copiously after gently cleaning it with appropriate concentrations of antiseptic soap (ideally, a 0.05% solution of chlorhexidine gluconate) to neutralize the detergent base of the antiseptics. In the realm of lavage solutions, phosphate-buffered saline (PBS) and Ringer's lactate solution seem safest [37].

Topical application of steroids slows wound healing by decreasing fibroblast proliferation and inhibits protein synthesis [41]. In leg wounds in horses, however, where exuberant granulation tissue tends to develop, the temporary use of topical steroids may be beneficial. A study found that topical application of fluoroprednisolone under bandages neutralized the stimulatory effect of the bandage on fibroplasia and significantly increased the speed of contraction and overall repair [42].

Age of wound

Although the age of the wound may not always specify the appropriate method of repair, it should be considered when selecting topical treatments and wound management techniques. Because of the many factors governing the rate of infection, no definitive interval can accurately predict the risk of infection in every situation. Thus, the "golden period," considered to be the 6 to 8 hours after injury, does not dependably determine whether primary closure should be attempted or not.

Acute wounds

Acute wounds are described as disruptions in the integrity of the skin that evolve through the healing process in a predictable and timely manner [6].

Repair and management of acute wounds thus depends on many of the factors discussed previously, such as degree of contamination, location, mechanism of onset, and characteristics of the wound itself.

Chronic wounds

Conversely, chronic wounds do not progress normally through the various phases of repair, usually as a consequence of underlying conditions [43]. As a result, the goal in such instances is to identify and resolve the causal factors so that healing can proceed. There are many sources of chronic inflammation in a wound, including necrotic tissue, foreign bodies, repetitive mechanical trauma, and the application of cytotoxic agents [5]. The horse is particular in this respect in that its inflammatory response to trauma inflicted to the limb does not resolve normally and becomes chronic [44,45]. Necrotic tissue and foreign bodies prolong inflammation because of the body's attempt to rid the area of the alien matter. Debridement of devitalized tissue is the most effective method to improve healing in these cases [32]. The misuse of wound dressings, bandages, and debridement techniques can be a source of repetitive mechanical trauma that retards healing because of persistent disruption of the new and tenuous cellular populations (epithelial and endothelial cells and fibroblasts) [32]. Ultimately, the goal of chronic wound therapy is to eliminate the causal agents and convert the wound environment to one that closely resembles that of the acute wound.

Other factors

Economic factors can certainly limit repair options based on the expense of different treatments and the use of the horse. Other aspects that influence wound repair include the temperament, health, and nutritional status of the horse. For example, research has shown that wounds of malnourished human beings have a higher incidence of infection and other complications that delay healing [6,32]. Similarly, in horses, poor health and conditions like malnutrition and protein and vitamin deficiencies as well as hormonal imbalances, although rare, significantly slow repair [5]. For example, protein intake is important in the recovery from severe injury, particularly burn wounds. Specifically, protein deficiencies can decrease fibroblast proliferation, angiogenesis, proteoglycan and collagen synthesis, and collagen remodeling [32]. Serum protein must be less than 2 g/dL before wound repair is impeded [46], however, and this is extremely uncommon in the horse. Vitamin A exerts beneficial effects on repair by enhancing epithelialization [47] and by positively influencing wound contraction [48,49]. Vitamin C, along with iron, acts as a cofactor during the production and cross-linking of collagen. Zinc is hypothesized to play a significant role in the synthesis of granulation and scar tissue as well as epithelialization [50].

Summary

The rate and outcome of wound healing are determined by many factors, some of which are already in effect when the horse is first presented to the veterinarian. A thorough understanding of wound healing principles, coupled with clear client communication, should enable the practitioner to minimize the number of additional factors that may exacerbate the initial situation.

References

[1] Smilanich RP, Bonnet I, Kirkpatrick JR. Contaminated wounds: the effect of initial management on outcome. Am Surg 1995;61(5):427–30.
[2] Page CP, Bohnen JMA, Fletcher JR, et al. Antimicrobial prophylaxis for surgical wounds; guidelines for clinical care. Arch Surg 1993;128:79–88.
[3] Stanley B. Management of the contaminated wound. In: Proceedings and Abstracts of the XXIst Congress of the World Small Animal Veterinary Association. Jerusalem, Israel: World Small Animal Veterinary Association; 1996. p. 245–51.
[4] Phillips TJ. Initial management of equine wounds: part II. Equine Vet Educ 1995;7(4):193–8.
[5] Knottenbelt DC. Handbook of equine wound management. Liverpool, UK: WB Saunders; 2003.
[6] Moy LS. Management of acute wounds. Dermatol Clin 1993;11(4):759–76.
[7] Jacobs KA, Leach DH, Fretz PB, et al. Comparative aspects of the healing of excisional wounds on the leg and body of horses. J Vet Surg 1984;13(2):83–90.
[8] Bertone A. Management of exuberant granulation tissue. J Vet Clin N Am Equine Pract 1989;5(3):551–6.
[9] Lindsay MA. Wound healing in horses: guidelines for classification. J Vet Med 1988;83: 387–95.
[10] Schwartz AJ, Wilson DA, Keegan KG, et al. Factors regulating collagen synthesis and degradation during second-intention healing of wounds in the thoracic region and distal aspect of the forelimb of horses. Am J Vet Clin 2002;63(11):1564–70.
[11] Theoret CL, Barber SM, Moyana TN, et al. Expression of transforming growth factor β1, β2, and basic fibroblast growth factor in full-thickness skin wounds of equine limbs and thorax. J Vet Surg 2001;30:269–77.
[12] Cochrane CA, Pain R, Knottenbelt DC. In-vitro wound contraction in the horse: differences between body and limb wounds. Wounds 2003;15(6):175–81.
[13] Berry DB II, Sullins KE. Effects of topical application of antimicrobials and bandaging on healing and granulation tissue formation in wounds of the distal aspect of the limbs in horses. Am J Vet Res 2003;64(1):88–92.
[14] Howard RD, Stashak TS, Baxter GM. Evaluation of occlusive dressings for management of full-thickness excisional wounds on the distal portion of the limbs of horses. Am J Vet Res 1993;54(12):2150–4.
[15] Bertone A. Principles of wound healing. J Vet Clin N Am Equine Pract 1989;5(3): 449–63.
[16] Orredson SU, Knighton DR, Scheuenstuhl H, et al. A quantitative in vitro study of fibroblast and endothelial cell migration in response to serum and wound fluid. J Surg Res 1983;35(3):249–58.
[17] Johnston DE. Tension relieving techniques. Plast Reconstr Surg 1990;20(1):67–80.
[18] Jones V, Harding K. Moist wound healing. In: Krasner DL, Rodeheaver GT, Sibbald RG, editors. Chronic wound care: a clinical source book for healthcare professionals. 3rd edition. Wayne, PA: HMP Communications; 2001. p. 245–52.

[19] Katz MH, Alvarez AF, Kirsner RS, et al. Human wound fluid from acute wounds stimulates fibroblast and endothelial cell growth. J Am Acad Dermatol 1991;25(6):1054–8.
[20] Hutchinson JJ, McGuckin M. Occlusive dressings: a microbiologic and clinical review. Am J Infect Control 1990;18(4):257–68.
[21] Wilson AM, McGrouther DA, Eastwood M, et al. The effect of burn blister fluid on contraction. Burns 1997;23(4):306–12.
[22] Atiyeh BS, Ioannovich J, Al-Anim CA, et al. Management of acute and chronic open wounds: the importance of moist wound environment in optimal wound healing. Curr Pharm Biotechnol 2002;3(3):179–95.
[23] Trengove NJ, Stacey MC, MacAuley S, et al. Analysis of the acute and chronic wound environments: the role of proteases and their inhibitors. Wound Repair Regen 1999;7(6): 442–52.
[24] Mendez MV, Raffeto JD, Phillips T, et al. The proliferative capacity of neonatal skin fibroblasts is reduced after exposure to venous leg ulcer wound fluid: a potential mechanism for senescence in venous ulcers. J Vasc Surg 1999;30(4):734–43.
[25] Wysocki AB, Staiano-Coico L, Grinnel F. Wound fluid from chronic leg ulcers contains elevated levels of metalloproteinases. J Invest Dermatol 1993;101(1):64–8.
[26] Dyson M, Young SR, Hart J, et al. Comparison of the effects of moist and dry wound conditions on the process of angiogenesis during dermal repair. J Invest Dermatol 1993;99: 729–33.
[27] Alvarez OM, Mertz PM, Eaglstein WH. The effect of occlusive dressings on collagen synthesis and re-epithelialization in superficial wounds. J Surg Res 1983;35:142–8.
[28] Madden MR, Nolan E, Finkelstein JL, et al. Comparison of an occlusive and a semi-occlusive dressing and the effect of the wound exudate upon keratinocyte proliferation. J Trauma Injury Infect Crit Care 1989;29(7):924–30.
[29] Holm C, Petersen JS, Gronboek F, et al. Effects of occlusive and conventional gauze dressings on incisional healing after abdominal operations. Eur J Surg 1998;164(3):179–83.
[30] Bowler PG. The 10(5) bacterial growth guideline: reassessing its clinical relevance in wound healing. Ostomy Wound Manage 2003;49(1):44–53.
[31] Edwards R, Harding KG. Bacteria and wound healing. Current Opin Infect Dis 2004;17: 91–6.
[32] Stotts NA, Wipke-Tevis DD. Co-factors in impaired wound healing. In: Krasner DL, Rodeheaver GT, Sibbald RG, editors. Chronic wound care: a source book for healthcare professionals. 3rd edition. Wayne, PA: HMP Communications; 2001. p. 265–73.
[33] Gift LJ, Debowes RM. Wounds associated with osseous sequestration and penetrating foreign bodies. J Vet Clin N Am Equine Pract 1989;5(3):695–708.
[34] Hashmito I, Nakanishi H, Shono Y, et al. Angiostatic effects of corticosteroid on wound healing of the rabbit ear. J Med Invest 2002;49:61–6.
[35] Kirsner RS, Eaglstein WH. The wound healing process. Dermatol Clin 1993;11(4):629–40.
[36] Madison JB, Gronwall RR. Influence of wound shape on wound contraction in horses. Am J Vet Res 1992;53(9):1575–8.
[37] Buffa EA, Lubbe AM, Verstraete FJM, et al. The effects of wound lavage solutions on canine fibroblasts. Vet Surg 1997;26:460–6.
[38] Sanchez IR, Swaim SF, Nusbaum KE, et al. Effects of chlorhexidine diacetate and povidone-iodine on wound healing in dogs. Vet Surg 1988;17(6):291–5.
[39] Rodeheaver G, Bellamy W, Kody M, et al. Bactericidal activity and toxicity of iodine-containing solutions in wounds. Arch Surg 1982;117(2):181–6.
[40] Lineaweaver W, Howard R, Souey D, et al. Topical antimicrobial toxicity. Arch Surg 1985; 120:267–70.
[41] Bodner NS, Kiss-Buris ST, Buris L. Novel soft steroids: effects on cell growth in vitro and on wound healing in the mouse. Steroids 1991;58(8):434–9.
[42] Barber SM. Second intention wound healing in the horse: the effect of bandages and topical corticosteroids. Proc Am Assoc Equine Pract 1990;35:107–16.

[43] Kane DP. Chronic wound healing and chronic wound management. In: Krasner DL, Rodeheaver GT, Sibbald RG, editors. Chronic wound care: a source book for healthcare professionals. 3rd edition. Wayne, PA: HMP Communications; 2001. p. 7–19.

[44] Wilmink JM, van Weeren PR, Stolk PWT, et al. Differences in second-intention wound healing between horses and ponies: histological aspects. Equine Vet J 1999;31:61–7.

[45] Wilmink JM, van den Boom R, Veenman JN, et al. Differences in polymorphonucleocyte function and local inflammatory response as a possible cause for differences in wound healing efficiency between horses and ponies. Equine Vet J 2003;35:561–9.

[46] Peacock EE. Wound repair. 3rd edition. Philadelphia: WB Saunders; 1984.

[47] Braungart E, Magdolen V, Degitz K. Retinoic acid upregulates the plasminogen activator system in human epidermal keratinocytes. J Invest Dermatol 2001;116(5):778–84.

[48] Varani J, Warner RL, Gharaee-Kermani M, et al. Vitamin A antagonizes decreased cell growth and elevated collagen-degrading matrix metalloproteinases and stimulates collagen accumulation in naturally aged human skin. J Invest Dermatol 2000;114:480–6.

[49] Xu G, Bochaton-Piallat ML, Andreutti D, et al. Regulation of alpha-smooth muscle actin and CRBP-1 expression by retinoic acid and TGF-beta in cultured fibroblasts. J Cell Physiol 2001;187(3):315.

[50] Tarnow P, Agren M, Steenfos H, et al. Topical zinc oxide treatment increases endogenous gene expression of insulin-like growth factor-1 in granulation tissue from porcine wounds. Scand J Plast Reconstr Hand Surg 1994;28:255–9.

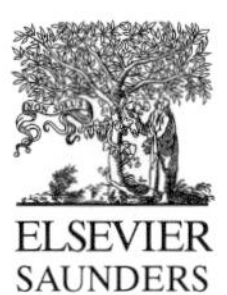
ELSEVIER
SAUNDERS

Vet Clin Equine 21 (2005) 45–62

VETERINARY
CLINICS
Equine Practice

Principles of Early Wound Management

David A. Wilson, DVM, MS

Department of Veterinary Medicine and Surgery, University of Missouri, Columbia, MO 65211, USA

Preserving life and preventing infection should be the primary objectives of the veterinarian to whom a horse with a traumatic injury is presented. A minor wound should not divert attention from more serious problems, such as hemorrhagic shock, exhaustion, or cerebral contusion associated with head injuries. Thus, a quick assessment of the wound should be followed by a thorough physical examination and acquisition of pertinent vital signs, bleeding should be controlled, and therapy should be directed at returning the patient to normal functional and cosmetic status with the shortest delay possible.

The overall health status should be assessed, because systemic infection; diseases of the liver, kidneys, or cardiovascular system; and endocrine imbalances may delay healing [1]. Although rarely a problem in horses, hypoproteinemia adversely affects wound healing by hindering fibroplasia, angiogenesis, remodeling, and overall tensile strength [2].

Initial examination

Time elapsed

Historically, the "golden period" of 4 to 12 hours has been considered the time during which primary closure can be accomplished with little risk of infection. Although this may be considered a rough guideline, the interval varies greatly as a result of other factors, such as the degree and type of contamination; the mechanism of injury; the degree of tissue trauma; the initial management and location of the wound; and the patient's overall condition, including nutritional and immunologic status.

E-mail address: wilsonda@missouri.edu

doi:10.1016/j.cveq.2004.11.005 **vetequine.theclinics.com**

Blood loss

Significant blood loss can impair wound healing. Although preliminary hematologic testing may help to determine the amount of blood lost, it must be interpreted in light of other factors, such as time since injury, heart and respiratory rates, mucous membrane color and capillary refill time, peripheral perfusion, and clinical assessment of hydration. Normovolemic anemia unrelated to malnutrition or chronic disease does not seem to affect wound healing until the packed cell volume (PCV) falls to less than 12%. If dehydration accompanies blood loss, resulting in a hypovolemic state, the result is vasoconstriction and reduced oxygen tension at the site of injury, increasing the risk of infection by slowing chemotaxis and phagocytosis. Supportive therapy should be instituted in the form of fluid therapy and blood transfusion, and the nutritional needs of the patient should be determined and addressed.

Prior treatment and vaccination status

Any previous therapy should be ascertained, because systemic and local treatments modify the course of repair. Horses with deep wounds, particularly puncture wounds, are more likely to develop tetanus. If a tetanus toxoid booster has not been administered within the last year, it should be done at this time and the patient should start receiving prophylactic penicillin therapy. Tetanus antitoxin should only be administered if the vaccination status is unknown because of the risk, primarily in adult horses, of developing serum hepatitis (Theiler's disease).

Mechanism of injury

The cause of injury influences the susceptibility of the wound to infection. Sharp lacerations caused by objects like metal, glass, and knives generally are resistant to infection. Conversely, more jagged wounds caused by barbed wire, sticks, nails, and bites are more susceptible because of the degree of soft tissue damage (Fig. 1). Soft tissue trauma from entanglement or entrapment or from impact with a solid object or a kick is more prone to infection because of the degree of soft tissue injury and resultant reduction in blood supply. The greater the energy on impact, the more severe is the soft tissue damage and the higher is the potential for vascular compromise. Indeed, wounds created by impact injury are reported to be 100 times more susceptible to infection than those caused by shear forces [3].

Patient restraint

The temperament of the horse occasionally affects the final outcome of an injury. It is more likely that daily care can be successfully completed on

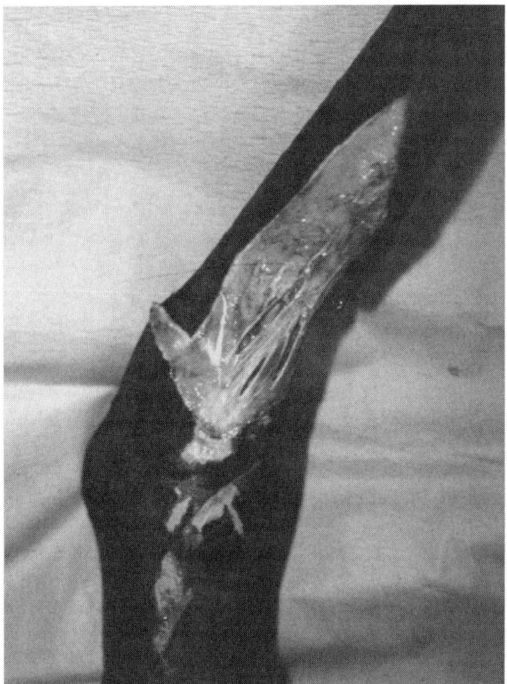

Fig. 1. A relatively clean degloving wound of the medial aspect of the metatarsus caused by a woven wire fence. The wound exposed the medial branch of the suspensory ligament.

compliant horses. Although initial evaluation and treatment can usually benefit from substantial chemical restraint, including general anesthesia, the subsequent daily care may not be afforded that luxury and wound management may suffer.

Tranquilizers should be used judiciously because of their potential for producing hypovolemia. The phenothiazine tranquilizers, such as acepromazine, should be avoided in hypovolemic patients because they cause peripheral vasodilation, which can result in a serious decrease in blood pressure, particularly in a horse that has significant blood loss and may be in shock.

Commonly, an α_2-adrenoreceptor agonist, such as xylazine or detomidine, provides sufficient sedation to complete a preliminary evaluation. If more sedation or analgesia is required, concurrent administration of an opioid, such as morphine or butorphanol, produces a combination (neuroleptanalgesia) that provides greater sedation and analgesia than can be achieved with either agent alone.

Visual appraisal

The location of the wound greatly influences its susceptibility to infection. For example, wounds involving the head region are more resistant to

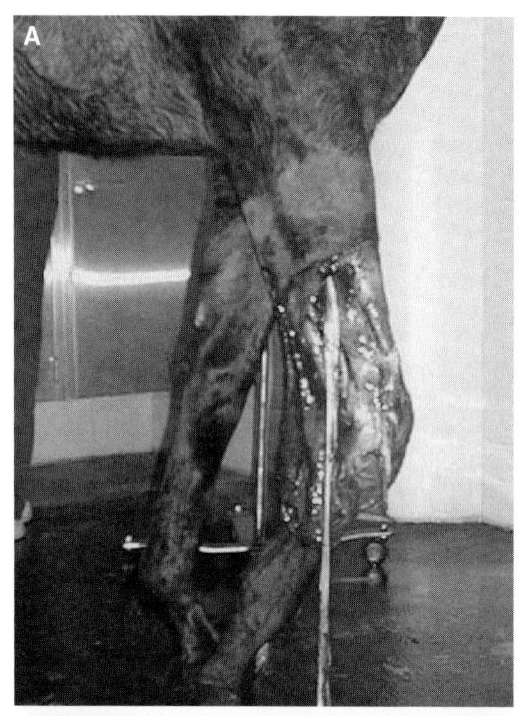
A

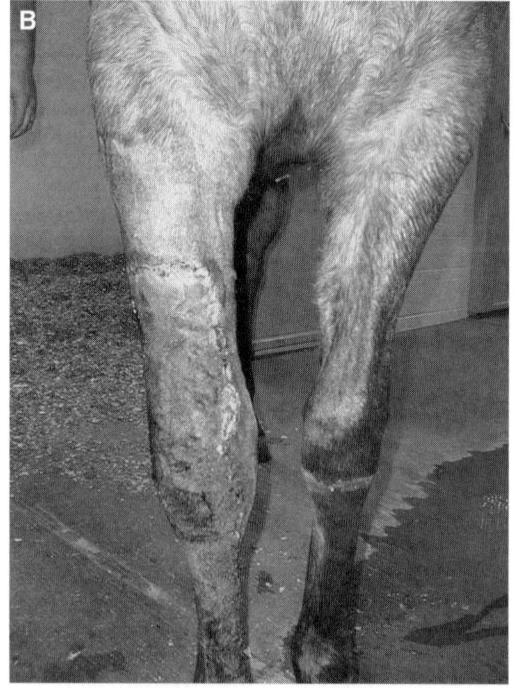
B

infection than those involving the distal extremities because they benefit from a better blood supply. Degloving wounds that encircle the limb and damage the periosteum and paratendon are more susceptible to infection and subsequent osteomyelitis or septic tendinitis because of compromise of the blood supply (Fig. 2). In these cases, soft tissue coverage of the site should be attained as soon as possible because of the increased risk of bone sequestration, tendon degeneration, and uncontrollable infection if the blood supply is not quickly returned [4]. Puncture wounds and even seemingly insignificant wounds of the limbs should be carefully evaluated for involvement of synovial structures. Open wounds are less likely to become infected compared with puncture wounds, whereas wounds with flaps that lack a good blood supply are more susceptible to infection. Blood supply can be assessed by several methods. Palpation may reveal that the tissues surrounding the wound are cool to the touch. The use of fluorescein dye has been reported, although it is not always practical. When specialized equipment is available, a vascular phase scintigraphic evaluation or Doppler ultrasonography may also be used to detect perfusion.

Wound infection results when the number of organisms reaches a concentration of 10^6 organisms per gram of tissue or per milliliter of fluid. Contaminated wounds with fewer organisms may become infected when foreign bodies are present (eg, wood, sutures, glove powder), excessive necrotic tissue is left in the wound, a hematoma develops, local tissue defenses are impaired (burn patients or immunosuppressed patients), or the vascular supply is compromised [1].

Blood and other body fluids can act as culture media for bacteria and can reduce the blood supply if the expanding fluid pressure within the dead space is sufficient. The presence of blood inhibits local tissue defenses and mechanically separates the wound edges. The presence of hemoglobin interferes with chemotaxis and the phagocytic ability of neutrophils. Furthermore, the ferric ion can increase the virulence and replication of organisms [1,5,6].

Wounds contaminated with dirt have a higher risk of infection because of specific infection-potentiating fractions (IPFs) found in the organic and inorganic components of soil [7]. These IPFs decrease the effect of white blood cells, decrease humoral factors, and neutralize antibodies. As few as 100 organisms can cause infection in the presence of IPFs. Wounds contaminated with feces, which are quite susceptible to infection, may contain up to 10^{11} organisms per gram [4]. Wounds contaminated with 10^9 microorganisms per gram of tissue develop infection in spite of antibiotic treatment [3].

Fig. 2. (*A*) Degloving laceration of the forearm involving the lateral digital extensor tendon. (Courtesy of J. Kramer, DVM, Columbia, MO.) (*B*) Attempts to close this wound should be made within 3 to 4 days to restore blood supply to decrease the risk of tendon degeneration and wound infection. (Courtesy of J. Kramer, DVM, Columbia, MO.)

Wound anesthesia

Many wounds can be cleaned and repaired in the standing horse. Although some head and upper neck wounds can be treated with mild sedation or tranquilization, wounds of the distal limb are often sensitive and frequently require neuroleptanalgesia and local anesthesia. Regional, perineural, or local anesthesia is useful for wounds of the distal extremities and head. Regional infiltration of a local anesthetic is used everywhere else. Ideally, the anesthetic should be infiltrated at a site distant from the wound. The location of the wound may limit the available options, however, and infiltration of the anesthetic agent through the wound margins or into the subcutaneous tissues through the skin adjacent to the wound margins may be the only viable options. Subsequent patient compliance suggests that infiltration through the wound margins is often the best option. Direct infiltration of the wound should only be performed after cleaning to minimize the chances of disseminating bacteria and possible foreign bodies deeper into the wound.

Generally, intralesional anesthesia with 2% concentrations of lidocaine or mepivacaine is effective and safe, although studies have inconsistently reported that it may inhibit collagen synthesis, platelet aggregation, and bradykinin-stimulated antiaggregation of platelets and may cause vasoconstriction and thrombosis in microvessels [8–12]. Adding epinephrine to the local anesthetic causes vasoconstriction and exacerbates these effects. Despite these controversies, local anesthetics are commonly used in surgical wounds to reduce postoperative pain, because advantages may well outweigh disadvantages.

Preparation of surrounding tissues

The objective in wound preparation is to reduce the contamination of a wound to obtain a "clean" field. The most important factor in delaying wound healing is the development of infection. Infections are classified as primary, in which the contamination occurs at the time of injury, or secondary, in which the contamination occurs through the suture line or through other portals (ie, drains, fistulas).

Before wound preparation, the wound should be protected by placing a sterile, water-soluble, lubricating jelly or sterile moist gauze sponges into the wound. A wide area of hair around the wound should be clipped. To prevent hair from falling into the wound, the hair may be dampened with water or lightly coated with a sterile, water-soluble lubricating jelly. Sponges used to pack the wound should be discarded and replaced by new ones after each stage of preparation. The clipped area should be scrubbed at least three times with antiseptic soap and rinsed between scrubs with sterile 0.9% saline solution. The wound bed itself should be gently cleansed with antiseptic soap and sterile gauze sponges, followed by copious lavage to neutralize the detergent base of the antiseptics.

Antiseptics for skin preparation

The two most commonly used surgical scrubs for skin preparation are povidone-iodine and chlorhexidine. Rinsing with saline or 70% isopropyl alcohol does not make a difference in the antimicrobial effect of povidone-iodine; however, alcohol reduces the residual effect and antiseptic quality of chlorhexidine [1]. Although uncommon, one disadvantage of povidone-iodine is a skin reaction, which seems more frequent after clipping, scrubbing, rinsing with 70% alcohol, spraying with povidone-iodine solution, and bandaging. Detergent forms of chlorhexidine should not be used around the eye, because exposure may lead to corneal edema and bulbous keratopathy [13–15].

The mechanical effect of scrubbing the wound with these antiseptic soaps can be helpful in removing debris and reducing bacterial concentration at the wound surface. There is a marked delay in wound healing if the soap is not thoroughly rinsed from the wound, however. Additionally, even though these antiseptics are effective, much of the bacterial population in the skin resides in protected hair follicles, sebaceous glands, and crevices of the lipid coat of the superficial epithelium.

Wound exploration: approaches

After the wound is cleaned and free of devitalized tissue and debris, it should be digitally explored using sterile gloves. A sterile probe is helpful in identifying the depth and margins of the wound. The probe can also be used to locate foreign bodies or, in conjunction with plain radiography, to determine if bone or other structures, such as tendons or ligaments are involved. Synovial fluid is identified by stringing the fluid between the thumb and forefinger; if the quality of the fluid is questionable, a sample should be submitted for cytologic examination and culture and sensitivity testing. To verify whether a synovial structure has been penetrated, a needle is placed in the synovial cavity at a site remote to the wound. If synovial fluid can be retrieved, it is submitted for cytology and culture and sensitivity testing. Sterile saline is then injected into the cavity, and if the joint capsule or tendon sheath has been violated, fluid escapes from the wound. In this case, the synovial structure is lavaged with 3 to 5 L of sterile saline or crystalloid solution. Intrasynovial instillation of antibiotics or 10% dimethylsulfoxide (DMSO) solution is also recommended. Plain film and contrast radiographs should be considered, as appropriate. Ultrasound examination can be used to document tendon and ligament injury, to locate and identify foreign bodies, and to identify gas accumulation and muscle separation. Arthroscopy can be helpful in identifying occult radiographic lesions, particularly those involving cartilage, and in identifying foreign bodies within the joint (eg, hair, dirt, wood).

Infection within a wound delays healing by mechanically separating the wound edges with exudate and reducing the vascular supply by mechanical pressure and the formation of microthrombi in small vessels surrounding the wound. Infection also increases cellular responses and consequently prolongs the inflammatory phase of repair. Finally, bacteria produce proteolytic enzymes that digest collagen and release endotoxins, which inhibit growth factor activity and collagen synthesis.

Wound lavage

Bacteria adhere to the wound surface by means of an electrostatic charge. Lavage cleans the wound of debris and reduces the bacterial numbers and IPFs. In addition, lavage stimulates peripheral microcirculation through its gentle massaging action, which may favor the formation of granulation tissue. Lavage is easy to perform, requires no special equipment, is cost-effective, and is well tolerated by most patients. Lavage solutions are most effective when delivered by a fluid jet of at least 8 psi [16]. Pressures of 10 to 15 psi are approximately 80% effective in removing IPFs and adherent bacteria from a wound [1]. Although this cannot be achieved by gravity flow or lavage with a bulb syringe, adequate pulsatile pressure can be attained in other ways, including forcefully expressing lavage solutions from a 35- or 60-mL syringe through an 18-gauge needle or by using a spray bottle or a WaterPik. The WaterPik delivers water at a rate of 40 to 50 mL/min at 10 to 15 psi at the low-intermediate setting and is effective for heavily contaminated wounds. Care must be taken not to drive contaminants deeper within the wound or inadvertently separate loose fascial planes. The ideal lavage solution should be sterile, isotonic, normothermic, nontoxic, and compatible with antibiotic or disinfectant medications that may be added. Isotonic crystalloids, such as normal saline or lactated Ringer's solution, meet these criteria and are the most commonly used solutions. In cases in which tap water must be used initially, a final lavage with sterile isotonic fluid may help to restore tissue normotonicity and reduce edema.

Wound lavage should also be considered for closed wounds. The advantages of flushing a closed wound include the dilution and mobilization of exudates and the delivery of medication. The disadvantages are that bacteria can readily be introduced into the wound and dead space may be created or expanded.

Wound debridement

The ideal goal of debridement is to obtain fresh clean wound margins and skin edges for primary closure. Although many wounds cannot be closed primarily, several types nonetheless require removal of contaminated tissues or foreign material before wound healing can efficiently progress. Debridement involves the removal of dead or damaged tissue, foreign bodies, and bacteria that compromise local defense mechanisms. The liberal removal of possibly contaminated fascia, fat, and muscle and the careful retention of bone, tendons, nerves, and major vessels should be of primary concern. Fascia, fat, and muscle all have excellent blood supplies and provide excellent media for the growth of contaminating organisms. Although skeletal muscle is not replaced, there are usually sufficient backup systems available to make up for the loss. Small pieces of bone that have lost their blood supply should also be removed.

Surgical debridement

Surgical debridement may be accomplished in a variety of ways (layered, staged, or en bloc). En bloc resection is probably the most effective method of surgical debridement. With this technique, the entire wound is excised at its margins, such that all wounded and contaminated tissue is removed. This method is mostly reserved for draining tracts. With layered debridement, tissue removal is started at the most superficial tissue layer and is continued into the depths of the wound. This systematic approach helps to prevent contamination of deeper tissues with debris from more superficial layers as debridement progresses. In most equine distal limb wounds, where tissue is at a premium, staged debridement is used over a number of days to avoid inadvertent removal of viable tissue. When performing staged debridement, the two governing criteria are color and attachment. White, tan, black, and green tissues as well as those that are poorly attached should be debrided. Tissues that are pink to dark purple in color and that are well attached should be left in place. Nonsurgical types of wound debridement include chemical or enzymatic, laser, bandage, or biosurgical therapy.

Enzymatic debridement

Tissue injury results in increased vascular permeability. Proteins leak from the vasculature into the wound, producing a surface coagulum that persists until primary closure of the wound edges is complete. This coagulum encompasses surface contaminants, preventing contact by topical or systemic antibiotics. Additionally, bacterial proliferation produces a biofilm that results in the same type of protective coagulum. Proteolytic enzymes function by degrading the coagulum and biofilm, exposing the bacteria to topical and systemic antibiotics.

Several varieties of enzymatic products are available and can be used with topical antibiotic therapy without inhibiting their activity. A few common enzyme preparations include pancreatic trypsin (Granulex; Bertek Pharmaceuticals, Research Triangle Park, NC), streptodornase or streptokinase of streptococcal bacterial origin (Varidase; Lederle Laboratories, Wayne, NJ), collagenases, proteases, and a combination of fibrinolysin and deoxyribonuclease (Elase; Fujisawa Health Care, Deerfield, IL) [17–23]. Recently, collagenases have been shown to have the highest proteolytic activity and the greatest likelihood of achieving a clean wound compared with other methods of nonsurgical wound debridement [24–26]. This form of debridement is useful when surgical debridement is contraindicated because it could result in damage to or removal of viable tissue that may be needed for reconstruction.

Laser debridement

Lasers have been used in a variety of ways to stimulate wound healing. Low-level laser therapy has been advocated to stimulate wound healing by shortening the inflammatory phase and enhancing the release of factors that stimulate the proliferative stage of repair [27]. Controlled studies have shown mixed results of low-level laser therapy using a gallium aluminium arsenide (GaAlA) or helium neon laser [28–34]. Increased collagen deposition and endothelial cell, fibroblast and myofibroblast proliferation have been shown to be the most significant effects of low-level laser therapy [30,34–36]. It has been postulated that attenuation of reactive oxygen species by neutrophils may contribute to the effects of low-level laser therapy [37].

Wound debridement requires higher power than that achieved for therapeutic purposes. A high-powered carbon dioxide laser has been shown in weanling pigs to be as effective as surgical sharp debridement for full-thickness burn wounds, with the advantages of being quicker, providing better hemostasis, and resulting in minimal debridement of the surrounding normal skin [31]. Although carbon dioxide and neodymium:yttrium aluminum garnet (Nd:YAG) laser surgery have been shown to delay the onset of healing compared with sharp scalpel surgery, the ultimate outcome is unchanged [38,39].

Bandage debridement

Debridement dressing includes adherent open-mesh gauze (eg, 4 × 4 gauze sponges) or wet-to-dry bandages using 4 × 4 mesh gauze or sheet cotton. In a recent study evaluating various methods of nonsurgical debridement, wet-to-dry dressings proved inferior to collagenase and fibrinolysin based on the likelihood of achieving a clean wound bed at 2 weeks and the cost of 1 month of treatment [25]. Furthermore, bandage debridement is contraindicated during the proliferative stage of repair, because the adherent bandages tend to damage new cellular populations.

Biosurgical debridement

Biosurgical debridement in the form of maggot therapy using sterile greenbottle fly larva (*Lucilia sericata*) has enjoyed resurgent worldwide popularity in human wound therapy [40–45]. The ability of these creatures to combat wound infection, including that caused by antibiotic-resistant strains of bacteria, has been well documented [42]. No significant risks or adverse events have been linked to the use of maggots, which seem to function by secreting proteolytic enzymes [43]. The foremost indication for biosurgical debridement seems to be in necrotic, infected, or chronic non-healing wounds, where maggots remove necrotic tissue, disinfect the wound, and promote granulation tissue formation [44]. Although maggots are occasionally present in naturally occurring equine wounds, only one report of maggot therapy for the successful treatment of a nonhealing wound is documented in the literature [45].

Wound closure

Priorities during wound closure are to curtail infection or contamination, minimize skin loss, and exert the least amount of tension possible on the suture line. Ideally, wounds should be managed by primary closure. Wounds amenable to primary closure include those of the head and upper body, flap wounds with a good blood supply, and recent minimally contaminated wounds of the extremities. Wounds with considerable skin loss or severe contamination or infection are generally not initially closed and may be allowed to heal by second intention. Delayed primary and delayed secondary closures are for wounds with significant contamination and considerable soft tissue damage, where additional time is required to prepare the wound for closure.

Primary closure, leading to first-intention healing, usually occurs after surgery or soon after injury. The golden period relates to the time required for multiplying bacteria to reach an infective level, considered to be 10^6 organisms per gram of tissue. This may be longer in clean wounds and considerably shorter in severely contaminated wounds. Ideally, primary closure is used for fresh minimally contaminated wounds with a good blood supply and not involving vital structures.

Delayed primary closure occurs 3 to 5 days after injury when the threat of infection has been controlled by the inflammatory and debridement phases of healing but before fibroplasia. Delayed primary closure is best used for severely contaminated, contused, or swollen wounds and for those involving a synovial structure. It is particularly useful in distal limb wounds, where contamination is a frequent problem.

Delayed secondary closure occurs more than 5 days after injury, once granulation tissue has begun forming. As with delayed primary closure, delayed secondary closure is used after several days of therapeutic care for contaminated wounds with compromised blood supply.

Second-intention healing consists of fibroplasia followed by wound contraction and epithelialization. Indications for second-intention healing include severe contamination or infection, considerable skin loss, excessive skin tension that precludes primary closure, and unavoidable motion like that occurring in the pectoral and gluteal regions. Second-intention healing is best used for wounds not located over a joint surface, those with an adequate vascular supply to the underlying soft tissues, and those with sufficient mobile skin to allow wound contraction.

Suture material and patterns and tissue adhesive

The suture material used to close skin incisions or lacerations influences wound healing. A general goal should be to choose a suture material that generates minimal tissue reactivity and is sufficiently strong for the intended purpose. All suture materials potentiate infection by acting as foreign bodies when placed in contaminated wounds. Natural materials (eg, catgut, silk, cotton, linen, collagen) are generally considered more reactive and weaker and have a variable rate of absorption. Synthetic absorbable sutures, such as polyglycolic acid (Dexon; Davis & Geck Division, American Cyanamid Co., Danbury, CT), polyglactin 910 (Vicryl; Ethicon, a Johnson & Johnson Company, Somerville, NJ), polydioxanone (PDS; Ethicon), polyglyconate (Maxon; Davis & Geck Division. American Cyanamid Co.), and poliglecaprone (Monocryl; Ethicon), have the distinct advantage of being absorbed at a constant rate by hydrolysis. Additionally, monofilament sutures are less reactive than twisted or braided materials. Synthetic nonabsorbable sutures, such as nylon (Ethylon; Ethicon), polypropylene (Prolene; Ethicon), and polyfilament polyamide, are generally considered to be less reactive than absorbable sutures. Polyfilament polyamide has characteristics that make it the least desirable synthetic nonabsorbable suture, such as losing 15% to 20% of its strength when wet and being associated with an increased incidence of suture sinus tract formation [46].

The suture pattern also can affect wound healing. Although the simple continuous pattern is the easiest to apply and provides the most uniform support, its design leads to reduced microcirculation to the wound margins and a single break can be disastrous. Comparatively, a simple interrupted pattern leads to less edema, does not exert a negative impact on the microcirculation, and encourages greater wound tensile strength after 5 and 10 days [46], although these positive effects are attenuated at later times [47–51]. The disadvantages of interrupted versus continuous patterns include the use of more suture material and increased overall time of placement. Interrupted suture patterns should be used when impaired healing is anticipated and excessive tension is present. Simple interrupted suture patterns cause less inflammation than vertical mattress and far-near-near-far patterns because of relatively less suture material in the incision line and fewer skin penetrations.

Sutures should be placed such that they just appose the wound edges. Loosely approximated wounds are stronger at 7, 10, and 21 days after surgery than wounds tightly secured with sutures [52], possibly because overtightening disrupts the microvascular circulation to the wound edges.

The placement of sutures may also affect wound healing. Wound edges weaken over time because of collagen lysis; therefore, sutures should be placed at least 0.5 cm from the margins. Additionally, although more sutures improve initial strength, the increased number of sutures compromises blood supply to the wound edges and stimulates an excessive tissue reaction and subsequent infection rate. Deep sutures should be placed only in fascial planes, tendons, and ligaments, because additional deep sutures are generally ineffective and cause excessive tissue reaction.

Tissue adhesives

Various tissue adhesives, such as cyanoacrylates, collagen gelatin, and fibrin glue, are used for primary wound closure [53–60]. Advantages include rapid and painless application, hemostatic and bacteriostatic properties, the provision of a water-resistant protective coating, no need for suture removal, and an acceptable cosmetic result [53,55]. Cyanoacrylates are used in numerous different tissues and have been evaluated in wounds of the distal limbs of horses [53]. It is generally thought that tissue adhesives may have some benefits in small incisions or wounds in which primary suture closure is indicated, whereas larger wounds are unlikely to benefit from tissue adhesives as a replacement for conventional suture material. Wounds healing by second intention may profit from tissue adhesive sprays after a healthy granulation tissue bed has formed [60].

Stents

A stent or tie-over bandage can be used to help obliterate dead space in wounds in which bandaging is not possible. This type of bandage protects the wound and may provide relief to the primary suture line as well as direct pressure over areas of dead space.

Management of dead space

Dead space allows the seepage and accumulation of blood and serum in a warm and moist environment that is ideal for bacterial proliferation, thus encouraging infection. Dead space may be dealt with by layered wound closure when adequate tissue is available, by compression bandages, by drainage, or by suture obliteration [61], although the latter may promote wound infection in contaminated wounds. Walking sutures can be used to advance a skin flap over the wound bed at the same time the dead space is eliminated.

Management of skin tension

Excess tension on a primary suture line is likely to complicate healing via local ischemia, cutting out of sutures, and wound disruption. Methods to decrease tension include undermining the surrounding skin and providing relief incisions. Although excessive undermining is deleterious, undermining up to 4 cm from the wound edge on distal limb wounds has not been associated with complications [62]. Relief incisions away from the wound margins can sometimes decrease tension. The relief incisions may be closed after the primary incision is closed or left to heal by second intention.

Tension suture patterns used to reduce the tension on the primary suture line are placed well back from the wound margins so that the blood supply is not compromised. Once the tension sutures are in place, the primary incision line is sutured to appose the wound edges. Widely placed vertical mattress sutures, with or without support using buttons, gauze, or rubber or polyethylene tubing, are effective in reducing tension on the primary suture line. Other tension suture patterns include horizontal mattress, far-near-near-far, and far-far-near-near patterns. Tension sutures with supports are used in regions that cannot be effectively bandaged (eg, upper body, neck), whereas no supports are used under bandages or casts, because pressure on the supports may cause tissue necrosis (Fig. 3). Tension sutures are removed in 4 to 10 days, depending on the appearance of the wound. Staggered removal is preferred, removing half of the sutures initially and the remaining half later.

Drains

Drains are used when there is a large dead space remaining after suture closure or there is sufficient tissue damage so that continued seepage of fluids can be expected. They can be therapeutic to remove existing fluid accumulation or prophylactic to ensure against fluid accumulation. Drains must be maintained in a sterile environment to decrease the chance of secondary infection. They should traverse the wound from a proximal to distal orientation, adjacent to but not directly underlying the suture line, and should exit from a separate incision adjacent to the wound edges to minimize the chances of retrograde infection. The drains should be sutured proximally and at their exit point.

Drains can be classified as active or passive. Active drains are closed-suction drains that function by negative pressure to suction out excess fluid or air, whereas passive drains, including Penrose drains or some form of rubber or polyethylene tubing, function by gravity or pressure differentials. The ideal drain is inert, soft, smooth, nonreactive, and radiopaque. The disadvantages of drains include the potential introduction of bacteria or foreign bodies into the wound, the care involved to maintain patency, and the potential irritation and resultant scar tissue and adhesion formation that

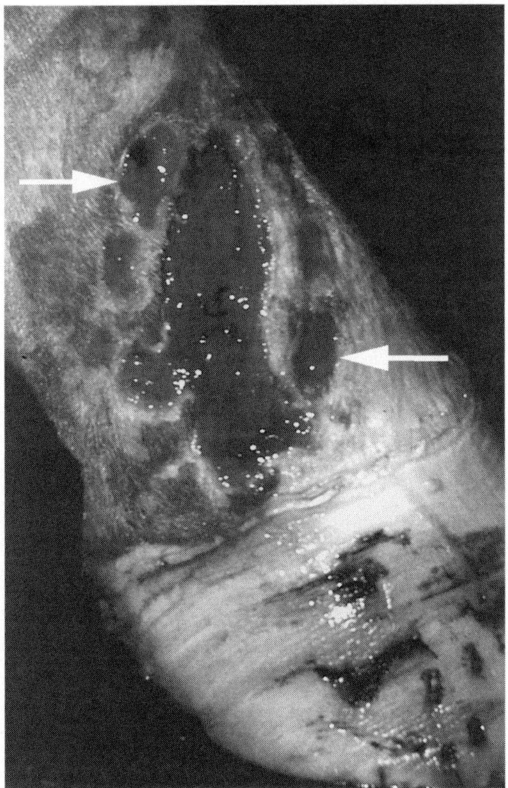

Fig. 3. Previously repaired pastern laceration showing evidence of skin necrosis secondary to bandages applied over tension suture supports. Three horizontal mattress sutures had been placed with polyethylene supports 2 weeks previously.

may occur as the result of a foreign body reaction. Drains should be removed after 2 to 3 days or when infection is controlled. The drainage is expected to change from an exudate to a transudate, and its quantity should gradually diminish to negligible levels during the 2- to 3-day period.

References

[1] Stashak TS. Selected factors that affect wound healing. In: Equine wound management. Philadelphia: Lea & Febiger; 1991. p. 2–35.

[2] Peacock EE Jr. Collagenolysis and the biochemistry of wound healing. In: Wound repair. 3rd edition. Philadelphia: WB Saunders; 1984. p. 102–40.

[3] Stashak TS. Current concepts in wound management in horses: parts I–III. In: Proceedings of the North American Veterinary Conference. Orlando (FL): North American Veterinary Conference; 2003. p. 231–7.

[4] Stashak TS. Principles of wound management and selection of approaches to wound closure. In: Equine wound management. Philadelphia: Lea & Febiger; 1991. p. 36–69.

[5] Bullen JJ, Spalding PB, Ward CG, et al. The role of Eh, pH and iron in the bactericidal power of human plasma. FEMS Microbiol Lett 1992;94(1–2):47–52.

[6] Ratledge C. Iron, mycobacteria and tuberculosis. Tuberculosis 2004;84(1–2):110–30.
[7] Swaim SF. Management of contaminated and infected wounds. In: Surgery of traumatized skin: management and reconstruction in the dog and cat. Philadelphia: WB Saunders; 1980. p. 119.
[8] Borg T, Modig J. Potential anti-thrombotic effects of local anaesthetics due to their inhibition of platelet aggregation. Acta Anaesthesiol Scand 1985;29(7):739–42.
[9] Grant GJ, Ramanathan S, Patel N, et al. The effects of local anesthetics on maternal and neonatal platelet function. Acta Anaesthesiol Scand 1989;33(5):409–12.
[10] Berntsen RF, Simonsen T, Sager G, et al. Therapeutic lidocaine concentrations have no effect on blood platelet function and plasma catecholamine levels. Eur J Clin Pharmacol 1992;43(1):109–11.
[11] Az-ma T, Hardian, Yuge O. Inhibitory effect of lidocaine on cultured porcine aortic endothelial cell-dependent antiaggregation of platelets. Anesthesiol 1995;83(2):374–81.
[12] Drucker M, Cardenas E, Arizti P, et al. Experimental studies on the effect of lidocaine on wound healing. World J Surg 1998;22:394–8.
[13] Hamill MB, Osato MS, Wilhelmus KR. Experimental evaluation of chlorhexidine gluconate for ocular antisepsis. Antimicrobial Agents Chemother 1984;26(6):793–6.
[14] Phinney RB, Mondino BJ, Hofbauer JD, et al. Corneal edema related to accidental Hibiclens exposure. Am J Ophthalmol 1988;106(2):210–5.
[15] Nasser RE. The ocular danger of Hibiclens (chlorhexidine). Plast Reconstr Surg 1992;89(1): 164–5.
[16] Baxter GM. Wounds and wound healing. In: Colahan PT, Merritt AM, Moore JN, et al, editors. Equine medicine and surgery. 5th edition. St. Louis: Mosby; 1999. p. 1801–8.
[17] Rodeheaver G, Marsh D, Edgerton MT, et al. Proteolytic enzymes as adjuncts to antimicrobial prophylaxis of contaminated wounds. Am J Surg 1975;129(5):537–44.
[18] Schwarz N. Wound cleansing with the enzyme combination fibrinolysin/deoxy-ribonuclease [in German]. Fortschr Med 1981;99(25):978–80.
[19] Noble TA, Carr DS, Gonzalez MF. Use of a trypsin, Peru balsam, and castor oil spray on the oral mucosa: case report and review of the literature. Pharmacotherapy 1989;9(6):386–8.
[20] Smith BA. The dressing makes the difference. Trial of two modern dressings on venous ulcers. Prof Nurse 1994;9(5):348, 350–2.
[21] Falabella AF, Carson P, Eaglstein WH, et al. The safety and efficacy of a proteolytic ointment in the treatment of chronic ulcers of the lower extremity. J Am Acad Dermatol 1998;39(5 Part 1):737–40.
[22] Carson SN, Wiggins C, Overall K, et al. Using a castor oil-balsam of Peru-trypsin ointment to assist in healing skin graft donor sites. Ostomy Wound Manage 2003;49(6):60–4.
[23] Nemoto K, Hirota K, Mrakami K, et al. Effect of Varidase (streptodornase) on biofilm formed by Pseudomonas aeruginosa. Chemotherapy 2003;49(3):121–5.
[24] Glyantsev SP, Adamyan AA, Sakharov Y. Crab collagenase in wound debridement. J Wound Care 1997;6(1):13–6.
[25] Mosher BA, Cuddigan J, Thomas DR, et al. Outcomes of 4 methods of debridement using a decision analysis methodology. Adv Wound Care 1999;12(2):81–8.
[26] Peter FW, Li-Peuser H, Vogt PM, et al. The effect of wound ointments on tissue microcirculation and leucocyte behaviour. Clin Exp Dermatol 2002;27(1):51–5.
[27] Mison M. Principles of traditional wound management. In: Proceedings of the American College of Veterinary Surgeons Veterinary Symposium. Bethesda (MD): American College of Veterinary Surgeons; 2003. p. 622–4.
[28] Kaneps AJ, Hultgren BD, Riebold TW, et al. Laser therapy in the horse: histopathologic response. Am J Vet Res 1984;45(3):581–2.
[29] Petersen SL, Botes C, Olivier A, et al. The effect of low level laser therapy (LLLT) on wound healing in horses. Equine Vet J 1999;31(3):228–31.
[30] Reddy GK, Stehno-Bittel L, Enwemeka CS. Laser photostimulation accelerates wound healing in diabetic rats. Wound Repair Regen 2001;9(3):248–55.

[31] Graham JS, Schomacker KT, Glatter RD, et al. Efficacy of laser debridement with autologous split-thickness skin grafting in promoting improved healing of deep cutaneous sulfur mustard burns. Burns 2002;28(8):719–30.

[32] Lucas C, Criens-Poublon LJ, Cockrell CT, et al. Wound healing in cell studies and animal model experiments by Low Level Laser Therapy; were clinical studies justified? A systematic review. Lasers Med Sci 2002;17(2):110–34.

[33] Lucas C, van Gemert MJ, de Haan RJ. Efficacy of low-level laser therapy in the management of stage III decubitus ulcers: a prospective, observer-blinded multicentre randomised clinical trial. Lasers Med Sci 2003;18(2):72–7.

[34] Medrado AR, Pugliese LS, Reis SR, et al. Influence of low level laser therapy on wound healing and its biological action upon myofibroblasts. Lasers Surg Med 2003;32(3): 239–44.

[35] Schindl A, Merwald H, Schindl L, et al. Direct stimulatory effect of low-intensity 670 nm laser irradiation on human endothelial cell proliferation. Br J Dermatol 2003;148(2):334–6.

[36] Vinck EM, Cagnie BJ, Cornelissen MJ, et al. Increased fibroblast proliferation induced by light emitting diode and low power laser irradiation. Lasers Med Sci 2003;18(2):95–9.

[37] Fujimaki Y, Shimoyama T, Liu Q, et al. Low-level laser irradiation attenuates production of reactive oxygen species by human neutrophils [see comment]. J Clin Laser Med Surg 2003; 21(3):165–70.

[38] Lippert BM, Teymoortash A, Folz BJ, et al. Wound healing after laser treatment of oral and oropharyngeal cancer. Lasers Med Sci 2003;18(1):36–42.

[39] Mison MB, Steficek B, Lavagnino M, et al. Comparison of the effects of the CO2 surgical laser and conventional surgical techniques on healing and wound tensile strength of skin flaps in the dog. Vet Surg 2003;32(2):153–60.

[40] Graner JLSK. Livingston and the maggot therapy of wounds. Mil Med 1997;162(4): 296–300.

[41] Sherman RA, Sherman J, Gilead L, et al. Maggot debridement therapy in outpatients. Arch Phys Med Rehabil 2001;82(9):1226–9.

[42] Thomas S, Jones M, Wynn K, et al. The current status of maggot therapy in wound healing. Br J Nurs 2001;10(22 Suppl):S5–8, S10, S12.

[43] Chambers L, Woodrow S, Brown AP, et al. Degradation of extracellular matrix components by defined proteinases from the greenbottle larva *Lucilia sericata* used for the clinical debridement of non-healing wounds. Br J Dermatol 2003;148(1):14–23.

[44] Horobin AJ, Shakesheff KM, Woodrow S, et al. Maggots and wound healing: an investigation of the effects of secretions from Lucilia sericata larvae upon interactions between human dermal fibroblasts and extracellular matrix components. Br J Dermatol 2003;148(5):923–33.

[45] Bell NJ, Thomas S. Use of sterile maggots to treat panniculitis in an aged donkey. Vet Rec 2001;149:768–70.

[46] Stashak TS. Selection of suture materials and suture patterns for wound closure. In: Equine wound management. Philadelphia: Lea & Febiger; 1991. p. 52–69.

[47] Fingland RB, Layton CI, Kennedy GA, et al. A comparison of simple continuous versus simple interrupted suture pattern for tracheal anastomosis after large-segment tracheal resection in dogs. Vet Surg 1995;24(4):320–30.

[48] Kirpensteijn J, Maarschalkerweerd RJ, van der Gaag I, et al. Comparison of three closure methods and two absorbable suture materials for closure of jejunal enterotomy incisions in healthy dogs. Vet Q 2001;23(2):67–70.

[49] Magee AA, Galuppo LD. Comparison of incisional bursting strength of simple continuous and inverted cruciate suture patterns in the equine linea alba. Vet Surg 1999;28(6): 442–7.

[50] Van Hoogmoed L, Snyder JR, Stover SM, et al. In vitro biomechanical comparison of the strength of the linea alba of the llama, using two suture patterns. Am J Vet Res 1996;57(6): 938–42.

[51] Weisman DL, Smeak DD, Birchard SJ, et al. Comparison of a continuous suture pattern with a simple interrupted pattern for enteric closure in dogs and cats: 83 cases (1991–1997). J Am Vet Med Assoc 1999;214(10):1507–10.
[52] Brunius U, Ahren C. Healing of skin incisions during reduced tension of the wound area. A tensiometric and histologic study in the rat. Acta Chir Scand 1969;135(5):383–90.
[53] Blackford J, Shires M, Goble D, et al. The use of N-butyl cyanoacrylate in the treatment of open leg wounds in the horse. Proc Am Assoc Equine Pract 1986;32:349–56.
[54] Yaron M, Halperin M, Huffer W, et al. Efficacy of tissue glue for laceration repair in an animal-model. Acad Emerg Med 1995;2:259–63.
[55] Liebelt EL. Current concepts in laceration repair. Curr Opin Pediatr 1997;9(5):459–64.
[56] Stark GB, Horch RE, Voigt M, et al. Biological wound tissue glue systems in wound healing [in German]. Langenbecks Archiv Chir Suppl Kongressbd 1998;115:683–8.
[57] Bruns TB, Worthington JM. Using tissue adhesive for wound repair: a practical guide to Dermabond. Am Fam Physician 2000;61(5):1383–8.
[58] Tritle NM, Haller JR, Gray SD. Aesthetic comparison of wound closure techniques in a porcine model. Laryngoscope 2001;111(11 Part 1):1949–51.
[59] Thomazini-Santos IA, Barraviera SRCS, Mendes-Giannini MJS, et al. Surgical adhesives. J Venom Anim Toxins 2001;7(2):159–71.
[60] Bello TR. Practical treatment of body and open leg wounds of horses with bovine collagen, biosynthetic wound dressing and cyanoacrylate. J Equine Vet Sci 2002;22(4):157–64.
[61] Trotter GW. Techniques of wound closure. Vet Clin N Am Equine Pract 1989;5(3):499–511.
[62] Bailey JV, Jacobs KA. The mesh expansion method of suturing wounds on the legs of horses. Vet Surg 1983;12(2):78–82.

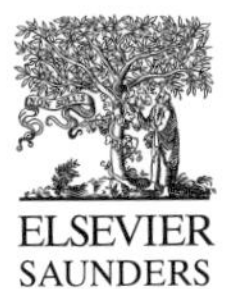
ELSEVIER
SAUNDERS

Vet Clin Equine 21 (2005) 63–75

VETERINARY
CLINICS
Equine Practice

Use of Antimicrobials in Wound Management

Gordon W. Brumbaugh, DVM, PhD

PO Box 248, Wellborn, TX 77881–0248, USA

Antimicrobial drugs have one broad indication, that is, to alter the microbial population in which they are placed. Antibacterial drugs are most frequently called to mind when the term *antimicrobial* is used; however, antifungal and antiparasitic medications are also classified as antimicrobial drugs. Each of these targets a selective population of organisms (microbes). It follows that each is indicated as a component of wound management only when its particular target organism(s) contributes to the formation of the wound or interferes with its repair. Determining the indication for use of these medications becomes a matter of clinical judgment, experience, and consideration of pertinent medical information. This article concentrates on antibacterial medication.

Determinants of wound infection

Classification of wounds according to their degree of contamination is discussed in more detail elsewhere in this issue. Each wound requires a different approach to antimicrobial treatment, which is loosely based on the wound classification system. Ideally, contamination should be controlled or managed so that bacterial invasion or infection is avoided. That may not always be possible, however, because horses are presented to veterinarians at various, and sometimes unknown, intervals after trauma. Because horses do not live in a sterile environment, wounds become contaminated with organisms present in the surroundings. *Staphylococcus aureus*, *Streptococcus pyogenes*, gram-negative aerobic enterics, and anaerobes are among the bacteria most frequently encountered in wounds [1–6]. Whether those organisms affect progression of the wound or interfere with healing is important. Mixed populations of bacteria are more common than are pure

E-mail address: gordon.brumbaugh@pfizer.com

doi:10.1016/j.cveq.2004.11.012 **vetequine.theclinics.com**

isolates. Opportunistic bacteria can be responsible for nosocomial infections, but the epidemiology of the latter in veterinary medicine may differ among bacteria [7]. Nevertheless, awareness of the existence of nosocomial infections, enacting preventive measures, and monitoring are valuable tools to reduce their occurrence.

Whether the wound becomes infected depends on many factors, including the inoculum size and pathogenicity of the contaminating bacteria, functional capacity of the host's defenses, and microenvironment of the wounded site [3,7–10]. The ability of bacteria to infect a wound depends on a critical level of contamination, which is usually considered to be greater than 10^5 organisms per gram of tissue, as well as their virulence and pathogenicity. Bacteria with thick capsules (eg, *S aureus*, *Klebsiella pneumoniae*, *S pyogenes*) are more resistant to phagocytosis. Those that produce cytotoxic exotoxins (eg, *Clostridium* spp, *S aureus*, *S pyogenes*) promote the microbes' habitation within tissue by creating more damage. In addition, during the process of bacterial degradation, lipopolysaccharide and/or protein complexes are liberated as endotoxins that can aberrantly activate the complement and coagulation pathways, which may cause systemic organ or immune dysfunction, and activate macrophages to liberate other inflammatory mediators and/or chemotaxins. Infection and complications of healing may be apparent within a few hours to several days after wound creation, which underlines the importance of careful monitoring of the condition and progress of the wound. Myonecrosis associated with clostridial organisms is a particularly devastating consequence of wounds or lacerations. Results of a recent study [11] suggest that intramuscular or inadvertent perivascular injections of commonly used medications can precede (6–72 hours) development of clostridial myonecrosis. If this type of minimal trauma can precipitate proliferation of clostridial organisms in a closed site, damaged tissues at sites of more extensive wounds should also be afforded attention.

Although the concept of a "golden period" for treatment of wounds has been questioned, timing of administration of antimicrobial medication is related to the particular therapeutic objective. If viewed as a time line beginning with the wounding incident, prevention or reduction of contamination is the objective during the first minutes to hours. For the next several hours or days, infection, invasion, or systemic effects may occur. As granulation tissue begins to fill an open wound or as repair progresses in a wound closed by first intention, systemic effects become less probable. During the first 7 to 10 days after wounding, progressive necrosis or damage may be observed and wounds on distal limbs of horses tend to increase in size [12]. When contraction then dominates healing and epithelialization progresses, antimicrobial treatment is directed at organisms that interfere locally with those processes rather than with systemic bacterial problems. Organisms like streptococci, which produce proteolytic exotoxins, are arguably more detrimental to healing than are aerobic gram-negative enterics.

The host's inflammatory response contributes to the microenvironmental condition of the wound and is important for infection control and healing [3,9]. In addition to bacteria, humoral components consisting of various amounts of enzymes, inflammatory mediators and cytokines, antibodies, and complement, to list a few, may be found in wounded and infected tissue. Neutrophils are the most rapidly appearing cellular component of inflammation and are followed by macrophages. These phagocytic cells are collectively responsible for most of the microscopic debridement and cleanup of the wound. Relative to other species, horses seem to mount a less intense and, in some cases, inefficient inflammatory response [9]. This may predispose them to infection of wounds, especially when other factors, such as massive tissue loss, excessive contamination, or the presence of a foreign body, are concomitant. Although the acute inflammatory response is desirable, accumulation of inflammatory debris (eg, blood clot, ischemic tissue, pockets of fluid and foreign material) at the site of infection may be detrimental to the host's defense mechanisms and create conditions favorable to bacterial infection. Much like the presence of a foreign body, accumulated debris may allow the establishment and persistence of infection with fewer bacteria than would be necessary if the wound were free of the debris or foreign body. For that reason, minimizing dead space, providing drainage, and physically reducing the amount of debris by lavage (physiologic crystalline solutions) and surgical debridement are critical aspects of wound management [3,4].

An open wound may serve as a portal of entry for aerobic gram-negative enteric organisms, leading to the development of bacteremia or septicemia [4] Attempts to prevent the development of bacteremia include lavaging and debriding the wound to remove organisms, thereby reducing the size of inoculum present. Antimicrobial drugs or antiseptics may be included in the lavage solution to assist in eliminating the inoculum chemically. Because the skin is breeched by a wound, the natural "barrier" to absorption is no longer present on exposed tissue of a wound. Application of medication directly to the exposed surface of a wound is not topical application as conventionally considered. Indeed, such application should be considered as modified subcutaneous or intramuscular administration, depending on the anatomic site exposed. The surface area to which the medication is applied may actually be considerably larger than that of conventional parenteral administration into the same tissues. That change alone can markedly increase the amount of medication absorbed systemically from the site of application. Consequences of that absorption should be considered in making a risk-benefit decision. Is the medication effective systemically? Does it contribute to adverse systemic reactions? If it is absorbed from the wound, is there a benefit to direct application? Drugs that are typically administered parenterally into those tissues should generally be well tolerated when applied directly. If the same drug is also administered systemically, the dose applied topically must be included in the total dose.

Burns are sterile for a short time after they are created. When a large dermal injury is created by a burn (or by any incident), loss of fluids and electrolytes can occur. Associated cardiovascular events can complicate or contribute to the adverse systemic effects of medications. Injury to tissue of the blunt "crush" type may also contribute to failure of some organs, although the trauma may not have resulted in an open wound. Cardiovascular, pulmonary, gastrointestinal, and renal insufficiencies may be inappropriately attributed to the medication or may reduce the amount of medication needed to induce adversity [13,14]. Those individual contributors must be considered in context.

Judicious use of antimicrobial drugs for management of wounds

An overarching principle to guide the use of antimicrobial drugs in treating wounds is that antimicrobial drugs are an adjunctive treatment and should be used to support healing. Antimicrobial drugs cannot debride the wound of damaged or avascular tissue, and they cannot produce angiogenesis, fibroplasia, contraction, or epithelialization. Those processes naturally proceed when or if bacterial interference is halted by the action of antimicrobial drugs.

The type of tissue having sustained trauma, extent of injury, and location and type of wound (eg, puncture, burn, open superficial lesion) dictate the appropriate antimicrobial therapy [4,14]. Tissues with relatively poor vascularity, such as tendons or ligaments, may undergo inflammatory or necrotic changes for several days after an injury occurs. As a result, trauma to periarticular ligamentous tissue may not originally penetrate the joint capsule, but within a few days, necrosis of damaged tissue may progress through the fibrous joint capsule and culminate in synovial infection. Recognition of that possibility, careful inspection and surgical debridement of the wound, monitoring of the wounded tissue, and prophylactic use of antimicrobial medication may help to prevent the development of septic arthritis from a simple periarticular desmitis. Conversely, antimicrobial drugs alone do not prevent the trauma-induced necrosis.

Clinical experience is valuable for monitoring healing of wounds and health of the tissues [3,4,12]. Physical characteristics of the wound, including color, odor, nature of drainage, and indicators of inflammation, as well as the general demeanor of the patient can be initial indicators of complications and signal the need for additional diagnostic support, such as isolation of bacteria and their respective antibiograms. Proper acquisition and submission of a sample for aerobic and possible anaerobic bacterial culture and sensitivity testing is crucial to identify the infecting organism and to provide specific data regarding drug efficacy. The surface of a granulating wound is expected to be contaminated, and discernment should be exercised when interpreting results. When a draining tract or chronic nonhealing wound is considered, the ideal sample may be deep to the surface and require surgical acquisition (ie, biopsy of bone, sequestrum, foreign body) [4]. Synovial fluid or tissue may be appropriate material for culture when synovial structures are wounded. Techniques to enhance the probability of isolating organisms may be used if the sample is processed in a particular manner or transported in special medium. These details can be learned by discussing the case with personnel at the receiving diagnostic laboratory before obtaining the sample. Some authors recommend requesting aerobic and anaerobic isolation procedures to be as diagnostically thorough as possible.

Although antimicrobials are necessary or helpful adjuncts in the treatment of many wounds, superinfection, adverse reactions, or the development of resistance, especially the gram-negative enterics, are serious side effects that may develop. The equine practitioner must understand the indications for use of antimicrobials and be familiar with the mechanisms of action of the most commonly used of these drugs [13]. Factors that contribute to the failure of antimicrobial therapy include a depressed immune system; lack of compliance with a treatment regimen; presence of a foreign body; drug interactions; antimicrobial antagonisms; drug resistance; incorrect dose, route, or frequency of administration of the drug; and incorrect diagnosis [3].

How to select and apply antimicrobial drugs depends on the contaminating organism(s) as well as the site of the wound (Tables 1 and 2). As mentioned previously, *S aureus*, *S pyogenes*, gram-negative aerobic enterics, and anaerobes are the bacteria most frequently encountered in traumatic wounds of horses. Infection of a wound is usually characterized by the exaggerated presence of redness, pain, and swelling along with a purulent discharge from the wound. The most common systemic changes associated with infection include fever and leukocytosis with a left shift. If there is no clinical improvement in the horse within 3 to 5 days of treatment with an antimicrobial drug selected in view of the most likely pathogen, the selection and administration regimen of the drug should be reviewed. Problems with treatment could include selection of an inappropriate antimicrobial, inadequate dose or inappropriate route, an abscess or a persistent infection that requires surgical drainage, a distant infection, a foreign body, or antimicrobial resistance [3].

Benzylpenicillin G, metronidazole, and chloramphenicol have consistently demonstrated the broadest activity against anaerobes. Other classes of antimicrobial drugs may contain individual representatives that have restricted activity against particular organisms, but reliance on those idiosyncrasies for initial treatment seldom leads to clinical success. β-Lactams, examples of which are penicillin and cephalosporin, are susceptible to degradation by the hydrolytic activity of bacterially produced β-lactamase(s). In some geographic areas more than others, anaerobes (particularly *Bacteroides* spp) that produce β-lactamases are relatively common.

Table 1
Suggested initial regimens for antimicrobial drugs in horses

Drug	Dose (mg/kg)	Route	Frequency
Amikacin sulfate	6.6	IM	q6–8h
	2 g + 200 mL saline	IU	q24 h for 3 days
Amoxicillin sodium	22	IM	q6–12h
Ampicillin sodium trihydrate	25–100	IV	q6h
	11–22	IM	q12h
Chloramphenicol	50	IV	q8h
	50	Orally	q6–8h
Gentamicin	3–5	IM	q6–8h
Metronidazole[a]	15–25	Orally	q6h
Oxacillin sodium	16–50	IM or IV	q8–12h
Oxytetracycline	4.4–5	IV	q12h
Penicillin G			
Potassum	12,500–100,000 IU/kg	IV or IM	q4h
Procaine	20,000–50,000 IU/kg	IM	q12h
Sodium	12,500–100,000 IU/kg	IV or IM	q4h
Ticarcillin	22–44	IV	q5h
	22–44	IM	q8h
Trimethoprim-sulfadiazine	15	IV	q8–12h

Abbreviations: h, hours; IM, intramuscular; IU, intrauterine; IV, intravenous; q, every.

[a] Anorexia may be an adverse effect exhibited when this regimen is used. Author suggests dosage regimen of 10 of 15 mg/kg twice daily.

Adapted from Brumbaugh GW. Rational selection of antimicrobial drugs for treatment of infections of horses. Vet Clin N Am Equine Pract 1987;3:191–220; with permission.

β-lactams can enter and remain effective in the microenvironment of anaerobic infections, but it may be necessary to administer the appropriate salt of the drug intravenously four or more times daily during the first few days of treatment to achieve and maintain adequate concentrations at the site of infection. Metronidazole is only active in its reduced state, which occurs in the low-redox microenvironment of anaerobic sites of infection rather than in circulation. Concentrations in circulation should not be expected to be in the reduced bioactive form and serve as a reservoir to provide drug to the site of infection. The pharmacokinetic relation of circulating concentrations of metronidazole to the patient's clinical response has not been established. Metronidazole may be administered orally or parenterally, and this author suggests that metronidazole be administered orally twice daily at a rate of 10 to 15 mg/kg of body weight. During the initial days of treatment, that dose may be administered three times daily or intravenously, but higher doses or more frequent administration may be associated with adverse effects of metronidazole on appetite and mentation that could be misinterpreted as signs of disease. That regimen for metronidazole is not the same as those recommended by other authors and is based on the reasons presented previously as well as clinical experience. Chloramphenicol is active in vitro against virtually all anaerobes. In the opinion of this author, the clinical response has not been as

Table 2
Systemic antimicrobials used to treat orthopedic infections in horses

Antimicrobial	Dosage	Combinations and indications
Penicillin	22,000–44,000 IU/kg 6–12h IV or IM	Combined with gentamicin, amikacin, ceftiofur, or trimethoprim-sulfas Gram-positive infections
Cefazolin (cephalosporin)	10 mg/kg q8h IV or IM	Can be used alone, usually combined with gentamicin or amikacin
Gentamicin	2.2 mg/kg q6–8h or 6–8 mg/kg q24h IV or IM	Combined with penicillin or a cephalosporin Gram-negative infections
Amikacin	7 mg/kg q8–12h or 14 mg/kg q24h IV or IM	Combined with penicillin or a cephalosporin Gram-negative infections
Ceftiofur	2 mg/kg q12h or 4–5 mg/kg q12h or 1 mg/kg q6h IV or IM	Can be used alone or combined with penicillin, variable dosage Good for *Staphylococcus* infections
Trimethoprim-sulfonamides	30 mg/kg q12h PO or 3–5 mg/kg q12h PO (based on trimethoprim)	Used alone or combined with penicillin, not recommended for initial treatment because of resistance
Metronidazole	15–25 mg/kg q6–8h PO IV, or rectally	Rarely used alone Anaerobic infections Anaerobic infections
Rifampin	5–10 mg/kg q12–24h PO	Always combined with other antimicrobials to avoid resistance Good for *Staphylococcus* and *Rhodococcus* infections
Erythromycin	25 mg/kg q6–8h PO	Used primarily with rifampin for *Rhodococcus* infections
Enrofloxacin	2–3 mg/kg q12h or 5 mg/kg q24h PO	Used alone for infections resistant to above antimicrobials, not recommended for foals

Abbreviations: h, hours; IM, intramuscular; IV, intravenous; PO, orally; q, every.

From Baxter GM. Instrumentation and techniques for treating orthopedic infections in horses. Vet Clin N Am Equine Pract 1996;12(2):303–35; with permission.

impressive when mixed bacterial populations are present, such as is often the case in wounds. Although no reason for that anecdotal impression has been proven, the symbiotic existence of those organisms may be a partial cause. Some organisms constitutively produce chloramphenicol acetyl transferase (CAT), which inactivates chloramphenicol. If organisms that are susceptible to chloramphenicol in vitro are present in the wound with other organisms that produce CAT, the former may be protected by the latter. This same scenario can occur when organisms susceptible to benzylpenicillin are present with other organisms that produce β-lactamase, such that the former may be protected by the β-lactamase produced by the symbiotic existence and may not respond to treatment with β-lactams susceptible to enzymatic degradation [12]. Lincosamides are quite effective against anaerobes but possess a reputation of being associated with lethal alteration of intestinal bacterial flora in horses, such that they are generally not considered for treatment of horses. They are mentioned here only because the author has had practitioners comment on the use of dilute solutions for wound lavage without the notorious disastrous colitis. Such use should be with caution.

Aminoglycosides are still considered the drugs of choice against aerobic gram-negative enteric bacteria. Extended-spectrum penicillins, second- or third-generation cephalosporins, and potentiated sulfonamides could also be considered for initial treatment. The susceptibility of those organisms is not predictable, and antibiograms should be used to guide selection of medication for subsequent use. When administered systemically, the aforementioned drugs distribute well into the extracellular fluid that bathes the wound, such that direct application may not be necessary. In the opinion of this author, treatment against *Pseudomonas* spp should always be formulated according to the results of antibiograms because of the unpredictable nature of susceptibility of that genus of bacteria. Mafenide or silver sulfadiazine has historically been used topically on burns to control *Pseudomonas* spp, but other choices may be warranted by results of antibiograms.

In the case of burn wounds, 1% silver sulfadiazine cream is one of the most widely used topical antimicrobials. It provides broad-spectrum antibacterial and antifungal activity in vitro and has been shown in other species to increase the rate of epithelialization compared with other topical medications, although this has not been confirmed in the horse [14,15].

Alternative modes of administration

In addition to more conventional modes of administration, regional infusion and/or perfusion of some antibacterial drugs, particularly aminoglycosides and β-lactams that distribute well into extracellular fluid compartments, is a useful technique for the treatment of some wounds [16–22]. The procedure is designed to maintain a high concentration of drug in the immediate blood supply of the area of interest or in the extracellular fluid in areas in which compromised perfusion prevents systemically administered drugs from reaching the site of the wound. By maintaining an optimal concentration gradient between perfusate and infected tissue for a longer time, more drug diffuses into the targeted tissue, thereby producing higher concentrations at the site of infection than could be achieved by using the drug systemically. The advantage of this technique is particularly attractive when there is a propensity of a drug to produce systemic adversities. The same objective may be accomplished by intraosseous infusions [16,17,23,24], intrasynovial injections [19,25], antimicrobial-impregnated polymethylmethacrylate implants [4,26], or implantable pumps [4]. Those techniques are progressively being refined for successful application to some equine patients, and the list of conditions for which they may be considered is growing. Commercialization of equipment and materials used for these techniques should assist their application to a wider range of patients. Good descriptions and case reports containing pertinent details should be reviewed by interested readers [16,18,19–24,26], because a thorough review of the subject is beyond the scope of this article. As with any procedure or technique, skill and confidence naturally follow experience, and if more than one approach is possible, selection of the most appropriate can be individualized.

Antiseptics

Antiseptics are a popular form of wound medication and are available as over-the-counter formulations as well as by prescription. Opinions abound regarding these products, and favorites are often established with little more than anecdotal evidence for support. Indeed, a common challenge for the equine practitioner lies in arguing in favor of or against the use of a particular product that is desired by the owner. Results of studies have shown and investigators have concluded that hygiene of the wound is a prerequisite to healing but that antiseptics seldom contribute any more to repair than do careful cleansing, lavage, and debridement [15].

Antiseptics, such as chlorhexidine diacetate, povidone-iodine, or hydrogen peroxide, are often added to lavage solutions in an effort to enhance the antimicrobial effect [27–30]. Although unequivocal data to support or refute their use are not available, to be of any benefit, the additive must be active against the targeted organism(s) and have no significant negative effects on healing of the wound. Tissues on which they are used, the liquid in which they are diluted, and concentrations of the respective antiseptic are important factors relating to the inherent risk of antisepsis versus irritation to the tissue. Although the inflammatory response is important to wound repair, any treatment that creates more insult should be avoided.

A 0.05% solution of chlorhexidine gluconate and a 1% povidone-iodine solution are effective and relatively nontoxic to the cellular components of the wound [28,29]. Although commonly used as a wound disinfectant, a 3% solution of hydrogen peroxide is only weakly bactericidal and is significantly toxic to fibroblasts in the wound [27]. If it is used, hydrogen peroxide should be employed only once at the time of the initial lavage of heavily contaminated wounds for its foaming action to help physically remove debris [30]. The exothermic and foaming actions are characteristics that cause many therapists not to use hydrogen peroxide in closed spaces.

Ancillary treatments

When skin is disrupted by wounding, the underlying tissues are exposed to hyperbaric conditions relative to those present under intact skin. This situation seems to be conducive to bacterial control and epithelial migration [31]. In contrast, it may be speculated that puncture wounds are more prone to anaerobic growth than are open wounds. It has been shown in other species that some ancillary treatments may improve the activity of medication or the response of the patient to wound infection. Hyperbaric chambers are now used for the treatment of wounds with poorly perfused tissues in small animal and human patients and are available for horses in some locales. As experience is gained in using that form of treatment for horses, the author expects broader application in equine medicine. When equipment for containment of the entire horse is not available, many simple forms of oxygen treatment are possible. Oxygen can be insufflated under an occlusive bandage to increase its tension immediately at the surface of a wound. The location of the wound is important, because placement of an adequate bandage is a prerequisite. Furthermore, this treatment is no longer applicable in the fibroblastic phase of repair, because the presence of granulation tissue precludes local infection and can be contraindicated in wounds of the limb, where fibroplasia may become excessive under a bandage. Recognizing the lack of objective guidelines for this type of ancillary treatment, attending veterinarians should use their experience in monitoring wounds to assist them in determining the duration of each treatment, the interval between treatments, and the overall duration of therapy. Appropriate safety measures should be undertaken when using oxygen to ensure protection of the patient and personnel.

The microenvironment of a wound is generally acidic, particularly when infected. The low pH can impede host defense mechanisms, the activity of some antimicrobial drugs (particularly aminoglycosides), and physiologic events involving cell migration and proliferation. The acid surface of a wound can be buffered with a physiologic solution of sodium bicarbonate (1.3% $NaHCO_3$). After cleaning the wound with saline (pH is usually acidic) or with water (variable pH), a final rinse with physiologic sodium bicarbonate may aid healing and the activity of antimicrobial drugs applied directly or administered systemically. The author has used and recommended this approach, which is adapted from respiratory pharmacologic procedures, with anecdotal benefit but could find no reports of studies in horses. Tris-EDTA has also been used to enhance the antimicrobial activity of aminoglycosides [32].

By preventing or treating infections of wounds, antimicrobials drugs diminish inflammation of the wound. Glucocorticosteroids are also used for this purpose, particularly in wounds of the distal limb in horses, where some phases of repair (eg, inflammation, fibroplasia) are persistent or excessive and lead to the development of exuberant granulation tissue, which hinders subsequent contraction and epithelialization. Diligence must be used in designing this ancillary treatment, however, because corticosteroids can ultimately retard and diminish the quality of wound repair.

Dimethylsulfoxide (DMSO) also attenuates clinical signs of inflammation [33–35]. Results of many studies have failed to provide support for clinical application of its multiple activities in vitro, however. DMSO did not enhance the effectiveness of 1% silver sulfadiazine against *Pseudomonas aeruginosa* when applied as a topical antimicrobial to thermal burn wounds [36], the antibacterial activity of tetracyclines in vitro [37], or the diffusion of trimethoprim or sulfamethoxazole in cerebrospinal fluid of horses [38]. Compared with a placebo, DMSO does not improve collagen biosynthesis, epidermal resurfacing, or the number or types of bacteria in superficial wounds [39]. No doubt as with antimicrobial drugs, when, how, and why to use DMSO may be more important than whether to use it.

Summary

Antimicrobial medication should be considered an adjunct to the general care of wounds rather than a substitute for lavage, drainage, or other physical care intended to promote healing. Judicious use is based on results of diagnostic procedures and the professional judgment of the attending veterinarian.

Organisms that contaminate or infect wounds of horses are similar to those that can affect human patients, such that personal hygiene and protection are important when caring for these equine patients, because attendants can easily be exposed to them. Although those organisms are considered to be ubiquitous, the inoculum that may be present on or in an infected wound may be substantially greater than that encountered during other daily activities of the veterinarian. Proper disposal of the bandage materials and personal protective clothing is important.

Bacterial resistance is one of many "survival tactics" of bacteria and has been an important clinical consideration for physicians and veterinarians since antimicrobial drugs were discovered. Controversies and insufficient understanding of bacterial resistance abound, however. The entirety of the subject is beyond the scope of this article, but it is important to the veterinary profession and for the formulation of wound management in horses. We and our animal patients live in a world populated by microbial organisms of various types. Resistance among bacteria is likely to continue to be a clinical consideration in the future as it has been during the past 60 to 70 years. As veterinarians, we must recognize the zoonotic nature of resistance and implement biosecurity procedures to protect ourselves, other people in contact with those pathogens, and our patients. We must also recognize the merits of judicious targeted use of antimicrobial drugs and apply appropriate principles during the course of professional care for the well-being of our animal patients.

References

[1] Cockbill SM, Turner TD. Management of veterinary wounds. Vet Rec 1995;136(14):362–5.

[2] Dinev D, Koichev K, Kolev K, et al. Etiology and chemotherapy of suppurative surgical infection in horses and cattle. Vet Med Nauki 1986;23(9):51–6.

[3] Dunning D. Surgical wound infection and the use of antimicrobials. In: Slatter D, editor. Textbook of small animal surgery. 3rd edition. Philadelphia: WB Saunders; 2003. p. 113–21.

[4] Baxter GM. Instrumentation and techniques for treating orthopedic infections in horses. Vet Clin N Am Equine Pract 1996;12(2):303–35.

[5] Silver IA. Some factors affecting wound healing. Equine Vet J 1973;5(2):47–51.

[6] Spurlock SL, Hanie EA. Antibiotics in the treatment of wounds. Vet Clin N Am Equine Pract 1989;5(3):465–82.

[7] Boerlin P, Eugster S, Gaschen F, et al. Transmission of opportunistic pathogens in a veterinary teaching hospital. Vet Microbiol 2001;82(4):347–59.

[8] Wilmink JM, van Herten J, van Weeren PR, et al. Retrospective study of primary intention healing and sequestrum formation in horses compared to ponies under clinical circumstances. Equine Vet J 2002;34(3):270–3.

[9] Wilmink JM, Veenman JN, van den Boom R, et al. Differences in polymorpho-nucleocyte function and local inflammatory response between horses and ponies. Equine Vet J 2003;35: 561–9.

[10] Southwood LL, Baxter GM. Instrument sterilization, skin preparation, and wound management. Vet Clin N Am Equine Pract 1996;12(2):173–94.

[11] Peek SF, Semrad SD, Perkins GA. Clostridial myonecrosis in horses (37 cases 1985–2000). Equine Vet J 2003;35(1):86–92.

[12] Schumacher J, Brumbaugh GW, Honnas CM, et al. Kinetics of healing of grafted and nongrafted wounds on the distal portion of the forelimbs of horses. Am J Vet Res 1992;53(9): 1568–71.

[13] Brumbaugh GW. Rational selection of antimicrobial drugs for treatment of infections in horses. Vet Clin N Am Equine Pract 1987;3(1):191–220.

[14] Brumbaugh GW. Antimicrobial therapy of adult horses with emergency conditions. Vet Clin N Am Equine Pract 1994;10(3):527–34.

[15] Berry DB II, Sullins KE. Effects of topical application of antimicrobials and bandaging on healing and granulation tissue formation in wounds of the distal aspect of the limbs in horses. Am J Vet Res 2003;64(1):88–92.

[16] Butt TD, Bailey JV, Dowling PM, et al. Comparison of 2 techniques for regional antibiotic delivery to the equine forelimb: intraosseous perfusion vs. intravenous perfusion. Can Vet J 2001;42(8).617–22.

[17] Scheuch BC, Van Hoogmoed LM, Wilson WD, et al. Comparison of intraosseous or intravenous infusion for delivery of amikacin sulfate to the tibiotarsal joint of horses. Am J Vet Res 2002;63(3):374–80.

[18] Murphey ED, Santschi EM, Papich MG. Regional intravenous perfusion of the distal limb of horses with amikacin sulfate. J Vet Pharmacol Ther 1999;22(1):68–71.

[19] Werner LA, Hardy J, Bertone AL. Bone gentamicin concentration after intra-articular injection or regional intravenous perfusion in the horse. Vet Surg 2003;32(6):559–65.

[20] Whitehair KJ, Blevins WE, Fessler JF, et al. Regional perfusion of the equine carpus for antibiotic delivery. Vet Surg 1992;21(4):279–85.

[21] Whitehair KJ, Adams SB, Parker JE, et al. Regional limb perfusion with antibiotics in three horses. Vet Surg 1992;21(4):286–92.

[22] Whitehair KJ, Bowersock TL, Blevins WE, et al. Regional limb perfusion for antibiotic treatment of experimentally induced septic arthritis. Vet Surg 1992;21(5):367–73.

[23] Kettner NU, Parker JE, Watrous BJ. Intraosseous regional perfusion for treatment of septic physitis in a two-week-old foal. J Am Vet Med Assoc 2003;222(3):346–50.

[24] Mattson S, Boure L, Pearce S, et al. Intraosseous gentamicin perfusion of the distal metacarpus in standing horses. Vet Surg 2004;33(2):180–6.
[25] Chan CC, Murphy H, Munroe GA. Treatment of chronic digital septic tenosynovitis in 12 horses by modified open annular ligament desmotomy and passive open drainage. Vet Rec 2000;147(14):388–93.
[26] Holcombe SJ, Schneider RK, Bramlage LR, et al. Use of antibiotic-impregnated polymethyl methacrylate in horses with open or infected fractures or joints: 19 cases (1987–1995). J Am Vet Med Assoc 1997;211(7):889–93.
[27] Lineweaver W, McMorris S, Soucy D, et al. Cellular and bacterial toxicities of topical antimicrobials. Plast Reconstr Surg 1985;75:394–6.
[28] Sanchez IR, Nusbaum KE, Swaim SF, et al. Chlorhexidine diacetate and povidone-iodine cytotoxicity to canine embryonic fibroblasts and Staphylococcus aureus. Vet Surg 1988;17:182–5.
[29] Sanchez IR, Swaim SF, Nusbaum KE, et al. Effects of chlorhexidine diacetate and povidone-iodine on wound healing in dogs. Vet Surg 1988;17:291–5.
[30] Swaim SF, Henderson RA. Small animal wound management. 2nd edition. Baltimore: Williams & Wilkins; 1997. p. 13–51.
[31] Singer AJ, Clark RAF. Cutaneous wound healing. N Engl J Med 1999;341:738–46.
[32] Ritchie BW, Wooley RE, Kemp DT. Use of potentiated antibiotics in wound management. Vet Clin Exot Anim 2004;7(1):169–89.
[33] Brayton CF. Dimethyl sulfoxide (DMSO): a review. Cornell Vet 1986;76(1):61–90.
[34] Welch RD, DeBowes RM, Leipold HW. Evaluation of the effects of intra-articular injection of dimethylsulfoxide on normal equine articular tissues. Am J Vet Res 1989;50(7):1180–2.
[35] Welch RD, Watkins JP, DeBowes RM, et al. Effects of intra-articular administration of dimethylsulfoxide on chemically induced synovitis in immature horses. Am J Vet Res 1991;52(6):934–9.
[36] Raskin DJ, Sullivan KH, Rappaport NH. The role of topical dimethyl sulfoxide in burn wound infection: evaluation in the rat. Ann NY Acad Sci 1983;411:105–9.
[37] Wooley RE, Gilbert JP, Shotts EF Jr. Antibacterial action of combinations of oxytetracycline, dimethyl sulfoxide, and EDTA-tromethamine on *Proteus, Salmonella*, and *Aeromonas*. Am J Vet Res 1982;43:130–3.
[38] Green SL, Mayhew IG, Brown MP, et al. Concentrations of trimethoprim and sulfamethoxazole in cerebrospinal fluid and serum in mares with and without a dimethyl sulfoxide pretreatment. Can J Vet Res 1990;54:215–22.
[39] Goldblum OM, Alvarez OM, Mertz PM, et al. Dimethyl sulfoxide (DMSO) does not affect epidermal wound healing. Proc Soc Exp Biol Med 1983;172(3):301–7.

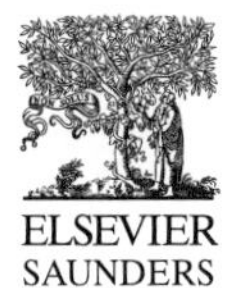
ELSEVIER
SAUNDERS

Vet Clin Equine 21 (2005) 77–89

VETERINARY
CLINICS
Equine Practice

Topical Treatments in Equine Wound Management

Andrew J. Dart, BVSc*,
Brad A. Dowling, BVSc,
Christine L. Smith, DVM

University Veterinary Centre Camden, Faculty of Veterinary Science, University of Sydney, Werombi Road, Camden, New South Wales 2570, Australia

Wound repair is a complex temporally and spatially coordinated series of cellular, molecular, physiologic, and biochemical events regulated by a delicately orchestrated cascade of mediators [1]. Damaged tissue is removed, and structural integrity is restored. Effective coordination of the healing process in horses, particularly of wounds involving the lower limb, is often problematic, resulting in chronic nonhealing wounds or exuberant granulation tissue that inhibits wound contraction and epithelialization. Various factors have been implicated, including poor blood supply, low oxygen tension and temperature, and an imbalance of mediators [1,2].

Numerous soluble mediators having a critical influence on repair belong to the cytokine family. Growth factors are a particular category of cytokines exerting primarily growth-inducing effects.

Role of growth factors

An adequate inflammatory response is a prerequisite for rapid and effective healing [3]. Compared with horses, ponies show a stronger initial inflammatory response characterized by higher in vivo production of chemoattractants and inflammatory mediators, particularly transforming growth factor (TGF)-β, tumor necrosis factor (TNF)-α, and interleukin (IL)-1 [4]. The result is a greater influx of leukocytes into the wound that further enhances the inflammatory process, leading to an earlier

* Corresponding author. University Centre Veterinary Centre PMB 4, Narellan Delivery Centre, Narellan, New South Wales 2570, Australia.

E-mail address: andrewd@camden.usyd.edu.au (A.J. Dart).

0749-0739/05/$ - see front matter
doi:10.1016/j.cveq.2004.11.003

demarcation of viable and nonviable tissue [4–7]. The initial weak inflammatory response in horses can contribute to a protracted inflammatory state characterized by persistently elevated concentrations of TGF-β1 [3,4,7].

Studies in horses and ponies show a peak in total TGFβ in the first 24 hours after wound creation [7,8]. This initial rise in TGFβ is attributed to the β1 and β2 isoforms, which are considered profibrotic [8,9]. A second rise in TGFβ occurs 5 to 9 days after wounding and is attributed to TGF-β3, the anti-inflammatory and antifibrotic isoform of TGFβ [10]. There is growing evidence that reciprocal regulation of TGF-β1 and TGF-β3 occurs, implying that a rapid decrease in TGF-β1 leads to a faster increase in TGF-β3, which ultimately moderates the inflammatory process [7,9]. In ponies and in wounds of the trunk in horses, TGF-β1 concentrations subside rapidly and are substantially reduced by 1 to 2 weeks after injury, which corresponds to the rise in TGF-β3 concentrations [7–9]. Although a recent study failed to establish in a significant manner the reciprocal role of TGF-β1 and TGF-β3 in modulating wound healing in distal limb wounds in horses, there was a consistent trend in the data to support a role for these isoforms in the production of exuberant granulation tissue [9]. In the presence of TGF-β1, angiogenesis and fibroplasia persist and delayed wound contraction and epithelialization lead to longer healing times in horses, particularly in wounds of the lower limb [3,4,7].

Wound contraction is delayed on the limb and in horses compared with ponies [5,11]. Although their exact contribution is unclear, myofibroblasts, a specialized contractile phenotype of fibroblast, have been attributed a role in wound contraction [12]. The myofibroblast's intrinsic contractility does not seem to differ between horses and ponies or between thoracic or limb wounds [6,13]. It is likely that the observed delay in wound contraction observed in the horse, particularly in limb wounds, is related to tissue environmental factors, such as blood supply and cytokine profiles during the inflammatory response, that ultimately influence the efficiency of myofibroblast activity [5,6,13].

Ultimately, an imbalance in the delicate equilibrium of cytokines and growth factors encourages exuberant granulation tissue production and delays wound contraction and epithelialization in wounds of the distal limb of the horse, leading to excessive scarring [7,14]. Manipulation of the cytokine profile or wound environment could potentially modulate the quality of repair and offers a window through which wound healing may be facilitated.

Topical application of growth factors

Several clinical studies using a variety of animal models suggest that growth factor therapy can accelerate healing of normal tissues and promote the repair of impaired wounds [14–17]. No single mediator can resolve all issues of repair or cover all vulnerabilities, however. As our knowledge of the role of such mediators broadens, cytokines, growth factors, and other biologic agents are likely to be used more specifically to target the particular promoters of healing [16].

Transforming growth factor-β

TGFβ was predicted to be of therapeutic value in the treatment of chronic, nonhealing, or slow-healing wounds over a decade ago and has been shown to increase granulation tissue and collagen formation as well as wound tensile strength when applied locally in some animal models of normal or impaired healing [16,18]. In limb wounds in horses, there were no beneficial effects of topical application of TGF-β1 during the early phases of wound healing when the inflammatory response is suboptimal [19].

There are at least five TGFβ isoforms, of which the first three (β1–β3) are expressed in mammals. Different roles and temporal patterns of the various isoforms, the site of the wound, and the timing of application of each isoform may have a bearing on the healing process. Differences in wound healing models, vehicle, timing, and frequency of application make it difficult to interpret findings, particularly across species.

Neutralization of TGF-β1 and TGF-β2 within human wounds produces an antiscarring effect, as does the use of antisense oligodeoxynucleotides against TGF-β1 mRNA [10,20]. There may be a future role for receptor antagonists in modulating wound healing in the horse, where the temporal and spatial regulation of TGFβ receptors in normal and pathologic wound repair has recently been described [21].

Platelet-rich plasma

Degranulating platelets release growth factors and substances associated with wound healing, including TGFβ, platelet-derived growth factor (PDGF), epidermal growth factor (EGF), TGFα, vascular endothelial growth factor (VEGF), platelet thromboplastin, thrombospondin, coagulation factors, calcium, serotonin, histamine, and hydrolytic enzymes [22]. Platelet-derived products offer an advantage over individual cytokines, because a large number of mediators are easily available in high concentrations when platelets are activated and the technology capitalizes on the synergistic or cumulative effects of cytokines [23]. Topical application of growth factors derived from platelets encouraged repair of previously nonhealing wounds in human patients [24].

A platelet-derived wound healing gel has been formulated from allergen-free homologous equine whole blood [15]. The platelet-rich plasma is packaged with a patented activator, and once activated, the gel is applied to the wound dressing for 3 to 7 days. Compared with control wounds, gel-treated wounds had a similar inflammatory response, accelerated epithelial differentiation, and more mature granulation tissue [15]. This study suggests that platelet-rich plasma might be an effective method of replacing essential growth factors, especially TGFβ and PDGF, in wounds of the distal limb, where an imbalance may exist [15].

Activated macrophage supernatant

Activated monocytes and the cytokines they produce have inhibitory and stimulatory effects on inflammation [25]. A rabbit peritoneal macrophage supernatant was shown to inhibit proliferation of equine, human, and rabbit fibroblasts in vitro [25,26], although no beneficial effects could be established in a standardized wound-healing model in ponies [27]. The failure to show an effect in vivo may be related to a number of factors, including the fact that wounds in ponies normally heal well; however, the in vitro effects suggest that further investigation and application may hold promise.

Growth hormone

Growth hormone is a small protein produced by the anterior pituitary gland that is responsible for the growth of most body tissues [28]. It regulates growth through hypertrophy, hyperplasia, or both as a result of tissue differentiation, cell proliferation, and protein synthesis [28]. Its effects may be mediated directly through interaction with target tissue receptors or indirectly through the production of somatomedins, particularly insulin-like growth factor (IGF)-1 [28]. Systemic treatment with recombinant growth hormone has been used in human patients with severe burn injuries and has enhanced rates of repair and patient survival in most studies [28]. It is suggested that the beneficial action of exogenously administered growth hormone on burn wounds may be related to the restoration of anabolic metabolism rather than to the stimulation of repair at the cellular level [28]. In some animal models of healing, growth hormone does stimulate granulation tissue formation and biomechanical wound strength [29], and a lack of efficacy has also been reported [30].

Equine recombinant growth hormone (Equigen; Pfizer Animal Health, Sydney, New South Wales, Australia) has recently become available, and the effects of daily systemic administration on a standardized model of distal limb wound healing were studied in horses [28]. No difference in overall wound healing time was found; however, treated wounds were found to retract further than untreated wounds initially and then to contract faster after treatment with growth hormone ceased. It was suggested that growth hormone might modulate the role of fibroblasts and myofibroblasts within the wound. Interestingly, in vitro studies have identified growth hormone as an inhibitor of TGFβ-induced myofibroblast differentiation [30].

A more thorough understanding of the complex effects of cytokines on the cellular activity within healing wounds may provide an opportunity to re-evaluate the potential of growth hormone therapy in normal or impaired wound healing.

Topical agents that may alter the wound environment

Solcoseryl

Solcoseryl (Solco Basle Ltd, Birsfelden, Switzerland) is a dialysate and ultrafiltrate derived from calf blood that has been shown to improve healing in animals and people [31]. It is protein-free and does not contain any appreciable concentrations of growth factors; however, it influences fibroblast proliferation and migration in vitro [32]. This suggests a growth factor–like action, perhaps via receptor stimulation [31]. Furthermore, Solcoseryl promotes differentiation of human monocytes into macrophages [33], which produce the numerous cytokines and growth factors affecting fibroblast proliferation, collagen synthesis, endothelial cell migration, and angiogenesis. Through whichever mechanism, Solcoseryl enhances the inflammatory reaction and subsequent migration and proliferation of fibroblasts.

Solcoseryl has recently been shown to stimulate healing of deep wounds of the trunk and limbs of horses for the first 4 weeks after wounding; after that time, it had an inhibitory effect [31]. Solcoseryl initially provoked a greater inflammatory response, faster formation of granulation tissue, and faster contraction; however, it inhibited healing through protraction of the inflammatory phase and inhibition of epithelialization [31]. These effects were more pronounced in horses, particularly in limb wounds, when compared with ponies, perhaps as a result of the weaker initial inflammatory response normally demonstrated by horses [5,38]. Indeed, studies suggest that Solcoseryl is more effective when wound healing is impaired or when culture conditions are suboptimal [34–36].

Solcoseryl should be applied as a thin film daily for the first few weeks after injury. After wound contraction slows and epithelialization becomes predominant, application should cease.

Ketanserin

Ketanserin (Vulketan gel; Janssen Animal Health, Beerse, Belgium) is a selective serotonin inhibitor that competitively antagonizes serotonin-induced vasoconstriction and platelet aggregation [37]. It has been shown to counter cutaneous skin flap necrosis in animals after systemic administration, reportedly by improving circulation [38]. It also antagonizes the serotonin-induced suppression of wound macrophages and thus allows a strong and effective inflammatory response to occur within wounds. This should translate into superior control of infection and better orchestration of the later phases of repair when the cytokines and growth factors released by the activated macrophages play an important role. Ischemic, diabetic, venous, scleroderma, and decubitus ulcers and thermal burns have all been treated with 2% topical ketanserin ointment with varying degrees of success [38,39]. It seems that efficacy is best in wounds with impaired circulation or at peripheral sites, suggesting that some value may be seen in distal limb wounds in horses.

A controlled field study was performed to determine the efficacy of ketanserin in preventing exuberant granulation tissue formation in equine lower limb wounds [40]. Vulketan gel was two to five times more likely to result in successful closure (by reducing infection and exuberant granulation tissue formation) than an antiseptic or a desloughing agent.

Tripeptide- and tetrapeptide-copper complexes

Glycyl-L-histidyl-L-lysine (-L-phenylalanine) tripeptide- and tetrapeptide-copper complexes (TCCs; Iamin-vet; Procyte, Redmond, WA) are chemoattractants for mast cells as well as monocytes and macrophages, stimulating several biologic activities during acute wound healing [41]. These compounds are thought to increase angiogenesis, collagen deposition, epithelialization, and wound proteases, ultimately improving the wound environment [41].

TCC is applied as a gel after wound debridement and lavage, starting in the late inflammatory phase and continuing through the proliferative phase. In one study in dogs, granulation tissue formed during treatment, although both complexes tended to become exuberant and interfere with epithelialization, which might pose a problem in the treatment of lower limb wounds in horses [42]. Given these findings and the fact that the medication seems to have the greatest effect on healing in the first 7 days [43], application in horses should be restricted to early in the healing process.

Maltodextrin

Maltodextrin (Intracell; Macleod Pharmaceutical, Fort Collins, CO) is a D-glucose polysaccharide available in a soluble powder form. Its hydrophilic properties extract fluid through the wound, cleansing contaminated and infected wounds and enhancing the absorption of tenacious exudates [41,44]. It seems to be chemoattractant for polymorphonuclear cells, lymphocytes, and macrophages and may yield glucose as an energy supplement for cell metabolism and healing [41,45]. In addition to reducing odor, exudate, swelling, and infection, it may enhance early granulation tissue formation and epithelial growth [41,46]. In the horse, maltodextrin has been suggested to reduce pain and swelling and to stimulate granulation tissue production and epithelialization when compared with conventional topical antimicrobials [47].

After debridement and lavage, a 5- to 10-mm layer of maltodextrin is applied over the wound under a nonadherent dressing [45]. An absorbent bandage and outer tertiary layer are then applied and changed daily. The wound should be thoroughly lavaged before applying a new layer of powder. Maltodextrin is best applied soon after injury and through the proliferative phase.

Live yeast cell derivative

Live yeast cell derivative or skin respiratory factor is a water-soluble extract from brewer's yeast found in an over-the-counter hemorrhoid medication (Preparation H; Whitehall Laboratories, New York, NY). It is reported to contain substances that increase wound oxygen consumption, angiogenesis, epithelialization, and collagen synthesis [48]. Live yeast cell derivative is recommended in wounds with healthy granulation tissue and in the proliferative phase of repair [48]. In horses, live yeast cell derivative has been suggested to prolong healing time by delaying epithelialization and inhibiting contraction [49], although favoring the formation of exuberant granulation tissue [50].

Corticosteroids

Corticosteroids halt the inflammatory response to injury and thus can be expected to retard wound healing [51]. The resultant carryover effect into the proliferative phase delays angiogenesis, fibroblastic proliferation, and the synthesis of extracellular matrix components. Ultimately, corticosteroids impair epithelialization, wound strength, and contraction [52]. Despite this, anecdotes and controlled trials report the positive effects of topical corticosteroids in the management of exuberant granulation tissue in distal limb wounds in horses [49,53].

These controversies no doubt arise because of wide variations among the compounds used, routes of administration and dosages, species, relation between the time of administration of the drug and the onset of trauma, duration of treatment, and criteria used to assess the effects on wound healing [49]. Until the complex matrix of factors that influence wound healing is better understood and the processes that lead to healing impairment are fully elucidated, it is probably premature to condemn the use of corticosteroids for wound management, particularly in lower limb wounds in the horse. Corticosteroids are not a treatment panacea, however, and their use must be weighed against the results of concurrent suppression of epithelialization and reduction in localized cell responses in general [51].

Aloe vera

Aloe vera gel, extracted from the mucilaginous central zone of the aloe vera leaf, contains 75 potentially active constituents [54]. Suggested effects include an ability to penetrate and anesthetize tissue, inhibit bacterial and fungal growth, act as an anti-inflammatory, and dilate capillaries to encourage blood flow [55]. With respect to wound repair, aloe vera gel may enhance contraction and breaking strength through increased collagen activity, particularly the production of type III (immature) collagen [55]. Its combination with 1% silver sulfadiazine counteracts the inhibitory effects of silver sulfadiazine used alone [56,57]. Despite these intriguing hypotheses and the fact that it is used extensively in human burn wounds, clinical use of aloe vera is supported primarily by anecdotal reports [54]. Until more conclusive evidence is available, it is hard to recommend the use of aloe vera in the treatment of wounds in horses.

Acemannan

As a topical wound medication, acemannan (Carravet; Veterinary Products Laboratories, Phoenix, AZ, or Carrasorb; Carrington Laboratories, Irving, TX) is available in a hydrogel and freeze-dried powder. It is a β(1,4)-linked acetylated mannan derived from the aloe vera plant that acts as a growth factor stimulating macrophages to enhance IL-1 and TNFα secretion [45]. IL-1 stimulates fibroblast proliferation and, combined with TNFα, stimulates angiogenesis, epidermal growth and motility, and collagen deposition [45]. It may also have a stabilizing effect on growth factors to prolong their effects on fibroplasia [51]. In a topical gel form, it enhanced contraction and epithelialization of paw wounds in dogs and stimulated granulation tissue formation over exposed bone [51]. Studies would suggest that the greatest effects may be seen during the first 7 days after injury, and it has been recommended for full-thickness burns, lacerations, dermal ulcers, and abrasions in horses and other domestic species [41,51]. The freeze-dried form is hydrophilic and may reduce tissue edema by absorbing fluid [45]. Debridement and lavage should take place before acemannan is applied to the wound and its borders. Bandages should be changed and new medication applied daily [51]. Application can continue through the inflammatory phase into the proliferative phase of healing [45].

Sugar and honey

Topical application of sugar seems to exert antimicrobial activity and enhance fibroplasia and epithelialization and thus to accelerate wound healing in people [58], and it is superior to treatment with antiseptics in animal wound models [59]. These effects may be related to the high osmolarity of the solution [60] as well as to other mechanisms, including chemoattraction of monocytes and macrophages and provision of an energy source [61].

Wounds should be lavaged and surgically debrided before applying a layer of sugar at least 1 cm thick, taking care to fill all crevices. A large amount of absorbent dressing should be laid over the sugar to absorb the fluid and then covered with secondary and tertiary layers. Baby diapers can provide an effective absorbant layer and prevent seepage during the first few days. Multiple bandage changes along with thorough lavage may be required in the first 24 to 48 hours in heavily contaminated, edematous, and infected wounds because of large volumes of fluid and exudate. Bandage changes can become less frequent when there is undissolved sugar remaining in the wound. When debridement is complete, a healthy granulation bed is present, and epithelialization has begun, sugar dressings may be stopped.

Honey seems to possess specific antimicrobial properties unrelated to its high osmolarity [62]. In addition to imparting a low pH that favors repair, it contains inhibin, an enzyme that generates hydrogen peroxide, and glucolactone and/or gluconic acid, which acts as a mild disinfectant and mild antibiotic, respectively. Honey also provides antioxidants, which protect wound tissues from the damage imparted by free oxygen radicals released from inflammatory cells [63].

Honey used for treatment of wounds should ideally be unpasteurized and not heated to greater than 37°C to prevent inactivation of glucose oxidase [62]. Wounds should initially be lavaged and debrided [64]. It is recommended to use honey at a rate of 30 mL for each 10-cm × 10-cm dressing pad [64]. The presence of honey does not diminish wound exudate, so dressings should be changed daily or when there is exudate on the outer layer.

Although honey has been suggested to increase the speed of healing by reducing inflammation, edema, and infection, thereby enhancing debridement of necrotic wounds and promoting angiogenesis, granulation tissue, and epithelialization [60,65], the scientific merit of these studies has been questioned. Certainly, inhibition of bacterial growth has been demonstrated in vitro [62]; however, honey is a natural product, so any effect could be influenced by the species of bee, geographic location, or processing and storage conditions [63,66,67]. In conclusion, the use of honey in wound management warrants further investigation.

Phenytoin

Phenytoin is a widely prescribed anticonvulsant used for the treatment of epilepsy. It has also been studied in the healing of pressure, venous stasis, and diabetic ulcers as well as traumatic wounds and burns in people [68]. Used topically, it seems to enhance healing without side effects, although the precise mechanism of action is unknown and controlled studies are limited [69]. It seems to be capable of enhancing gene expression of PDGF in macrophages and monocytes [69]. Furthermore, it may promote healing through stimulation of fibroblast proliferation and angiogenesis, facilitation of collagen deposition and maturation, decrease of collagenase activity, and antagonism of glucocorticoid activity [70]. Phenytoin is suggested to provide rapid pain relief, decrease wound exudate and bacterial contamination by acidifying the environment, and increase blood supply and granulation tissue production when compared with conventional saline dressings, with an overall favorable effect on healing [70,71]. It is applied as a powder to the clean debrided surface of the wound, which is then bandaged. To date, any effect of phenytoin on equine wound healing has not been studied.

Maggots (biosurgery)

Medicinal maggots secrete digestive enzymes that selectively dissolve necrotic tissue, disinfect the wound, actively promote granulation tissue production, and stimulate wound healing [72,73]. Sterile maggots are bred specifically for biosurgery; a single maggot is reported to consume up to 75 mg of necrotic tissue per day [74]. Studies have suggested that maggot therapy is significantly more effective than other conventional nonsurgical forms of therapy at debriding chronic pressure ulcers [72]. Favorable effects have also been reported with their use in soft tissue infections, chronic open wounds related to cancer therapy, and osteomyelitis [74]. Despite the fact that maggots require an optimal temperature, oxygen supply, and moist wound milieu, 91.2% of doctors and patients expressed a favorable opinion of biosurgery [74].

The exact mechanism by which maggots stimulate repair is unclear, but it may be that the maggots consume or inactivate inhibitory proteases and cytokines [72] or secrete stimulatory ones [75]. Furthermore, larval extracts and secretions seem to enhance fibroblast motility, thereby enhancing spread through the extracellular matrix and subsequent fibroplasia [73].

Disinfected fly larvae are applied to the wound at a density of five to eight per square centimeter. A hole matching the wound dimension cut into a self-adhesive hydrocolloid dressing prevents maggots from crawling onto the intact skin and absorbs wound secretions. The wound is then covered with a porous sheet, such as nylon stockinette, which is glued to the dressing to trap the maggots in the wound. The dressing is covered by a pad of light gauze and replaced every 4 to 8 hours to remove exudate. Maggots are applied for two 48-hour cycles each week, and the wounds are dressed with saline-moistened gauze dressings during the intervening periods. The combination of hydrogels and maggots has been investigated; however, it was found that different hydrogels had variable effects on larval development or mortality [74].

References

[1] Theoret CL. Growth factors in pathologic wound repair in horses. Compend Contin Educ Pract Vet 2001;23:479–82.

[2] Knottenbelt DC. Equine wound management: are there significant differences in healing at different sites on the body? Vet Dermatol 1997;8:273–90.

[3] Wilmink JM, Van Weeren PR, Stolk PW, et al. Differences in second intention wound healing between horses and ponies: histological aspects. Equine Vet J 1999;31:61–7.

[4] Wilmink JM, Veenman JN, van den Boom R, et al. Differences in polymorphonucleocyte function and local inflammatory response between horses and ponies. Equine Vet J 2003;35: 561–9.

[5] Wilmink JM, Stolk PW, Van Weeren PR, et al. Differences in second intention wound healing between horses and ponies: macroscopic aspects. Equine Vet J 1999;31: 53–60.

[6] Bacon Miller C, Wilson DA, Keegan KG, et al. Growth characteristic of fibroblasts isolated from the trunk and distal aspect of the limb of horses and ponies. Vet Surg 2000;29:1–7.
[7] Van den Boom R, Wilmink JM, Okane S, et al. Transforming growth factor-β levels during second-intention healing are related to the different course of wound contraction in horses and ponies. Wound Repair Regen 2002;10:188–94.
[8] Theoret CL, Barber SM, Moyana TN, et al. Expression of transforming growth factor β1, β3 and basic fibroblast growth factor in full-thickness skin wounds of equine limbs and thorax. Vet Surg 2001;30:269–77.
[9] Theoret CL, Barber SM, Moyana TN, et al. Preliminary observations on the expression of transforming growth factors β1 and β3 in equine full thickness skin wounds healing normally or with exuberant granulation tissue. Vet Surg 2002;31:266–73.
[10] Shah M, Foreman DM, Ferguson MWJ. Neutralization of TGF β1 and TGF β2 to cutaneous rat wounds reduces scarring. J Cell Sci 1995;108:985–1002.
[11] Jacobs KA, Leach DH, Fretz PB, et al. Comparative aspects of the healing of excisional wounds of the leg and body of horses. Vet Surg 1984;12:83–90.
[12] Swaim SF, Hinkle SH, Bradley DM. Wound contraction: basic and clinical factors. Compend Contin Educ Pract Vet 2001;23:20–34.
[13] Wilmink JM, Nederbrag H, van Weeren PR, et al. Differences in wound contraction between horses and ponies: the in vitro contraction capacity of fibroblasts. Equine Vet J 2001;33: 499–505.
[14] Schwartz AJ, Wilson DA, Keegan KG, et al. Factors regulating collagen synthesis and degradation during second-intention healing of wounds in the thoracic region and the distal aspect of the forelimb in horses. Am J Vet Res 2002;63:1564–70.
[15] Carter CA, Jolly DG, Worden CE, et al. Platelet rich plasma gel promotes differentiation and regeneration during equine wound healing. Exp Mol Pathol 2003;74:244–55.
[16] Ksander GA, Chu GH, McMuillin H, et al. Transforming growth factors-β1 and β2 enhance connective tissue formation in animal models of dermal wound healing by secondary intent. Ann NY Acad Sci 1990;593:135–7.
[17] Robson MC, Mustoe TA, Hunt TK. The future of recombinant growth factors in wound healing. Am J Surg 1998;176:80–2.
[18] Ashcroft GS, Yang X, Glick AB, et al. Mice lacking Smad 3 show accelerated wound healing and an impaired local inflammatory response. Nat Cell Biol 1999;1:260–6.
[19] Steel CM, Robertson ID, Thomas J, et al. Effect of topical rh-TGF-β-1 on second intention wound healing in horses. Aust Vet J 1999;77:734–7.
[20] Choi BM, Kwak HJ, Jun CD, et al. Control of scarring in adult wounds using antisense transforming growth factor β1 oligodeoxynucleotides. Immunol Cell Biol 1996;74:144–50.
[21] De Martin I, Theoret CL. Spatial and temporal expression of types I and II receptors for transforming growth factor β in normal equine and dermal wounds. Vet Surg 2004;33:70–6.
[22] Harrison P, Cramer EM. Platelet α-granules. Blood Rev 1993;7:52–62.
[23] Sanchez AR, Sheridan PJ, Kupp LI. Is platelet-rich plasma the perfect enhancement factor? A current review. Int J Oral Maxillofac Implants 2003;18:93–103.
[24] Knighton DR, Ciresi K, Fiegel VD, et al. Stimulation of repair in chronic, nonhealing, cutaneous ulcers using platelet-derived wound healing formula. Surg Gynecol Obstet 1990; 170:56–60.
[25] Renz H, Gong JH, Schmidt A, et al. Release of tumour necrosis factor-α from macrophages: enhancement and suppression are dose-dependently regulated by prostaglandin E2 and cyclic nucleopeptides. J Immunol 1988;141:2388–93.
[26] Concannon MJ, Barrett BB, Adelstein EH, et al. The inhibition of fibroblast proliferation by a novel monokine: an in vitro and in vivo study. J Burn Care Rehabil 1993;14:141–7.
[27] Wilson DA, Adelstein EH, Keegan KG, et al. In vitro and in vivo effects of activated macrophage supernatant on distal limb wounds in ponies. Am J Vet Res 1996;57:1220–4.
[28] Dart AJ, Creis L, Jeffcott LB, et al. The effect of equine recombinant growth hormone on second intention wound healing in horses. Vet Surg 2002;31:314–9.

[29] Seyer-Hansen M, Andreassen TT, Oxlund H. Strength of colonic anastomoses and skin incisional wounds in old rats—influence by diabetes and growth hormone. Growth Horm IGF Res 1999;9:254–61.
[30] Thorey IS, Hinz B, Hoeflich A, et al. Transgenic mice reveal novel activities of growth hormone in wound repair, angiogenesis and myofibroblast differentiation. J Biol Chem 2004;279:2667–84.
[31] Wilmink JM, Stolk PWTh, van Weeren R, et al. The effectiveness of the haemodialysate Solcoseryl for second intention wound healing in horses and ponies. J Vet Med 2000;47: 311–8.
[32] Schreier T, Degen E, Baschong W. Fibroblast migration and proliferation during in vitro wound healing. Res Exp Med 1993;193:195–205.
[33] Spessato P, Dri P, Baschong W, et al. Effect of a protein-free dialysate from calf blood on human monocyte differentiation in vitro. Arzneimittelforschung 1993;43:747–51.
[34] Jochle W, Hamm D. Effects of topical treatment with Solcoseryl and its fraction 3 on wound healing after burns and surgical lesions in horses. In: May SR, Dogo G, editors. Care of the burn wound. Basel: Karger; 1983. p. 83–9.
[35] Liebich HG, Hamm W, Jochle W. Histological evaluation of wound healing in horses treated with the protein-free haemodialysate Solcoseryl and its hexosylceramide fraction. J Vet Med 1988;35:84–95.
[36] Marichy J, Eyraud J. The wound healing effect of Solcoseryl ointment in the treatment of children with burns. Acta Ther 1984;10:107–17.
[37] Lawrence CM, Matthews JNS, Cox NH. The effect of ketanserin on healing of fresh surgical wounds. Br J Dermatol 1995;132:580–6.
[38] Rooman RP, Janssen H. Ketanserin promotes wound healing: clinical and preclinical results. Prog Clin Biol Res 1991;365:115–28.
[39] Roelens P. Double-blind placebo-controlled study with topical 2% ketanserin ointment in the treatment of ulcers. Dermatologica 1989;178:98–102.
[40] Engelen M, Besche B, Lefay MP, et al. Effects of ketanserin on hypergranulation tissue formation, infection, and healing of equine lower limb wounds. Can Vet J 2004;45: 144–9.
[41] Swaim SF, Riddell KP, McGuire JA. Effects of topical medication on the healing of open pad wounds in dogs. J Am Anim Hosp Assoc 1992;28:1–4.
[42] Swaim SF. Advances in wound healing in small animal practice: current status and lines of development. Vet Dermatol 1997;8:249–57.
[43] Swaim SF, Bradley DM, Spano JS, et al. Evaluation of multipeptide-copper complex medications on open wound healing in dogs. J Am Anim Hosp Assoc 1993;29:519–25.
[44] Swaim SF. Emergency wound management. In: Proceedings of the Fifth International Veterinary Emergency Critical Care Symposium. 1996. p. 638–42.
[45] Swaim SF, Gillette RL. An update on wound medications and dressings. Compend Contin Educ Pract Vet 1998;20:1133–44.
[46] Silvetti AN. The antimicrobial effect of maltodextrin NF in the healing of chronic wounds and ulcers including pressure ulcers. In: Proceedings of the Symposium of Advances in Wound Care Medical and Research Forum into Wound Repair. 1995. p. 70.
[47] Thomas S, Hay P. Fluid handling properties of hydrogel dressings. Ostomy Wound Manage 1995;41:54–9.
[48] Liptak JM. An overview of topical management of wounds. Aust Vet J 1997;75:408–13.
[49] Blackford JT, Blackford LW, Adair HS. The use of antimicrobial glucocorticosteroid ointment on granulating lower leg wounds in horses. Proc Am Assoc Equine Pract 1991;37: 71–7.
[50] Bigbie RB, Schumacher J, Swaim SF, et al. Effects of amnion and live yeast cell derivative on second intention wound healing in horses. Am J Vet Res 1991;52:1376–82.
[51] Swaim SF, Hendersen RA. In: Small animal wound management. 2nd edition. Baltimore: Williams & Wilkins; 1997. p. 53–85.

[52] Lawrence WT. Clinical management of nonhealing wounds. In: Cohen IK, Diegelmann RF, Linblad WJ, editors. Wound healing: biochemical and clinical aspects. Philadelphia: WB Saunders; 1992. p. 541–61.
[53] Barber SM. Second intention wound healing in the horse: the effect of bandages and topical corticosteroids. Proc Am Assoc Equine Pract 1989;35:107–16.
[54] Atherton P. Aloe vera revisited. Br J Phytotherapy 1998;4:176–83.
[55] Heggars JP, Kucukelebi A, Listengarten D, et al. Beneficial effect of aloe on wound healing in an excisional wound model. J Altern Complement Med 1996;2:271–7.
[56] Gallagher J, Gray M. Is aloe vera effective for healing chronic wounds. J Wound Ostomy Contin Nurs 2002;30:68–71.
[57] Muller MJ, Hollyoak MA, Maoveni Z, et al. Retardation of wound healing by silver sulfadiazine is reversed by aloe vera and nystatin. Burns 2003;29:834–6.
[58] Knutson RA, Merbitz LA, Creekmore MA, et al. Use of sugar and povidone-iodine to enhance wound healing: five years experience. South Med J 1981;74:1329–35.
[59] Molan PC, Cooper RA. Honey and sugar as a dressing for wounds and ulcers. Trop Doct 2000;30:249–51.
[60] Moore OA, Smith LA, Campbell F, et al. Systematic review of honey as a wound dressing. BMC Complement Altern Med 2001;1:2–7.
[61] Kamat N. Use of sugar as a dressing for wounds and ulcers. Trop Doct 2000;3:1.
[62] Cooper RA, Molan PC, Harding KG. Antibacterial activity of honey against strains of Staphylococcus aureus from infected wounds. J R Soc Med 1999;92:283–5.
[63] Tonks AJ, Cooper RA, Jones KP, et al. Honey stimulates cytokine production from monocytes. Cytokine 2003;21:242–7.
[64] Matthews K, Binnington AG. Wound management using honey. Compend Contin Educ Pract Vet 2002;24:53–60.
[65] Molan PC. Potential of honey in the treatment of wounds and burns. Am J Clin Dermatol 2001;2:13–9.
[66] Allen KL, Molan PC, Reid GM. A survey of the antibacterial activity of some of New Zealand honeys. J Pharm Pharmacol 1991;43:817–22.
[67] Willix DJ, Molan PC, Harfoot CG. A comparison of the sensitivity of wound infecting species of bacteria to the antibacterial activity of Manuka honey and other honey. J Appl Bacteriol 1992;73:388–94.
[68] Muthukumarasamy MG, Sivakumar G, Manoharan G. Topical phenytoin in diabetic foot ulcers. Diabetes Care 1991;14:909–11.
[69] Talas G, Brown RA, McGrouther DA. Role of phenytoin in wound healing—a wound pharmacology perspective. Biochem Pharmacol 1999;57:1085–94.
[70] Carneiro PMR, Nyawawa ETM. Topical phenytoin versus eusol in the treatment of non-malignant chronic leg ulcers. East Afr Med J 2004;80:124–9.
[71] Pendse AK, Sharma A, Sodani A, et al. Topical phenytoin in wound healing. Int J Dermatol 1996;32:214–7.
[72] Sherman RA. Maggot versus conservative debridement therapy for the treatment of pressure ulcers. Wound Repair Regen 2002;10:208–15.
[73] Horobin AJ, Shakesheff KM, Woodrow S, et al. Maggots and wound healing: an investigation of the effects of secretions from Lucilia sericata larvae upon interactions between human dermal fibroblasts and extracellular matrix components. Br J Dermatol 2003;148:923–31.
[74] Wollina U, Kerte K, Herold C, et al. Biosurgery in wound healing—the renaissance of maggot therapy. J Eur Acad Dermatol Venereol 2000;14:285–91.
[75] Mumcouglu KY, Miller J, Ioffe-Upensky I, et al. The potential of maggots to secrete cytokines in vitro. In: Proceedings of the Fifth International Conference on Biotherapy, Wurzburg, Germany, 2000. p. 23.

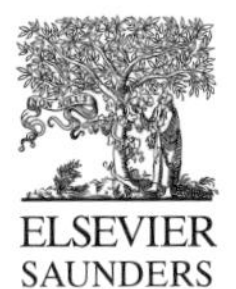
ELSEVIER
SAUNDERS

Vet Clin Equine 21 (2005) 91–104

VETERINARY
CLINICS
Equine Practice

Use of Dressings and Bandages in Equine Wound Management

Jorge H. Gomez, MVZ, MS*, R. Reid Hanson, DVM

Department of Clinical Sciences, College of Veterinary Medicine, Auburn University, 1500 Wire Road, Auburn, AL 36849, USA

Horses often suffer wounds in relation to their habitat, their use, and their natural instinct. Massive tissue loss, excessive skin tension, contamination, and infection make it difficult to treat some of these wounds by primary closure and first-intention healing. Wounds that heal by second intention are often managed with a dressing that covers the wound, providing protection from further trauma and contamination, absorbing excess exudate, and stimulating repair.

First- and second-intention repair of wounds on the limbs of horses is often delayed because of swelling, which results from chronic inflammation, and excessive movement at the site of the wound. Soft and rigid bandages are frequently used to control swelling, provide coaptation, and immobilize an area to minimize disruption of the fragile newly formed tissue. Bandages are usually composed of three layers: a primary or contact layer, often referred to as a "dressing"; a secondary or intermediate layer; and a tertiary or outer layer.

Dressings

Categories

The perfect dressing provides and maintains a moist environment and an adequate gaseous exchange at the wound surface that favors the proliferative phase of repair, particularly epithelialization. The dressing should also protect the wound from infection by acting as a bacterial shield and should provide thermal insulation. An ideal dressing occludes dead space, permits atraumatic removal of excessive exudate from the wound surface, and is easy to manipulate and nonantigenic [1].

* Corresponding author.
E-mail address: gomezjh@auburn.edu (J.H. Gomez).

doi:10.1016/j.cveq.2004.11.004 ***vetequine.theclinics.com***

Dressings can be classified as synthetic, semisynthetic, or biologic (Table 1). Synthetic dressings are composed of man-made fabric or plastic materials in the form of gauze, films, sprays, foams, and gels. Semisynthetic dressings are a combination of synthetic and biologic products. Biologic dressings are obtained from natural sources and include amnion, allografts, and xenografts as well as bioengineered tissues composed of various proteins (particularly collagen) or cultured wound-healing cells (primarily fibroblasts and keratinocytes). Biologic dressings often exert a beneficial effect on the wound in addition to providing protective covering.

According to their ability to adhere to a wound, dressings are also classified as adherent or nonadherent. According to their ability to permit passage of exudate and vapors, dressings are further classified as occlusive, semiocclusive, or nonocclusive (permeable). Occlusive dressings are impermeable to water vapor, fluid, and oxygen, thus providing an environment that favors proliferation of anaerobic bacteria. Because occlusive dressings encourage the formation of exuberant granulation tissue in equine wounds [2], it is recommended to restrict their use to the first 6 to 48 hours after

Table 1
Dressing categories

Dressings	Origin	Significant features
Fabric materials		
Release pad	Synthetic	Nonadherent
Telfa pad		Nonocclusive
Petrolatum-impregnated gauze		
Xerofoam	Synthetic	Nonadherent
Adaptic		Nonocclusive
Silver-impregnated gauze		
Silverlon	Synthetic	Low adherence
Acticoat		Antimicrobial properties
Hydrogels		
Solugel	Synthetic	Nonadherent Occlusive
Hydrocolloids		
Hydrofiber	Synthetic	Self-adherent Occlusive
Polyurethane		
Opsite	Synthetic	Nonadherent Semiocclusive
Calcium alginate		
Kaltostat	Semisynthetic	Adherent Nonocclusive
Processed collagen		
Vet BioSist	Biologic	Adherent Occlusive
Amnion	Biologic	Adherent Occlusive
Allograft	Biologic	Adherent Occlusive

injury. Conversely, semiocclusive dressings, which are permeable to oxygen and gases but not to fluids, provide a moist environment that favors wound epithelialization, which requires aerobic metabolism. Finally, nonocclusive dressings are permeable to fluid and oxygen in both directions.

Dressings may play an active role in wound healing. A dressing should be selected according to the condition of the wound and to the current phase of repair. The use of adherent dressings should be restricted to the initial inflammatory and debridement phases because they facilitate removal of debris and excess exudate but may damage fragile tissues formed in subsequent phases. Wide mesh fabrics accomplish this function and can be applied as a wet-to-dry dressing in wounds with thick exudate and as a dry-to-wet dressing in wounds with an abundant volume of fluid [3]. A gauze dressing pad and secondary gauze wrap impregnated with 0.2% polyhexamethylene biguanide antiseptic as an antimicrobial are now available to veterinarians. These dressings have been found effective in substantially reducing the amount of *Pseudomonas aeruginosa* and *Staphylococcus epidermidis* that penetrates bandages from topical contamination [4].

During the proliferative and remodeling phases of repair, nonadherent dressings are favored. They may have an absorptive layer that facilitates draining of exudate and a petrolatum layer that permits easy dressing changes without disrupting new epithelium.

Particular materials

Nonadherent dressings (Release pad; Johnson & Johnson, Arlington TX) or petrolatum-impregnated gauze (Xerofoam; Tyco International, Argyle, NY) is frequently used to cover wounds on horses. These nonocclusive dressings are most useful when applied during the proliferative phase of repair. They are available in different sizes and easy to remove once exudate has saturated their absorption capacity. A study demonstrated that the use of nonadherent gauze pads on limb wounds of horses led to significantly reduced healing times, production of wound exudate, and development of exuberant granulation tissue compared with that obtained with synthetic semiocclusive or fully occlusive dressings [2].

Silver chloride–coated dressings (Silverlon; Argentum Medical LLC, Lakemont, GA) are reputed to have a broad antibacterial spectrum [5] and are the dressing of choice in the treatment of burn wounds in human patients [6]. The dressings, available in pads and packing strips for deep wounds, are used from the inflammatory phase into the proliferative phase of repair. The authors have used Silverlon dressings in clinical equine practice, where they seem effective in controlling infection.

Hydrogels are three-dimensional, water-swollen, cross-linked structures that seem to promote healing by providing a biocompatible environment while increasing the moisture content of necrotic tissue and favoring collagenase production, thus facilitating debridement. They can also act as carriers for antimicrobial agents, growth factors, and other biologically active molecules [7]. Clinical trials in people suggest that hydrogels are superior to more conventional forms of dressings in some wounds [8]. Solugel is a commercially available mixture of 25% propylene glycol, 0.6% saline, and a gelling agent (Solugel; Johnson & Johnson). In an equine model, Solugel did not seem to have any beneficial effect on the healing of small full-thickness limb wounds [9]. Because hydrogels promote repair by enhancing debridement, it is possible that the model may have limited the opportunity to demonstrate the reported advantages of Solugel on more traumatically induced wounds. Indeed, clinical assessment has suggested some beneficial effect in naturally occurring wounds.

Hydrocolloid dressings, composed of a hydrophobic polymer bound to hydroactive particles (carboxymethylcellulose) that react with surface exudate or water vapor from the wound to form a semisolid gel, are occlusive and usually self-adherent [1]. These dressings provide a low oxygen content and moist environment for migration and proliferation of cells, particularly keratinocytes and are thus credited with facilitating epithelialization, at least in human beings. Unfortunately, a study performed in the horse showed no benefits in using hydrocolloid dressings in the management of limb wounds [2].

Calcium alginate dressings are made of a natural fiber derived from seaweed. They possess hemostatic properties and promote fibroplasias [10]. Wounds suitable to be covered with a calcium alginate dressing must produce enough fluid to transform the calcium alginate into a gel-like substance so as to avoid desiccation and excessive scarring [11].

Polyurethane dressings are highly conformable, nonadherent, and semiocclusive. The foam can be used to absorb exudate from the wound, thereby decreasing tissue maceration; simultaneously, they maintain a moist environment while, with the sheet form (Opsite; Smith & Nephew, Indianapolis, IN), exudating pools beneath the dressing. These dressings can be used in the early inflammatory phase as well as in the proliferative phase of repair because they do not adhere to the regenerating tissue and leave it undisturbed at bandage changes. In heavily exuding wounds, these dressings should be replaced frequently to increase comfort, whereas the frequency of dressing change decreases as healing progresses and less fluid is produced by the wound [12].

Silicone dressings are used as an effective alternative to intra-lesional corticosteroids, surgical excision, laser surgery, and cryosurgery for the management of excessive scarring in man. It appears that this type of synthetic, non-adherent, and fully occlusive dressing surpasses other modalities in decreasing the amount of scar tissue while exerting no negative side effects. In a recent study performed in wounds of the distal limbs of horses, the silicone dressing surpassed a conventional permeable, non-adherent dressing in preventing the formation of exuberant granulation tissue and improving tissue quality [13].

Collagen dressings are commercially available in the form of sheets, mats, powders, gels, sponges, and laminates [14]. The benefits of these dressings relate to enhanced inflammation and hemostasis [15] and the provision of a collagen scaffold thought to accelerate fibroplasia and epithelialization. Topically applied bovine collagen gel and a collagen membrane were found to yield equivocal results when experimentally evaluated in equine wounds [16,17].

A lyophilized, porcine-derived, small intestinal or vesical submucosa product is available for use as a primary layer in wound management (Vet Bio-Sist; Cook Veterinary Products, Bloomington, IN). It contains collagen (types I, III, IV, V, VI, and VII), fibronectin, hyaluronan, chondroitin sulfate A, heparan, and heparin sulfate as well as various growth-enhancing cytokines. The product acts as a scaffold and is gradually replaced by host tissue with characteristics of normal adjacent tissue. It has been used clinically [18] and experimentally [19] in horses, with no apparent advantages over a traditional synthetic nonadherent pad [19].

Amniotic membrane has been used for the treatment of large skin wounds and burns in human patients since the early 1900s. It is also useful as a temporary dressing in the preparation of wounds for skin grafts and as a bandage for skin graft donor sites. Amnion is essentially a layer of epithelial cells overlying a matrix containing a large amount of collagen and scattered fibroblasts [20]. Amnion adheres and conforms to the surface of the wound and reduces pain. Its occlusive nature prevents the loss of fluids, electrolytes, and proteins from the wound surface and helps to control bacterial contamination [21]. Studies in horses suggest that wounds of the distal limb treated with amnion heal significantly faster, with greater epithelialization and decreased formation of exuberant granulation tissue [22,23], although controversy exists [2].

Amnion should be separated from the chorionic portion of the placenta near the convergence of umbilical vessels shortly after parturition. It should then be lavaged and debrided of any gross contaminants before being placed in a sterile container containing 2% povidone-iodine and saline solution and refrigerated. Within 24 hours, the amnion can be cut into smaller segments, which are washed in 2% povidone-iodine and saline, then sterile physiologic saline, and finally 0.25% acetic acid. After the final wash, the dressing is frozen at −20°C in a 0.25% acetic acid solution indeterminately or refrigerated for a maximum of 4 to 6 weeks [22].

Cutaneous autografts are the most physiologically normal dressings available; however, their quantity is limited. Conversely, an allograft refers to a skin graft transferred between members of the same species and represents the temporary wound dressing of choice for burn wounds in human patients. Allografts are more effective than other biologic or synthetic dressings in promoting rapid wound healing and arresting infection. Indeed, although the cells within the allograft do not survive long term, the graft provides a biologic wound environment that prevents desiccation, induces angiogenesis, and enhances fibroplasia and epithelialization [24,25].

Allografts used to treat skin defects can be split thickness or full thickness. Split-thickness allografts are obtained from the ventral aspect of the abdomen of cadavers, whereas full-thickness allografts can be obtained from the cranial pectoral region of a standing and sedated horse. In the case of the latter, subcutaneous tissue should be removed before grafting to optimize vascularization of the allograft. Aseptic technique should be used in preparing and collecting the skin [26]. Graft fenestration yields many advantages, including the ability to expand the graft, and permits medications to be in contact with the wound as well as facilitating drainage and the avoidance of dead space separating the graft from the wound bed [27].

Allograft revascularization relies on the presence of healthy granulation tissue in the wound bed. The initial binding of the graft to the granulation bed is accomplished with fibrin [28] in a manner analogous to that occurring in autografts. Proliferating vessels from the recipient bed penetrate this fibrin layer within the first 48 hours after grafting to anastomose with graft vessels within 4 to 12 days [29]. Unlike xenografts, allografts seem to cause a minimal antigenic reaction even when applied repeatedly [25,30].

Adherence of the allograft to the wound determines the success of the procedure because it allows revascularization and precludes suppuration beneath the dressing. Moreover, adherence can reduce pain and limit infection, increasing acceptance of the graft and, consequently, optimizing the rate of healing [31]. Fibrin glue is used to improve adhesion between the graft and the granulation bed, especially in areas in which movement is difficult to avoid [32].

Harvested allografts can be used immediately or can be stored frozen, refrigerated, or glycerolized for later use [33]. Fresh skin has a better ability to survive after grafting than does skin that has been previously refrigerated, frozen, or dried [34]. Although cryopreservation is simpler and of superior longevity compared with refrigeration, the latter yields better results on grafting. Storage solutions should provide a physiologic concentration of electrolytes, nutrients, and buffers so as to ensure graft preservation, although air must also be present within the container to provide oxygen for cellular metabolism [35]. The graft can be refrigerated for 4 to 6 weeks.

Preparation of the wound bed and application of the allograft resemble what is described for conventional autografting. Allografts can be applied repeatedly in successive "crops" after the preceding graft has been absorbed, leaving a clean granulation base [36].

Tissue engineering has generated commercially available cultured epithelial allografts (Apligraft; Organogenesis, Canton, MA) that seem to provide a potent healing stimulus to the wound bed, possibly via the release of cytokines or other mediators that stimulate the formation of extracellular matrix [37,38]. According to this premise, it is suggested that cutaneous allografts may enhance wound healing by providing a skin substitute and by adding stimulatory cytokines to the wound environment [39].

The use of porcine cutaneous xenografts in the management of large wounds in human patients arose from the need for a substitute biologic dressing because of the short supply of cadaveric skin. Like allografts, xenografts decrease bacterial colonization of the wound through adherence and promotion of angiogenesis at the recipient bed. Clinical comparisons have nonetheless shown that porcine xenografts are inferior to allografts because they adhere less tightly, allowing higher bacterial counts in the wound, and cause a more intense immunologic response, often leading to rejection [30,40]. Equine wounds treated with porcine xenografts, however, did not form exuberant granulation tissue and healed faster than control wounds [41], suggesting some benefit in this form of therapy if allografts are not available.

Bandages

Bandages are usually made of natural or synthetic materials applied consecutively over the primary contact layer. Commonly, equine bandages are composed of a secondary layer and a tertiary layer that maintain the dressing in place. The main purpose of the secondary (intermediate) layer is to absorb deleterious agents (eg, serum, blood, exudate, bacteria, necrotic debris) from a wound. This layer should be thick enough to collect absorbed moisture, pad the wound against trauma, and splint it to prevent excessive motion. Materials used in the secondary layer are elastic gauze and cotton pads, which must be carefully applied to conform to the shape of the leg.

The tertiary layer is usually composed of materials stiffer than those used for the secondary layer. The purpose of this outer layer is to hold the previous layers in place, prevent contamination and trauma, provide coaptation to minimize swelling of the limb with a consequent increase in tension at the wound edges, and decrease the range of motion. This final layer should be porous yet waterproof. Elastic self-adhesive bandages (Vetrap; 3M Animal Care Products, St. Paul, MN) are frequently used as the tertiary layer. The tertiary layer must be applied with constant pressure that is gradually increased as the bandage is wrapped in a distal-to-proximal direction. The most proximal and distal aspects of the cotton pad (secondary layer) are initially left uncovered to avoid pressure points that may affect circulation within intact skin. As a final step, the proximal and distal ends are covered with an adhesive band that adheres to the outer layer and the skin. This is done to prevent penetration of foreign bodies (eg, shavings, dirt) between the skin and the bandage, which may cause skin sores and wound contamination.

Special bandaging techniques

Some anatomic particularities must be considered when applying bandages and dressings on horses. Wounds involving the superficial deep flexor tendon (SDFT), deep digital flexor tendon (DDFT), hoof and pastern area, carpus, hock, head, and trunk require special techniques to hold the bandages in place and to avoid long-term complications associated with bandaging.

Hoof and pastern

Wounds of the coronary band and the pastern are subjected to a significant amount of motion that favors proliferation of granulation tissue and consequent delays in repair. A cast applied with the horse sedated or under general anesthesia is the authors' preferred method to manage wounds of this area. A nonadherent synthetic dressing is applied over the wound and is secured with elastic gauze. A roll of brown gauze is used to wrap the hoof and the pastern. A double layer of stockinette is applied from the bottom of the hoof to 4 to 5 cm past the planned proximal end of the cast. At the proximal aspect of the pastern, a 2- to 3-cm wide band of orthopedic felt is applied to the circumference of the leg over the stockinette and maintained in place with adhesive tape. In the standing and sedated horse, three to four rolls of 7.5-cm fiberglass cast tape are applied starting from 1 cm below the proximal edge of the orthopedic felt and rolling down to the bottom of the foot, without covering the sole. After 3 to 4 minutes (enough time for the cast to harden), the hoof is picked up and two to three rolls of 10-cm fiberglass cast are applied to the bottom of the hoof to cover the sole and the hoof wall. Immediately after casting, an acrylic protector (Technovit; Jorgensen Laboratories, Loveland, CO) is applied to the bottom of the cast to minimize wear on weight bearing. The cast is left in place for 10 to 14 days; at that time, the wound is re-examined. If necessary, a new cast can be applied at that time.

Tendon and ligament injury

Injuries to the SDFT and the DDFT require special bandaging techniques to decrease tension on the wound edges and permit adequate healing. Lesions affecting more than 50% of the SDFT, DDFT, or both should be immobilized with the fetlock fixed in partial flexion. A fiberglass cast is applied from the bottom of the hoof to the proximal aspect of the metacarpus or metatarsus. A wedge of wood or a folded roll of fiberglass tape placed on the bottom of the hoof elevates the heel and improves weight bearing. For injuries affecting the hind limbs, a Kimzey splint (Kimzey, Woodland, CA) keeps the fetlock in partial flexion and avoids complications associated with the prolonged use of a cast, while enabling open wound management.

Carpus

Bandaging the carpus requires special care to avoid placing excessive pressure over the medial and lateral tuberosities of the radius or over the accessory carpal bone, because these prominent and superficial structures are predisposed to the development of pressure sores. An adhesive primary dressing is preferred. A cotton pad may be used as a secondary layer, from which a plug of cotton is removed over the prominence to minimize pressure. An adhesive bandage applied in a figure-eight fashion, starting from proximal to distal and avoiding the prominence, is recommended as a tertiary layer. Alternatively, a "donut" of stockinette can be used over the secondary layer to encircle the prominence and thereby redistribute pressure from the tertiary layer to the periphery of the bony prominence, which is much less prone to pressure necrosis.

Hock

One of the most challenging areas to bandage is the hock. The conformation and the combination of forces that allow flexion and extension (ie, reciprocal apparatus) impose some important considerations when applying a bandage to this area. Horses are more reluctant to accept a contraption in this region and frequently disrupt the bandages because of exaggerated flexion. The primary and secondary layers should be applied, avoiding excessive pressure over the point of the hock (calcaneal tuberosity), using the same techniques as described for the carpus. The tertiary layer, a figure-eight bandage, is applied starting with complete loops on the distal aspect of the tibia and continuing down with figure-eight loops below and above the point of the hock (Fig. 1). The authors use a thick cotton bandage as a secondary layer on the distal aspect of the leg from the coronary band to the most proximal aspect of the metatarsus. This helps to prevent slippage of the hock bandage and, by decreasing the range of motion of the fetlock, restricts movement. Applying a rigid bandage or splint to the distal limb with the fetlock in partial flexion significantly decreases the range of motion of the hock, thereby increasing survival time of the bandage and allowing optimal wound healing.

Head wounds

It is sometimes necessary to cover wounds of the head. A custom-made stockinette with perforations for the ears and eyes is suitable for this purpose. To cover wounds that require some pressure (ie, enucleation, sinus flap), a figure-eight self-adhesive bandage is wrapped above and below the eyes and around the circumference of the nasal bones and the mandible (Fig. 2). Horses are usually tolerant of this type of bandage.

Trunk wounds

Stent or "tie over" bandages are suitable to cover wounds of the trunk. This is achieved by placing loops of heavy nonabsorbable suture material (no. 1 or 2) through the skin 3 cm apart and parallel to the wound edges. The bandage

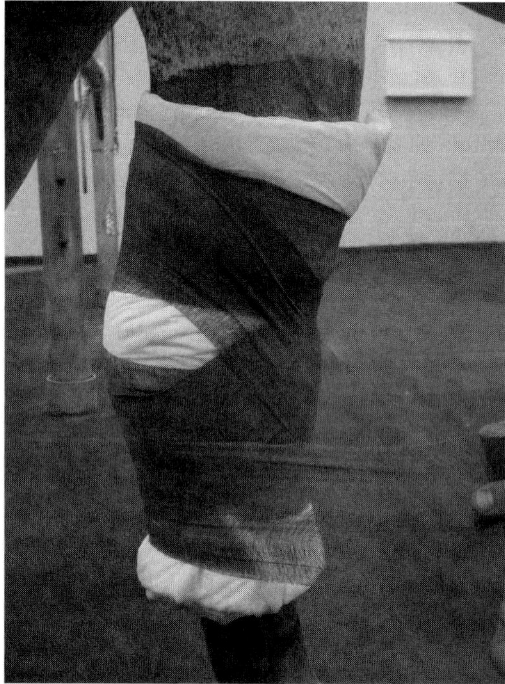

Fig. 1. Bandage of the hock.

that is applied to cover the wound is maintained in place by lacing umbilical tape through the previously created suture loops. The bandage can be changed as frequently as necessary. This type of bandage prevents retraction of the wound edges, keeps the wound free of contaminants, and provides a moist environment that is conducive to healing.

Casts and splints

Casts and splints are frequently used to immobilize wounds on the distal aspect of the limb. Wounds involving extensor or flexor tendons; wounds over the fetlock, carpal, and tarsal joints; and lacerations over the pastern, coronary band, and heel bulbs often heal more quickly and with less scarring when the leg is immobilized.

Fiberglass is preferred over plaster of Paris because of its greater strength and durability. Casts of various lengths are used according to the location of the injury. A hoof cast that covers only the hoof and the pastern is recommended for wounds involving the hoof wall, coronary band, heel bulbs, or pastern region. For wounds involving the fetlock or the extensor and flexor tendons, application of a half-limb cast that extends from the bottom of the hoof to the most proximal aspect of the metacarpus or

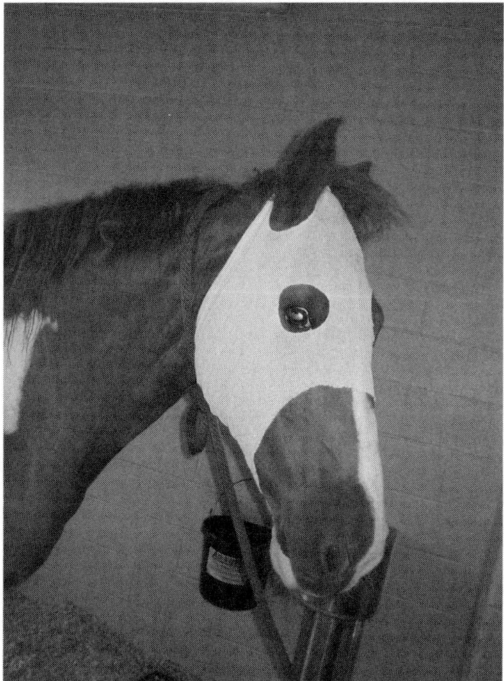

Fig. 2. Stockinette used to cover a wound on the head of a horse.

metatarsus is recommended. Tube casts from the most distal aspect of the metacarpus or tarsus to the most proximal aspect of the radius or tibia are suitable to manage wounds over the carpal and tarsal joints.

Bandage casts are useful to manage wounds that need long-term immobilization yet frequent monitoring. To construct a bandage cast,

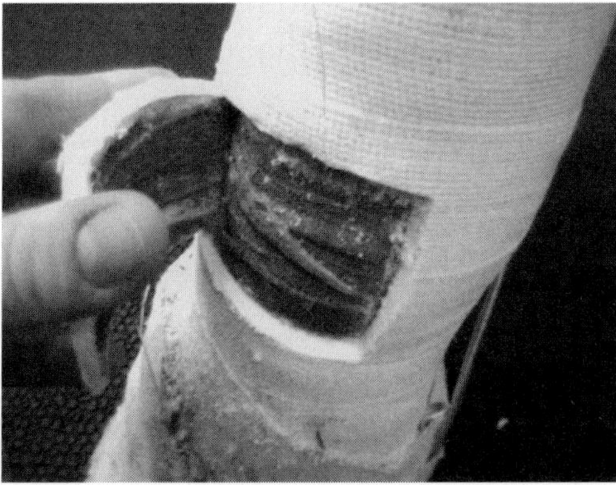

Fig. 3. Bandage cast. A window was created to monitor a wound on the dorsal aspect of the fetlock.

primary, secondary, and tertiary layers are applied over the wound. Several rolls of fiberglass cast material are then applied over the bandage to increase its strength and ensure immobilization (Fig. 3). This final coat can then be split into halves for wound treatment and dressing changes. After rebandaging the wound, the two parts of the cast are reapplied and fixed with commercially available elastic tape.

Alternatively, distal limb immobilization to protect lacerations of the extensor and flexor tendons can be provided with custom-made polyvinyl chloride (PVC) splints or with a commercially available metal splint (Kimzey). These splints allow frequent monitoring of the wound and dressing changes while providing adequate immobilization of the involved tissues.

Cast sores are a common complication of fiberglass casts. An increase in lameness, fever, poor appetite, and low fecal output may signal the presence of cast sores, and the cause should be investigated immediately.

References

[1] Purna SK, Babu M. Collagen based dressings—a review. Burns 2000;26:54–62.

[2] Howard RD, Stashak TS, Baxter GM. Evaluation of occlusive dressings for management of full-thickness excisional wounds on the distal portion of the limbs of horses. Am J Vet Res 1993;54:2150–4.

[3] Stashak TS. Update—wound dressings and other topical wound agents: parts I and II. In: Proceedings of the North American Veterinary Conference. 2003. O'Fallon(IL): Veterinary Software Publishing, Inc. p. 238–9.

[4] Swaim SF, Bohling MW. Mise au point sur les récents développements en gestion des plaies chez les animaux de compagnie. Med Vet QC 2003;33:99–103.

[5] Adams AP, Santschi EM, Mellencamp MA. Antibacterial properties of a silver chloride-coated nylon wound dressing. Vet Surg 1999;28:219–25.

[6] Holder IA, Durkee P, Supp AP, et al. Assessment of silver-coated barrier dressing for potential use with skin grafts on excised burns. Burns 2003;29:445–8.

[7] Thomas S, Hay P. Fluid handling properties of hydrogel dressings. Ostomy Wound Manage 1995;41:54–9.

[8] Smith RA, Rushbourne J. The use of Solugel™ in the closure of wounds by secondary intention. Primary Intention 1994;1:14–7.

[9] Dart AJ, Creis L, Jeffcott B, et al. Effects of a 25% propylene glycol hydrogel (Solugel) on second intention wound healing in horses. Vet Surg 2002;31:309–13.

[10] Swaim SF, Gillete RL. An update on wound medication and dressings. Compend Contin Educ Pract Vet 1998;20:1133–44.

[11] Limova M. Evaluation of two calcium alginate dressings in the management of venous ulcers. Ostomy Wound Manage 2003;49(9):26–33.

[12] Horch RE, Stark B. Comparison of the effect of a collagen dressing and a polyurethane dressing on the healing of split thickness skin graft (STSG) donor sites. Scand J Plast Reconstr Hand Surg 1998;32:407–13.

[13] Ducharme-Desjarlais M, Céleste CJ, Lepault É, et al. Effect of a silicone-containing dressing on exuberant granulation tissue formation and wound repair in the horse. Am J Vet Res 2005, in press.

[14] Balasubramani M, Ravi T, Babu M. Skin substitutes: a review. Burns 2001;27:534–44.

[15] Shettigar UR, Jagannathan R, Natarajan R. Collagen film for burn dressings reconstituted from animal intestines. Artif Organs 1982;6:256–60.
[16] Yvorchuk-St. Jean K, Gaughan E, St. Jean G, et al. Evaluation of a porous bovine collagen membrane bandage for management of wounds in horses. Am J Vet Res 1995;56:1663–7.
[17] Bertone A, Sullins KE, Stashak TS, et al. Effect of wound location and the use of topical collagen gel on exuberant granulation tissue formation and wound healing in the horse and pony. Am J Vet Res 1985;46:1438–44.
[18] Brehm W, Wampfler B, Imhof A, et al. Experiences with the application of VET BIO SIS T in equids. In: Vezzoni A, Houlton J, Schramme M, editors. Proceedings of the 10th Annual European Society of Veterinary Orthopaedics and Traumatology Congress, Munich, 2000. p. 130.
[19] Gomez JH, Schumacher J, Lauten SD, et al. Effects of 3 biologic dressings on healing of cutaneous wounds on the limbs of horses. Can J Vet Res 2004;68:49–55.
[20] Trelford J, Trelford M. The amnion in surgery, past and present. Am J Obstet Gynecol 1979; 137:833–45.
[21] Walker A, Cooney D, Allen J. Use of fresh amnion as a burn dressing. J Pediatr Surg 1977; 12:391–5.
[22] Bigbie R, Schumacher J, Swaim S, et al. Effects of amnion and live yeast cell derivative on second-intention healing in horses. Am J Vet Res 1991;52:1376–82.
[23] Goodrich L, Moll D, Crisman M, et al. Comparison of equine amnion and a nonadherent wound dressing material for bandaging pinch-grafted wounds in ponies. Am J Vet Res 2000; 61:326–9.
[24] Qaryoute S, Mirdad I, Abu Hamail A. Usage of autograft and allograft skin in treatment of burns in children. Burns 2001;27:599–602.
[25] Moerman E, Middelkoop E, Mackie D, et al. The temporary use of allograft for complicated wounds in plastic surgery. Burns 2002;28(Suppl):S13–5.
[26] Gresham R, Perry V, Thompson V. Practical methods of short-term storage of homografts. Arch Surg 1963;87:417–21.
[27] Druecke D, Streintraeser L, Homman H, et al. Current indications for glycerol-preserved allografts in the treatment of burn injuries. Burns 2002;28:26–30.
[28] Burlesson R, Eiseman B. Nature of the bond between partial-thickness skin and wound granulations. Surgery 1972;72:315–22.
[29] Schumacher J, Hanselka D. Skin grafting of the horse. Vet Clin North Am Equine Pract 1989;5:591–614.
[30] May SR. The effects of biological wound dressings on the healing process. Clin Mater 1991;8: 243–9.
[31] Tavis MJ, Thornton JW, Harney JH, et al. Graft adherence to de-epithelialized surfaces. Ann Surg 1976;184:594–600.
[32] Dhennin Ch, Desbois I, Yassine A, et al. Utilization of glycerolized skin allografts in severe burns. Burns 2002;28:21–5.
[33] Bravo D, Rigley T, Gibran N, et al. Effect of storage and preservation methods on viability in transplantable human skin allografts. Burns 2000;26:367–78.
[34] Heslop B, Shaw J. Early vascularization of syngeneic, allogeneic and xenogeneic skin grafts. Aust NZ J Surg 1986;56:357–62.
[35] Hurst L, Brown D, Murray KA, et al. Prolonged life and improved quality for stored skin grafts. Plast Reconstr Surg 1984;73:105–9.
[36] Brown J, Fryer M, Zaydon T. A skin bank for postmortem homografts. Surg Gynecol Obstet 1955;101:401–12.
[37] Kirsner R, Falanga V, Eaglstein W. The biology of skin grafts as pharmacologic agents. Arch Dermatol 1993;129:481–3.
[38] Oshima H, Inoue H, Matzukasi K, et al. Permanent restoration of human skin treated with cultured epithelium grafting—wound healing by stem cell based tissue engineering. Hum Cell 2002;15:118–28.

[39] Spence RJ, Wong L. The enhancement of wound healing with human skin allografts. Surg Clin N Am 1977;77:731–45.

[40] Fiala T, Lee W, Hong H, et al. Bacterial clearance capability of living skin equivalent, living dermal equivalent, saline dressing, and xenograft dressing in the rabbit. Ann Plast Surg 1993; 30:516–9.

[41] Diehl M, Ersek R. Porcine xenografts for treatment of skin defects in horses. J Am Vet Med Assoc 1980;177:625–8.

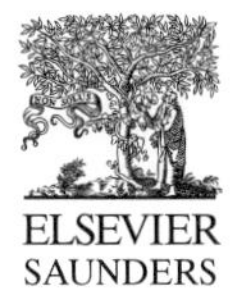

ELSEVIER
SAUNDERS

Vet Clin Equine 21 (2005) 105–123

VETERINARY
CLINICS
Equine Practice

Management of Burn Injuries in the Horse

R. Reid Hanson, DVM

Department of Clinical Sciences, College of Veterinary Medicine, J.T. Vaughan Hall, Auburn University, Auburn, AL 36849, USA

Burns are uncommon in horses, with most occurring as a result of barn fires. Thermal injuries may also result from contact with hot solutions, electrocution or lightening strike, friction (eg, rope burns), abrasions, radiation therapy, and chemicals (eg, improperly used topical drugs, maliciously applied caustic agents) [1,2].

Most burns are superficial, easily managed, and inexpensive to treat and heal in a short time. Serious burns, however, can result in rapid severe burn shock or hypovolemia with associated cardiovascular changes. Smoke inhalation and corneal ulceration also are of great concern [1,2]. Management of severe and extensive burns is difficult, expensive, and time-consuming. The large surface area of the burn dramatically increases the potential for loss of fluids, electrolytes, and calories. Burns covering up to 50% or more of the body are usually fatal, although the depth of the burn also influences mortality. Massive wound infection is almost impossible to prevent because of the difficulty of maintaining a sterile wound environment. Long-term care is required to prevent continued trauma, because burn wounds are often pruritic and self-mutilation is common. Burned horses are frequently disfigured, preventing them from returning to full function. Therefore, before treatment, the patient must be carefully examined, with particular attention paid to cardiovascular function, pulmonary status, ocular lesions, and the extent and severity of the burns. The cost of treatment as well as the prognosis should be thoroughly discussed with the owner [1–4].

Classification of burns

Burns are classified by the depth of the injury [1–3]. First-degree burns involve only the most superficial layers of the epidermis. These burns are

E-mail address: hansorr@auburn.edu

0749-0739/05/$ - see front matter
doi:10.1016/j.cveq.2004.11.006 *vetequine.theclinics.com*

painful and characterized by erythema, edema, and desquamation of the superficial layers of the skin. The germinal layer of the epidermis is spared, and the burns heal without complication (Fig. 1) [4]. Second-degree burns involve the epidermis and can be superficial or deep. Superficial second-degree burns involve the stratum corneum, stratum granulosum, and a few cells of the basal layer. Tactile and pain receptors remain intact. Because the basal layers remain relatively uninjured, superficial second-degree burns heal rapidly with minimal scarring within 14 to 17 days [5]. Deep second-degree burns involve all layers of the epidermis, including the basal layers. These burns are characterized by erythema and edema at the epidermal-dermal junction, necrosis of the epidermis, accumulation of white blood cells at the basal layer of the burn, eschar (slough produced by a thermal burn) formation, and minimal pain (Fig. 2) [1,3]. The only germinal cells spared are those within the ducts of the sweat glands and hair follicles. Deep second-degree wounds may heal spontaneously in 3 to 4 weeks if care is taken to prevent further dermal ischemia, which may lead to full-thickness

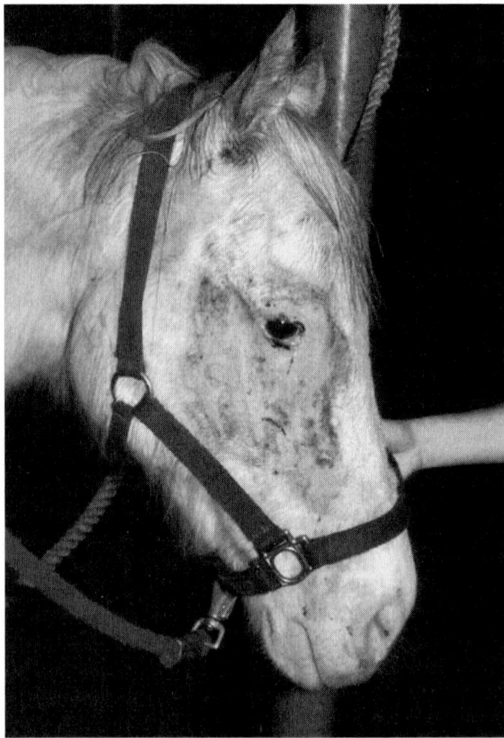

Fig. 1. First-degree burn of the right facial and periocular area. This type of burn involves only the most superficial layers of the epidermis. These burns are painful and characterized by erythema, edema, and desquamation of the superficial layers of the skin. The germinal layer of the epidermis is spared, and the burns heal without complication.

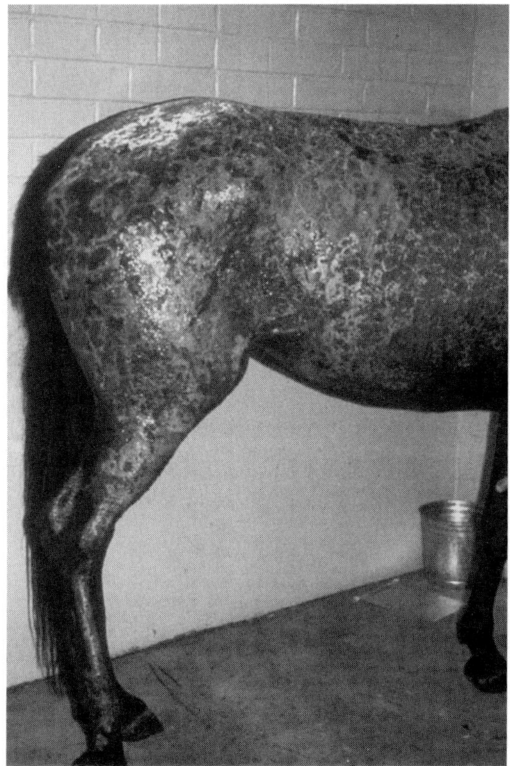

Fig. 2. Deep second-degree burn of the right dorsum and right hind limb. Deep second-degree wounds may heal spontaneously in 3 to 4 weeks if care is taken to prevent further dermal ischemia, which may lead to full-thickness necrosis.

necrosis. In general, deep second-degree wounds, unless grafted, heal with extensive scarring [6]. Third-degree burns are characterized by loss of the epidermal and dermal components, including the adnexa. The wounds range in color from white to black (Fig. 3). There is fluid loss and a marked cellular response at the margins and deeper tissue, eschar formation, lack of pain, shock, wound infection, and possible bacteremia and septicemia. Healing is by means of contraction and epithelialization from the wound margins or acceptance of an autograft. These burns are frequently complicated by infection. Fourth-degree burns involve all the skin and underlying muscle, bone, ligaments, fat, and fascia (Fig. 4) [7].

Mechanism of burn injury

The extent of tissue destruction is dependent on the temperature of the heat source, duration of exposure, blood supply, and local environment of the wound [7]. At the initial injury, there are three levels of injury: the

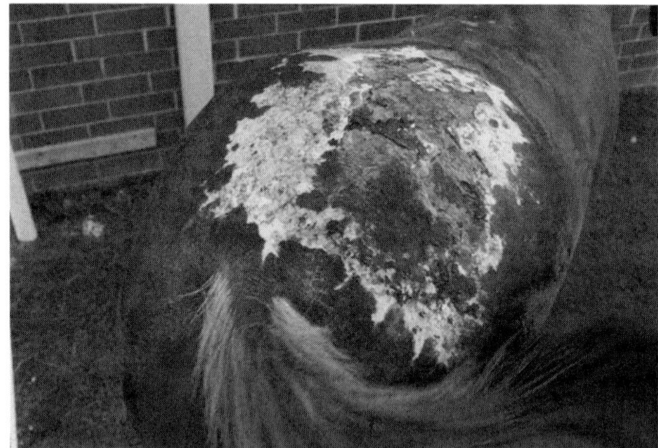

Fig. 3. Third-degree burn of the dorsal gluteal region incurred during a barn fire as a result of hot asphalt roof shingles falling on the horse. The central burn area is surrounded by deep and superficial second-degree burns.

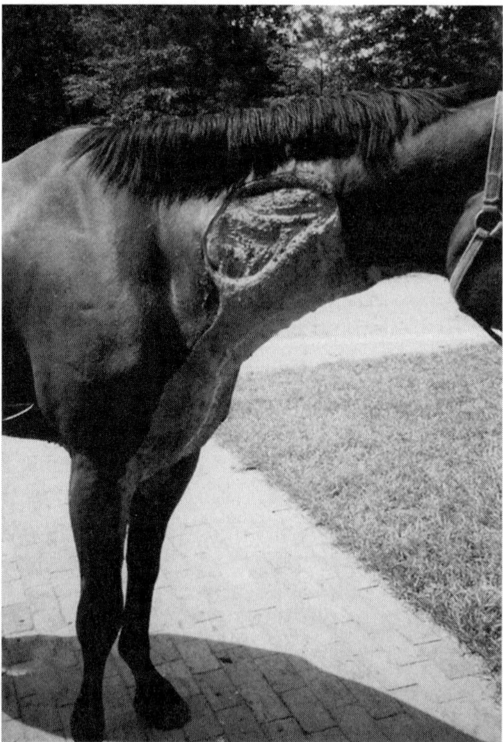

Fig. 4. Fourth-degree burn of the right cervical neck region and pectoral area. Fourth-degree burns involve all layers of the skin as well as underlying muscle, bone, ligaments, fat, and fascia.

central zone of coagulation, the intermediate zone of vascular stasis, and the outer zone of hyperemia. The central zone of coagulation corresponds to the area that was closest to the heat source. At temperatures higher than 45°C, protein denaturation exceeds the capacity for cellular repair and cell death ensues [6]. The severity of injury decreases radially from this center as heat is dissipated (Fig. 5). Adjacent to the coagulation core is an intermediate zone of vascular stasis caused as dermal vessels thrombose during the initial 24 hours after injury. The damaged cells in this zone survive only under ideal circumstances. The use of heparin and thromboxane inhibitors may moderate the amount of tissue damage in this zone [8–10]. The outer region is the zone of hyperemia; the epidermis is lost, but the dermis remains intact. Cellular recovery in this area is rapid. In human beings, the total body surface area affected and the depth of the injury correlate highly with the degree of morbidity and mortality associated with thermal injury [6].

Pathophysiology of burn injury

After severe burns, there is a dramatic cardiovascular effect termed *burn shock*, which resembles hypovolemic shock. A dramatic increase in local and systemic capillary permeability occurs as a result of heat and the release of cytokines, prostaglandins, nitric oxide, vasoactive leukotrienes, serotonin, histamine, and oxygen radicals [11]. Local tissue damage results from massive protein coagulation and cellular death. In the immediate area of the burn, arteries and venules constrict and capillary beds dilate. Capillary wall permeability is increased in response to vasoactive amines released as a result of tissue damage and inflammation. These vascular responses result in fluid, protein, and inflammatory cells accumulating in the wound. There is vascular sludging, thrombosis, and dermal ischemia, resulting in further

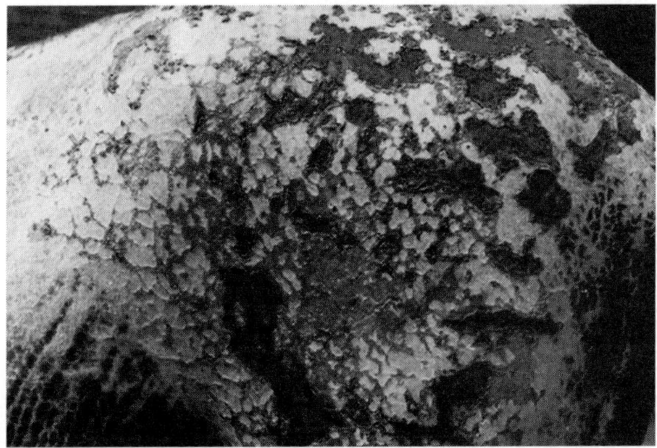

Fig. 5. Deep second-degree burn of the right hind limb. The central burn area is surrounded by less severe skin burns, illustrating the dissipating radiating effects of the heat and damage to the skin.

tissue damage. Tissue ischemia continues for 24 to 48 hours after injury and is caused by the local release of thromboxane A_2. Before any change in blood or plasma volume, there is a dramatic drop in cardiac output attributable to circulating levels of myocardial depressant factors [12]. Fluid loss into the extravascular space leads to an acute reduction in blood volume. With reductions in blood volume and cardiac output, peripheral and pulmonary vascular resistance increases, peripheral tissue perfusion decreases, and organ failure ensues [11,12].

The extent of fluid loss parallels the severity of the burn. Fluid losses result in increased heat loss from evaporation and an increased metabolic rate. The heat loss is in part responsible for the increased oxygen consumption and metabolic rate as the horse tries to generate heat. Depletion of fat stores and some endogenous protein supplies are two means by which metabolic compensation is achieved. In turn, this hypermetabolic rate leads to weight loss, a negative nitrogen balance, and delayed wound healing. Thus, the nutritional condition of the patient before injury is a prime prognostic consideration.

In burn injury, the vascular compartment remains permeable to proteins up to 15 nm in size, including albumin [13,14]. With moderate thermal injury, up to two times the total plasma albumin pool can be lost from the vascular compartment [15]. Loss occurs through the open wound and into the vascular space. Protein concentration can reach 3 g/dL in the extracellular fluid, which is sufficient to cause large fluid shifts because of osmotic pressure differences [16,17]. The resultant burn edema is clinically recognized within 60 minutes of injury [18].

Accompanying the fluid and protein shifts are electrolyte disturbances. Immediately after a burn, hyperkalemia may occur because of cellular disruption and potassium leakage [19]. When counterbalanced by increased mineralocorticoid secretion, the urinary sodium/potassium ratio is reversed and a subsequent potassium deficit may develop 3 to 5 days after injury [20]. Simultaneously, hypernatremia may result as sodium is reabsorbed after restoration of vascular membranes [21]. During replacement therapy, frequent determinations of protein concentrations, circulatory volume, and electrolyte concentrations are indicated [19–21].

Anemia is not usually a significant concern immediately after a burn. Anemia can, however, become a progressive problem in patients with burns exceeding 30% of the total body surface area [22]. An early anemia resulting from red cell hemolysis and splenic sequestration may be present but is often masked by hemoconcentration. Initial anemia is caused by the immediate destruction of red blood cells by heat and wound hemorrhage [23]. Subsequently, erythrocyte loss occurs from intravascular and extravascular removal of damaged cells as well as during eschar removal [21]. Thrombocytopenia may result from platelet aggregation on damaged capillary endothelium. If damage is extensive, a hemorrhagic diathesis may result from exhaustion of clotting factors.

Immunoglobulin levels in the serum drop, with the lowest values at 2 days after a burn. Serious defects in neutrophil function, such as an inefficient chemotaxis, and impaired phagocytic rate and bactericidal capacity have also been observed in severely burned horses. In addition to destruction of the mechanical barrier of the skin, decreased neutrophil chemotaxis and bactericidal properties, defective fibronectin, and complement opsonization, a decrease in IgG concentration often results. Their combined effect results in a compromised host that is prone to infection [24,25].

Metabolic rate increases in a curvilinear fashion proportional to the size of the thermal injury exceeding 10% of the total body surface area. This causes an increase in body core temperature from 1°C to 2°C and increases in oxygen consumption, fat degradation, and protein and glucose use [26–28]. Caloric expenditure and protein catabolism are greater in burn injury than in any other physiologic stress state. In patients with burns exceeding 30% of the total body surface area, energy expenditure doubles and fuel substrates are metabolized at two to three times the normal rate [29]. To avoid the rapid depletion of skeletal muscle, delayed wound healing, and impaired cellular defense mechanisms, caloric and protein intakes must be adjusted to maintain body weight [26,29,30]. Environmental temperatures should be kept between 28°C and 33°C to minimize the metabolic expenditure required to maintain the elevated core temperatures [26,30,31].

Pathophysiology of inhalation injury

Inhalation injury is a common sequela of closed-space fires and develops through three mechanisms: direct thermal injury, carbon monoxide poisoning, and chemical insult. Direct thermal injury causes edema and obstruction of the upper airway, but because of the efficient heat exchange capacity of the nasopharynx and oropharynx, superheated air is cooled before entering the lower respiratory tract [32].

Carbon monoxide interferes with oxygen delivery in several ways [33]. It has a 230 to 270 times greater affinity for oxygen, thus shifting the oxygen-hemoglobin curve to the left. The resultant carboxyhemoglobin is incapable of oxygen transport. Carbon monoxide also binds to myoglobin, thereby impairing oxygen transport to muscles [34,35]. Carbon monoxide is excreted by the lungs at a rate related to ambient oxygen tensions. In room air, carbon monoxide has a half-life of 3 to 4 hours. An increase in oxygen tension promotes the dissociation of carbon monoxide and hemoglobin; thus, 100% oxygen therapy reduces the half-life to 30 to 40 minutes. Hyperbaric oxygen therapy at 2.5 atm further decreases the half-life to 22 minutes [36].

Chemical insult depends on the material that was burned [32,37]. Combustion products, such as hydrogen cyanide, hydrochloric acid, phosgene, sulfuric acid, and aldehydes, may induce severe tracheobronchitis when combined with the moisture in the airways. Initially, only erythema may be present, but chemical injury continues as long as chemical-covered carbon particles remain attached to the airway mucosa, with particle size determining where damage occurs within the respiratory tree (Fig. 6). Combustion products cause increased pulmonary artery pressure, peribronchial edema, mucosal sloughing, bronchoconstriction, decreased mucociliary transport and bacterial clearance, and altered surfactant action [35,38]. Subsequently, significant pulmonary ventilation/perfusion mismatches may develop [34,39].

Pulmonary infection is a potential complication in every smoke inhalation patient. Alveolar macrophages, as the primary cellular defense in the lung, are increased in number after the injury but have decreased phagocytic and bactericidal functions [40–42]. Susceptibility to pulmonary infection, pulmonary edema, and lung dysfunction increases greatly in patients that also have cutaneous thermal injury. The interrelation between inhalation and surface burns is unclear but seems to be additive [40–42]. Major cutaneous burns alone have been reported to cause pulmonary dysfunction in as many as 25% of patients, whereas inhalation injury increases the morbidity and mortality rates for a given cutaneous thermal injury [34,38,43,44].

Physical examination findings

Because heat is slow to dissipate from burn wounds, it is often difficult to evaluate the amount of tissue damage accurately in the early phase of injury. The extent of the burn depends on the size of the area exposed, whereas the

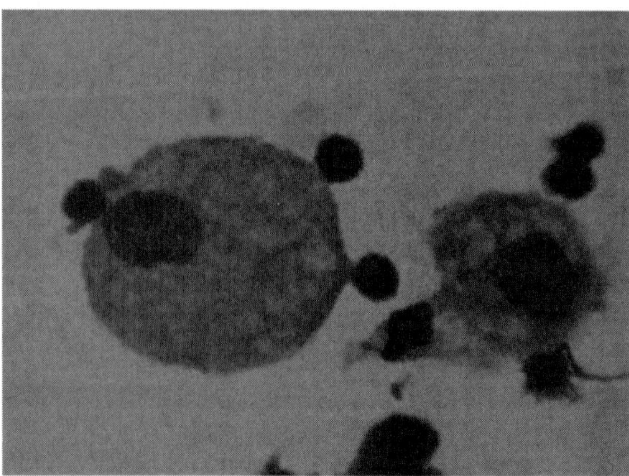

Fig. 6. Carbon particles associated with alveolar macrophages in the bronchoalveolar lavage as a result of inhalation smoke injury. Chemical injury continues as long as chemical-covered carbon particles remain attached to the airway mucosa, with the size of the particles determining where damage occurs within the respiratory tree.

severity relates to the maximum temperature the tissue attains and the duration of overheating. This explains why skin injury often extends beyond the original burn [45].

A complete physical examination should be performed on any burned animal before the wound is evaluated. Only after the patient's condition is stable should the burn wound be assessed. Physical criteria used to evaluate burns include erythema, edema and pain; blister formation; eschar formation; presence of infection; body temperature; and cardiovascular status [45]. In general, erythema, edema, and pain are favorable signs because they indicate that some tissue is viable, although pain is not a reliable indicator for determining wound depth [45]. Often, time must elapse to allow further tissue changes so that an accurate evaluation of burn severity can be made (Fig. 7).

Burns are most commonly seen on the back and face. Erythema, pain, vesicles, and singed hair are present depending on the extent of the injury. Increases in heart and respiratory rates are present in association with abnormal discoloration of mucous membranes. The burned horse may have blepharospasm, epiphora, or both, which signify corneal damage. Coughing may indicate smoke inhalation, whereas a fever signals or confirms a systemic response.

The percentage of total body surface area involved usually correlates with mortality, whereas the depth of the burn determines morbidity [16]. The rule of nine is used commonly in human beings to evaluate the total body surface area involved. Using this method, an approximate extent of the burn can be used to estimate the prognosis. Each forelimb represents 9%, each hind limb represents 18%, the head with the neck represents 9%, and the thorax and abdomen each represent 18% of body surface area [4]. Special attention should be taken to identify injury to major vessels of the lower limbs and the presence of eye, perineal, tendon sheath, and joint involvement. Initial laboratory data, including complete blood cell count, clotting profile, serum chemistry, urinalysis, arterial blood gas, carbon monoxide concentration, chest radiograph, and bronchoalveolar lavage, are helpful in the initial evaluation [7].

Laboratory findings may reveal a low total protein with anemia that may be severe and steadily progressive. Hemoglobinuria may be present. Hyperkalemia may be present initially, but hypokalemia is more likely later in the course of the condition and may often be associated with fluid therapy.

Although specific guidelines do not exist for burned large animals, euthanasia should be recommended for animals with deep partial-thickness to full-thickness burns involving 30% to 50% of the total body surface area [20,46]. The availability of adequate treatment facilities, cost of treatment, and pain experienced by the horse during long-term care should be considered when deciding whether or not to treat. Because convalescence may take up to 2 years, euthanasia is often an acceptable alternative [47].

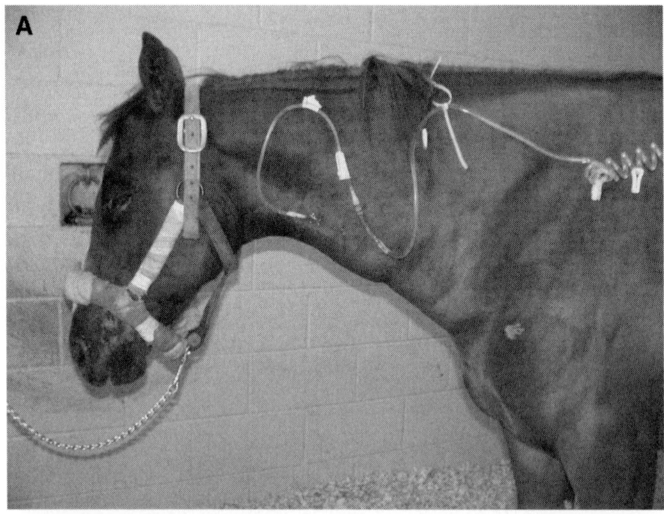

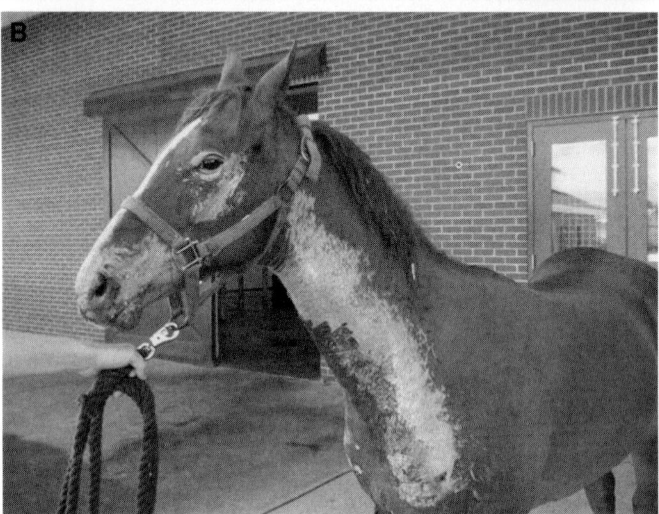

Fig. 7. (*A*) Severe burn edema along the ventral neck region in a horse 24 hours after burn injury caused by a barn fire. (*B*) The extent of the burn is more evident after the skin has sloughed because of the latent thermal injury to the skin.

Treatment of pulmonary injury

Maintenance of airway patency, adequate oxygenation and ventilation, and stabilization of hemodynamic status are the cornerstones of therapy for smoke inhalation injury. Early intervention and respiratory support are essential even before the diagnosis of respiratory injury is confirmed. Nasal or tracheal insufflation with humidified 100% oxygen counteracts the effects of carbon monoxide and facilitates clearance by decreasing the half-life of carbon monoxide in the blood. Oxygen insufflation rates of 15 to 20 L/min can be achieved through a tracheostomy and should be continued until the patient is able to maintain normal oxygenation. Humidification can relieve excessive airway drying or mucous plugging. Nebulizing with N-acetylcysteine and heparin and the use of humidified air can reduce the formation of pseudomembranous casts and aid in the clearance of airway secretions [35,39,44,48]. Nebulized dimethylsulfoxide (DMSO) helps to decrease lung fluid formation [39,44]. The β-adrenergic agonist albuterol can be aerosolized to reduce bronchospasm. DMSO and heparin may protect against airway damage caused by smoke [49–52]. Maintenance of optimal fluid status is essential; patients with concurrent surface burns and inhalation injury require 2 mL per percentage of burns per kilogram more fluid than those with cutaneous burns alone to support adequate cardiac and urine output [53].

Antibiotics and corticosteroids do not influence survival rates and should not be routinely administered to smoke inhalation patients. Systemic antimicrobials are indicated only for proven infections, the incidence of which increases 2 to 3 days after smoke inhalation. Intramuscular penicillin is effective against oral contaminants colonizing the airway. If signs of respiratory disease worsen, a transtracheal aspiration sample should be submitted for culture and sensitivity testing and the antibiotic regimen adapted accordingly [49,53].

Patients with suspected significant smoke inhalation should be observed closely for several hours and hospitalized in the presence of extensive burns. Therapy should be adjusted based on the clinical response and the results of serial blood gas analyses, complete blood cell counts, chest radiographs, airway endoscopy, and cultures. Successful treatment depends on continuous patient reassessment and early aggressive patient care.

Treatment of burn shock

With burn shock, large volumes of balanced electrolyte solution are generally the fluid of choice unless serum electrolyte analysis dictates otherwise. In patients with burns exceeding 15% of the total body surface area, intravenous fluid therapy is required to avoid circulatory collapse [54]. Inadequate fluid resuscitation results in decreased renal and gastrointestinal perfusion that could lead to gastrointestinal bacterial translocation and sepsis [55]. Administration of isotonic fluids at a rate of 2 to 4 mL/kg for each percentage of surface area burned is recommended, but fluid resuscitation is best titrated to maintain a stable and adequate blood pressure [26]. An alternative is to use hypertonic saline solution, 4 mL/kg, with plasma, hetastarch, or both, followed by additional isotonic fluids. If there has been smoke or heat inhalation injury, crystalloids should be limited to the amount that normalizes circulatory volume and blood pressure. The same continued rate of administration of electrolyte solutions after the resolution of burn shock results in edema in excess of any improvement in cardiovascular dynamics [56]. Plasma at a rate of 2 to 10 L is an effective albumin source as well as an exogenous source of antithrombin III for coagulopathies. One should carefully monitor the hydration, lung sounds, and cardiovascular status during fluid administration.

Flunixin meglumine (0.25–1.0 mg/kg administered intravenously every 12–24 hours) and pentoxifylline (8.0 mg/kg administered intravenously every 12 hours) are effective analgesics and improve blood flow in the small capillary networks. DMSO (1 g/kg administered intravenously) for the first 24 hours may decrease inflammation and pulmonary edema. If pulmonary edema is present and is unresponsive to DMSO and furosemide treatment, dexamethasone can be administered intravenously once at a dose of 0.5 mg/kg.

Nutritional needs

Assessment of adequate nutritional intake is performed with a reliable weight record. Weight loss of 10% to 15% during the course of illness is indicative of inadequate nutritional intake. Nutritional support can include parenteral and enteral routes, with the latter being superior [44]. Early enteral feeding not only decreases weight loss but maintains intestinal barrier function by minimizing mucosal atrophy. This reduces bacterial and toxin translocation and subsequent sepsis [44].

Gradually increasing the grain, adding fat in the form of vegetable oil (4–8 oz), and offering free-choice alfalfa hay increase caloric intake. An anabolic steroid may be used to help restore a positive nitrogen balance. If smoke inhalation is a concern or there is evidence of burns around the face, the hay should be soaked in water and fed on the ground with good ventilation provided [45].

Wound care

First-degree burns are generally not life threatening and are simply managed. Topical therapy in the form of cool compresses, cold-water baths, and wound coverings may provide relief. Pain control can be accomplished with nonsteroidal anti-inflammatory drugs or narcotics.

Second-degree burns are associated with vesicles and blisters. These vesicles should be left intact for the first 24 to 36 hours after formation, because blister fluid provides protection from infection and the presence of a blister is less painful than the denuded exposed surface. After this interval, the blister is partially excised and an antibacterial dressing is applied to the wound or an eschar is allowed to form [1,2,16].

Third-degree burns can be difficult to manage. The patient's condition should be stabilized as rapidly as possible before undertaking wound management. Destruction of the dermis leaves a primary collagenous structure called an eschar. Dry exposure is a treatment method that operates according to the principle that bacteria do not thrive on a dry surface. The goals of therapy are to keep the wound dry and protected from mechanical trauma. Heat and water loss from the uncovered wound, however, is a disadvantage.

There are several methods to treat burn wounds in the horse, and the choice depends on the extent and location of the injury. Full-thickness burns can be managed by occlusive dressings (closed technique), continuous wet dressings (semiopen technique), eschar formation (exposed technique), or excision and grafting [45].

The closed method uses occlusive artificial dressings. Wound cleansing and debridement are performed at each of the frequent dressing changes. Temporary dressings can, by adhering to the underlying wound bed, decrease the bacterial population, decrease heat and water loss, protect the bed of granulation tissue, and hasten wound healing. With large burns, however, frequent bandage changes and debridement can be painful and extensive bandaging may not be feasible or affordable in some animals [45].

With the semiopen method, the eschar is left in place but is kept covered with an antimicrobial-soaked dressing. The dressing provides protection against trauma, bacterial contamination, and evaporative losses. The wet dressings enhance eschar removal [45].

With the open technique the wound is left exposed to the air to form its own biologic barrier composed of exudate, collagen, and layers of dead skin known as the burn eschar. The eschar does not prevent bacterial contamination or heat or water evaporation, and the depth of tissue destruction may be marginally increased during the drying process. The eschar is covered with an antibacterial agent twice daily. Wound contraction does not occur while the eschar is intact [6]. The eschar is sloughed by bacterial collagenase activity with in 4 weeks [57]. The exposed bed can then be grafted or allowed to contract.

Eschar excision and grafting are useful for smaller burns but cannot be used for large burns because of lack of donor skin. Commercially available xenografts (porcine skin) can be used to cover large defects after excision; however, the cost can be prohibitive [1,16]. Eschar excision and open treatment are not practical for extensive burns in horses because of the likelihood of environmental contamination and massive losses of fluid and heat [45]. Therefore, the most effective and practical therapy for large burns in horses is the open method, leaving the eschar intact, with continuous application of antibacterial agents [1,2,45,58].

Initially, the surrounding hair should be clipped and the wound debrided of all devitalized tissue [16]. Attempts should be made to cool the affected skin using an ice or cold-water bath. Copious lavage with a sterile 0.05% chlorhexidine solution should be performed [16]. A water-based antibiotic ointment should be applied liberally to the affected areas to prevent heat and moisture loss, protect the eschar, prevent bacterial invasion, and loosen necrotic tissue and debris. This slow method of debridement allows removal of necrotic tissue as it is identified, thereby preventing possible removal of healthy germinal layers by mistake. The eschar is allowed to remain intact with gradual removal, permitting it to act as a natural bandage until it is ready to slough.

Dry flakes or sheets of a sterile starch copolymer are available and form a moldable gel when mixed with water. This material absorbs 30 times its weight in exudate, prevents further eschar formation by keeping tissues moist, and does not interfere with topical antibiotics, which can be applied before the gel or mixed with the gel.

Although bacterial colonization of large burns in horses is not preventable, the wound should be cleansed two or three times daily and a topical antibiotic reapplied to reduce the bacterial load to the wound Occlusive dressings should be avoided because of their tendency to produce a closed-wound environment that may encourage bacterial proliferation and delay healing.

Systemic antibiotics do not favorably influence wound healing, fever, or mortality and can encourage the emergence of resistant microorganisms. Additionally, circulation to the burned areas is often compromised, making it highly unlikely that parenteral administration of antibiotics can achieve therapeutic levels at the wound. Short-term prophylactic intravenous antibiotic therapy may be indicated in the immediate postburn period if quantitative biopsy cultures or a more rapid slide dilution method yields more than 100,000 cells per gram of tissue [59].

The most commonly used topical antibacterial for the treatment of burns is silver sulfadiazine in a 1% water miscible cream (Par Pharmaceutical, Spring Valley, NY). It is a broad-spectrum antibacterial agent able to penetrate the eschar. Silver sulfadiazine is active against gram-negative bacteria, especially *Pseudomonas*, with additional effectiveness against *Staphylococcus aureus*, *Escherichia coli*, *Proteus*, Enterobacteriaceae, and *Candida albicans* [16,45,56]. It causes minimal pain on application but must be used twice a day because it is inactivated by tissue secretions. Although pseudoeschar formation that may preclude wound evaluation, transient leukopenia, skin hypersensitivity, and the development of bacterial resistance have all been reported in human beings, silver sulfadiazine has few systemic effects and provides good results in the horse [45,56,60].

Aloe vera is a gel derived from a yucca-like plant and has antithromboxane and antiprostaglandin properties [61]. It is reported to relieve pain, decrease inflammation, stimulate cell growth, and kill bacteria and fungi. Although used successfully in the acute treatment of burns, it may actually delay healing once the initial inflammatory response has resolved [61]. Aloe vera and silver sulfadiazine are good first choices in antibiotic therapy for burns and are used extensively in human medicine.

Other effective topical antimicrobials include nitrofurazone (Furacin; Phoenix Pharmaceuticals, St. Joseph, MO), mafenide acetate, chlorhexidine

(Nolvasan; Fort Dodge Animal Health, Fort Dodge, IA), povidone-iodine (Betadine; Purdue Frederick Co., Norwalk, CT), and gentamicin sulfate ointment (Gentamicin sulfate ointment USP; Clay-Parks Labs, Bronx, NY). Nitrofurazone has a fairly narrow range of antibacterial activity, resistance can develop, and it does not penetrate the eschar well. Chlorhexidine is active in vitro against a number of gram-positive vegetative bacteria, yeasts, and dermatophyte fungi but has questionable effectiveness against gram-negative organisms. Because of its cationic nature, chlorhexidine binds strongly to skin, mucosa, and other tissues and is thus poorly absorbed. Chlorhexidine can be applied as a cream or solution. Povidone-iodine causes some patient discomfort but is effective against bacteria, yeast, and fungi. Its hyperosmolality causes severe hypernatremia and acidosis because of water loss [56], such that it should not be used on extensive burns where systematic absorption is likely. Immune system depression has also been reported in human patients [62]. Gentamicin is excellent for serious gram-negative infections but should be used only in selected cases, because resistance can develop and it may be nephrotoxic in patients with renal problems. Topical aqueous antibacterial preparations have also been used to treat burns. The solution (mixture of nitrofurazone, glycerin, and distilled water) can be applied to the wound as a mist from a spray bottle several times a day [1]. The nitrofurazone kills bacteria, whereas the moisture loosens the eschar and promotes debridement. Other agents that are occasionally used include neomycin, bacitracin, and polymyxin B. Their use is generally associated with the rapid development of bacterial resistance and systemic toxicity. They are not recommended for routine use in long-term wound care [60].

It is appropriate to change antibacterial creams according to clinical results. In large burns, quantitative wound biopsy analysis is advantageous. Wound flora densities of more than 10^5 organisms per gram of tissue predispose the patient to bacterial invasion of healthy tissue [57]. Preventing conversion of superficial wound sepsis to full-thickness infection with the risk of systemic sepsis is accomplished by administering local antibiotics. The use of systemic antibiotics is not recommended because they are ineffective in penetrating the avascular eschar, where the risk of contamination is greatest [60].

Many burned equine patients are pruritic, and measures must be taken to prevent self-mutilation of the wound. Reserpine can be effective in decreasing the urge to scratch by successfully breaking the itch-scratch cycle.

Skin grafts

Burns heal slowly, and many weeks may be required for the wound to close by means of granulation, contraction, and epithelialization. Closure of the burn wound by primary suturing or skin grafting after eschar removal allows for more rapid healing and superior pain relief and prevents loss of heat, water, and protein-rich exudate from the wound surface. Burns involving only the superficial dermis heal well within 3 weeks and do not need grafting. Conversely, deep partial-thickness wounds require several months to heal, during which time bacterial contamination of the wound develops. Second-intention healing results in a thin and hairless epithelium that is vulnerable to trauma. Excision, followed by grafting, of the wound is recommended in these cases. Full-thickness grafts from a cadaver donor can be used early in the clinical course of the burn to encourage healing, whereas split-thickness autogenous mesh grafts can be applied once healthy granulation tissue has formed. Early excision and grafting may also benefit horses that do not tolerate daily wound debridement and cleansing.

Complications

Healing burn wounds are pruritic [2,45]. Significant self-mutilation through rubbing, biting, and pawing can occur if the horse is not adequately restrained or medicated. Usually, the most intense pruritic episodes occur in the first weeks during the inflammatory phase of repair and during eschar sloughing. To prevent extreme self-mutilation, the animal must be cross-tied and/or sedated at this time. Other complications include habronemiasis, keloid-like fibroblastic proliferations, sarcoids, and other burn-induced neoplasia [2,47]. Hypertrophic scars, which commonly develop after deep second-degree burns, generally remodel in a cosmetic manner without surgery within 1 to 2 years. Because scarred skin is hairless and often depigmented, solar exposure should be limited. Chronic nonhealing areas should be excised and autografted to prevent neoplastic transformation. Delayed healing and poor epithelialization, complications of second-intention healing, may limit the return of the animal to its previous use (Fig. 8).

Summary

Extensive thermal injuries in horses can be difficult to manage. The large surface of the burn dramatically increases the potential for loss of fluids, electrolytes, and calories. Burns are classified by the depth of injury: first-degree burns involve only the most superficial layers of the epidermis; second-degree burns involve the entire epidermis and can be superficial or deep; third-degree burns are characterized by loss of the epidermal and dermal components; and fourth-degree burns involve all the skin and underlying muscle, bone, and ligaments. Burns cause local and systemic effects. Routine use of systemic antibiotics is not recommended in burn patients. Topical medications should be water based, be easily applied and removed, not interfere with wound healing, and be readily excreted or metabolized. Weight loss of 10% to 15% during the course of illness is

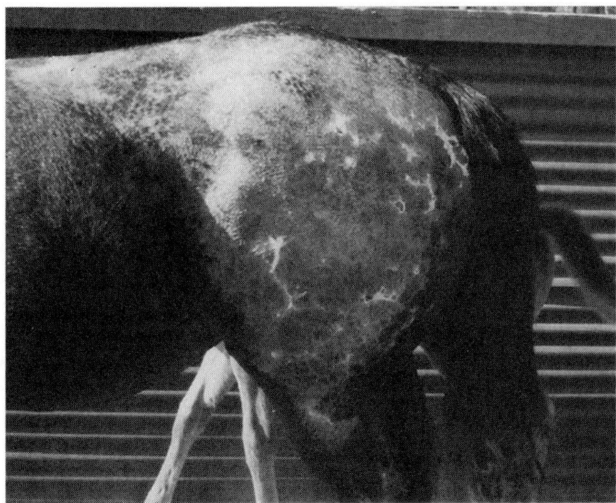

Fig. 8. Horse that sustained deep second- and third-degree burns of the dorsum and left hind limb 7 months previously. The entire wound has epithelialized. The skin is thin and brittle because of lack of sufficient subcutaneous tissue.

indicative of inadequate nutritional intake. Gradually increasing the grain, adding fat in the form of vegetable oil, and offering free-choice alfalfa hay increase caloric intake.

References

[1] Fubini SL. Burns. In: Robinson NE, editor. Current therapy in equine medicine 2. Philadelphia: WB Saunders; 1987. p. 639–41.

[2] Fox SM. Management of a large thermal burn in a horse. Compend Contin Educ Pract Vet 1988;10:88–95.

[3] Baxter GM. Management of burns. In: Colahan PT, Mayhew IG, Merritt AM, et al, editors. Equine medicine and surgery. 4th edition. Goleta: American Veterinary Publication; 1991. p. 1843–7.

[4] Warden GD. Outpatient care of thermal injuries. Surg Clin N Am 1987;67:147–57.

[5] Robson MC, Heggars JP. Pathophysiology of the burn wound. In: Carvajal HF, Parks DH, editors. Burns in children—pediatric burn management. St. Louis: Year Book Medical Publishers; 1988. p. 27–32.

[6] Harvey JS, Watkins GM, Sherman JT. Emergent burn care. South Med J 1984;77:204–14.

[7] Provost PJ. Thermal injuries. In: Auer JA, Stick JA, editors. Equine surgery. 2nd edition. Philadelphia: WB Saunders; 1999. p. 179–86.

[8] Robson MC, Kucan JO, Paik KI, et al. The effects of heparin and dermal ischemia after burning. Burns 1979;5:260–4.

[9] Bietner R, Chem-Zion M, Sofer-Bassukevitz Y. Therapeutic and prophylactic treatment of skin burns with several calmodulin antagonists. Gen Pharmacol 1989;20:165–73.

[10] Robson MC, Del Baccaro EJ, Heggers JP, et al. Increasing dermal perfusion after burning by decreasing thromboxane production. J Trauma 1980;20:722–5.

[11] Carleton SC. Cardiac problems associated with burns. Cardiol Clin 1995;13(2):257–62.

[12] Asch MJ. Systemic and pulmonary hemodynamic changes accompanying thermal injury. Ann Surg 1973;178:218–21.

[13] Dernling RH. Fluid replacement in burned patients. Surg Clin N Am 1987;67:15–30.
[14] Dernling RH, Mazess RB, Witt RM, et al. The study of burn wound edema using dichromatic absorptiometry. J Trauma 1978;18:124–8.
[15] Birke G, Lihjedahl SO, Plantin LO, et al. Studies of burns XI: the distribution and losses through the wound of ^{131}I albumen measured by whole body counting. Acta Chir Scand 1968;134:27–36.
[16] Fox SM. Management of thermal burns, part 1. Compend Contin Educ Pract Vet 1985;7: 631–42.
[17] Curreri PW, Richmond D, Marvin J, et al. Dietary requirements of patients with major burns. J Am Diet Assoc 1974;65:415–7.
[18] Till GO, Guilds LS, Mahroughi M. Role of xanthine oxidase in thermal injury of skin. Am J Pathol 1989;135:195–202.
[19] Pruitt BA. Fluid and electrolyte replacement in the burned patient. Surg Clin N Am 1978;58: 1291–312.
[20] Johnston DE. Burns: electrical, chemical and cold injuries. In: Slatter D, editor. Textbook of small animal surgery. Philadelphia: WB Saunders; 1985. p. 516–33.
[21] Baxter CR. Fluid volume and electrolyte changes if the early post burn period. Clin Plast Surg 1974;1:693–703.
[22] Birdsell DC, Birch JR. Anemia following thermal burns: a survey in 109 children. Can J Surg 1971;14:345–50.
[23] Baars S. Anemia of burns. Burns 1979;6:1–8.
[24] Alexander JW, Wixson D. Neutrophil dysfunction and sepsis in burn injury. Surg Gynecol Obstet 1970;130:431–8.
[25] Hansbrough JF, Zapata O, Sirvent RI, et al. Immunomodulation following burn injury. Surg Clin N Am 1987;67:69–92.
[26] Herndon DN, Curreri PW, Abston S. Treatment of burns. Curr Probl Surg 1987;24:341–97.
[27] Wilmore DW, Long JM, Mason AD. Catecholamines: mediator of the hypermetabolic response to thermal injury. Ann Surg 1974;180:653–69.
[28] Herndon DN, Wilmore DW, Mason AD. Development and analysis of a small animal model simulating the human post burn hypermetabolic response. J Surg Res 1978;25:394–403.
[29] Curreri PW, Luterman A. Nutritional support of the burn patient. Surg Clin N Am 1978;58: 1151–6.
[30] Gamelli RL. Nutritional problems of the acute and chronic burn patient. Arch Dermatol 1988;124:756–9.
[31] Markley K, Smallman E, Thorton SW, et al. The effect of environmental temperature and fluid therapy on mortality and metabolism of mice after burn and tourniquet trauma. J Trauma 1973;13:145–60.
[32] Peter WJ. Inhalation injury caused by the products of combustion. Can Med Assoc J 1981; 125:249–52.
[33] Young CJ, Moss J. Smoke inhalation: diagnosis and treatment. J Clin Anesth 1989;1(5): 377–86.
[34] Cahalane M, Demling RH. Early respiratory abnormalities from smoke inhalation. JAMA 1984;251:771–3.
[35] Fein A, Leff A, Hopewell PC. Pathophysiologic and management of the complications resulting from fire and inhaled products of combustion: review of the literature. Crit Care Med 1980;8:94–8.
[36] Mayes RW. ACP Broadsheet No 142: measurement of carbon monoxide and cyanide in blood. J Clin Pathol 1993;46(11):982–8.
[37] Walker HL, McLeod CG, McManus WF. Experimental inhalation injury in the goat. J Trauma 1981;21:962–4.
[38] Herndon DN, Traber DL, Niehaus GD. The pathophysiology of smoke inhalation injury in a sheep model. J Trauma 1984;24:1044–51.

[39] LaLonde C, Demling R, Brain J. Smoke inhalation injury in sheep caused the particulate phase, not the gas phase. J Appl Physiol 1994;77:15–22.
[40] Loke J, Paul E, Virgulto JA, et al. Rabbit lung after acute smoke inhalation. Arch Surg 1984; 119:956–9.
[41] Fick RB, Paul E, Reynolds E. Impaired phagocytic and bacteriocidal function of smoke exposed rabbit alveolar macrophages. Chest 1980;78:516.
[42] Demarest GB, Hudson LD, Altman LC. Impaired alveolar macrophage chemotaxis in patients with acute smoke inhalation. Am Rev Respir Dis 1979;119:279–86.
[43] Demling RH, Will JA, Belzer FO. Effect of major thermal injury on the pulmonary microcirculation. Surgery 1978;83:746–51.
[44] Nguyen TT, Gilpin DA, Meyer DA. Current treatment of severely burned patients. Ann Surg 1996;223:14–25.
[45] Geiser D, Walker RD. Management of large animal thermal injuries. Compend Contin Educ Pract Vet 1985;7(Suppl):S69–78.
[46] Fox SM, Goring RI, Probst CW. Management of thermal burn injuries. Part II. Compend Contin Educ Pract Vet 1986;8:439–44.
[47] Schumacher J, Watkins JP, Wilson JP, et al. Burn induced neoplasia in two horses. Equine Vet J 1986;18:410–3.
[48] Lloyd E, MacRae WR. Respiratory tract damage in burns. Br J Anaesth 1971;43:365–79.
[49] Muller MJ, Herndon DN. The challenge of burns. Lancet 1994;343:216–20.
[50] Brown M, Desai M, Traber LD. Dimethylsulfoxide with heparin in the treatment of smoke inhalation injury. J Burn Care Rehabil 1988;9(1):22–5.
[51] Cox CS Jr, Zwischenberger JB, Traber DL, et al. Heparin improves oxygenation and minimizes barotrauma after severe smoke inhalation in an ovine model. Surg Gynecol Obstet 1993;176(4):339–49.
[52] Kimura R, Traber L, Herndon D, et al. Ibuprofen reduces the lung lymph flow changes associated with inhalation injury. Circ Shock 1988;24(3):183–91.
[53] Herndon DN, Barrow RE, Traber DL, et al. Extravascular lung water changes following smoke inhalation and massive burn injury. Surgery 1987;102(2):341–9.
[54] Harvey JS, Watkins GM, Sherman RT. Emergent burn care. South Med J 1984;77:204–14.
[55] Deitch EA. Nutritional support of the burn patient. Crit Care Clin 1995;11:735–50.
[56] Orsini JA, Divers TJ. Burns and acute swelling. In: Orsini JA, Divers TJ, editors. Manual of equine emergencies. 2nd edition. Philadelphia: WB Saunders; 2003. p. 300–4.
[57] Heimbach DM. Early burn excision and grafting. Surg Clin N Am 1987;67:93–107.
[58] Scarratt WK. Cutaneous thermal injury in a horse. Equine Pract 1984;6:13–7.
[59] Ollstein RN, McDonald C. Topical and systemic antimicrobial agents in burns. Ann Plast Surg 1980;5:386–92.
[60] Monafo WW, Freedman B. Topical therapy for burns. Surg Clin N Am 1987;67:133–45.
[61] Swaim SF. Topical wound medications: a review. J Am Vet Med Assoc 1988;190:1588–93.
[62] Ninneman JL, Stein MD. Induction of suppressor cells by burn treatment with povidone-iodine. J Burn Care Rehab 1980;1:12–8.

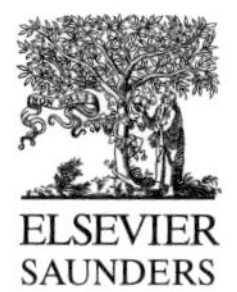
ELSEVIER
SAUNDERS

Vet Clin Equine 21 (2005) 125–144

VETERINARY
CLINICS
Equine Practice

Skin Grafts and Skin Flaps in the Horse

David G. Bristol, DVM

College of Veterinary Medicine, North Carolina State University, 4700 Hillsborough Street, Raleigh, NC 27606, USA

"It is a good horse that never stumbles."—C.H. Spurgeon. *John Ploughman's Talk*, 1869

Unfortunately, horses do stumble, and given the size, strength, and rapid response to "fight or flight" situations that horses exhibit, it is not surprising that they are frequently the victims of self-inflicted trauma. Although wounds on the neck and trunk tend to heal well by primary closure or secondary healing, those on the limbs, parts of the head, and perineum often present special challenges. Contracture near any body orifice can result in complications, whereas the general deficit of wound contraction and excessive production of granulation tissue impair healing of limb wounds. The use of reconstructive skin flaps or skin grafts can dramatically modify the final outcome of healing of these wounds, leading to a more cosmetic and functional result. This article reviews the indications for, classification of, and clinical approach to the use of skin flaps and grafts. Application of skin expansion techniques and artificial skin substitutes is also briefly discussed.

Indications and contraindications for skin grafting

Many wounds encountered in equine practice are detected shortly after their occurrence and can be treated by primary closure. For wounds in which primary closure is impossible, wound contraction and epithelialization close surprisingly large wounds of the neck, thorax, and abdomen without the need for grafts. Skin grafting is indicated primarily for wounds in which extensive loss of tissue results in an insufficient amount of skin for closure, wounds in which excessive granulation tissue formation prevents wound contraction, and wounds in which contraction and epithelialization

E-mail address: david_bristol@ncsu.edu

doi:10.1016/j.cveq.2004.11.007 ***vetequine.theclinics.com***

are insufficient to close the defect or may result in contracture. Contracture is the loss of normal elasticity and function of a structure, often an orifice or a joint, as a result of excessive wound contraction. For example, contraction of wounds near the eye can result in the inability to close the palpebrae and subsequent exposure keratitis. Fibrosis of wounds on the flexion surface of joints may prevent full extension but is rarely encountered in horses.

The healing of grafts to the recipient site is referred to as "take," and most contraindications to grafting derive from conditions leading to a poor take of the grafts. To survive, grafts must be transplanted to areas with a good local vascular supply. Free grafts do not survive if transplanted directly to exposed bone, tendon, or fat. Grafts should not be placed in an infected wound bed, and a bacterial count of 10^5 per gram of tissue is associated with graft failure. Some bacterial species (*Pseudomonas* spp) result in large amounts of exudate that can physically displace small grafts from the recipient bed. Others produce proteolytic enzymes that digest the fibrin initially holding the grafts in place [1–4].

Another contraindication to grafting is a lack of trained individuals to provide quality aftercare. Although some skin grafting procedures are technically simple to perform, aftercare is often the key to success. Grafted sites must be closely monitored for signs of infection and treated quickly should it occur. Granulation tissue may continue to proliferate and require debridement or topical medical therapies. Bandages must be changed regularly and applied appropriately. Bandages that are too tight prevent adequate perfusion of the grafts, with subsequent necrosis. Bandages that are too loose and move over the wound surface can physically dislodge the grafts.

Classifications of skin flaps and grafts

Numerous types of skin flaps and grafts can be used to close skin defects, and several methods of defining the type of flap or graft exist. In general, skin flaps have an intact blood supply, whereas skin grafts require neovascularization.

Local flaps come from adjacent skin, whereas distant flaps come from nonadjacent skin. In equine medicine, the most commonly used flap is a local advancement flap, where adjoining skin is advanced over the wound. If the flap is created without regard to the underlying vascular patterns, it is termed a *random pattern flap*. Although the viable length of a random pattern flap increases in proportion to its width [5], the ratio varies with the vascularity of the region. Thus, longer survival lengths can be expected for flaps of the same width in highly vascular areas, such as the face and perineum, than for those in less vascular regions. If the vascular pattern is identified and preserved during elevation of a flap, it is termed an *axial pattern flap*. A Doppler ultrasound stethoscope (Fig. 1) or other ultrasound device can be used to detect and map the flap vasculature before surgery. The flap is harvested with meticulous care to preserve the blood supply.

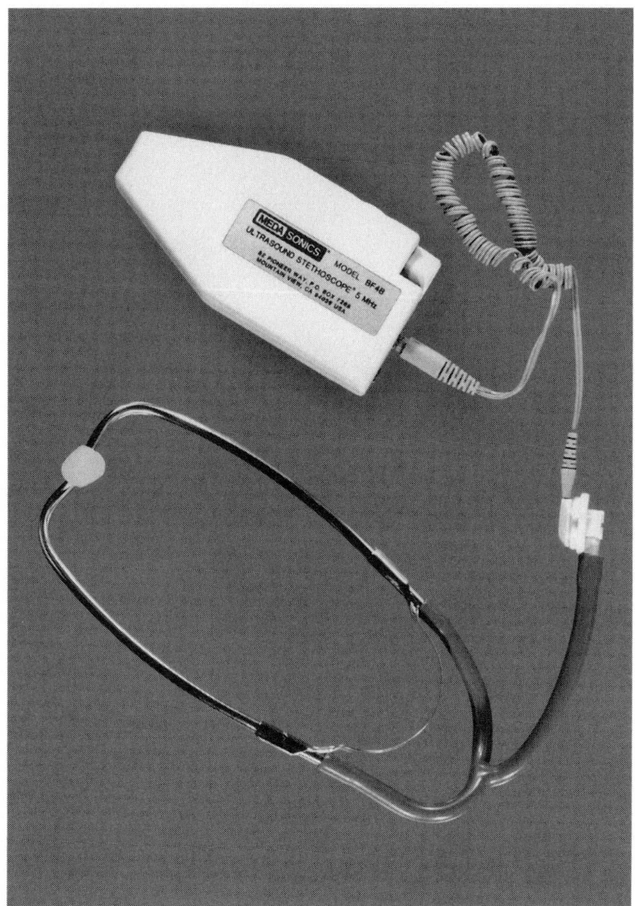

Fig. 1. Doppler ultrasound stethoscope used to define arterial supply to an axial pattern skin flap.

(Figs. 2–4). Free flaps are axial pattern distant flaps that are divided from their original blood supply. The vascular pedicle of the flap is transected, and an anastomosis between the primary artery and vein of the flap and an artery and vein at the recipient site is performed. The flap is then sutured to the recipient site. These are more commonly used in companion animals.

Flaps can also be classified according to how they are moved over a defect. Advancement flaps are pulled straight along their length to cover a defect, whereas rotational flaps are moved in an arcuate manner over a defect. Transposition flaps are advanced or rotated over intervening skin to cover a defect (see Fig. 3).

Skin grafts are defined by their thickness. Split-thickness grafts contain epidermis and a variable thickness of dermis. Thin split-thickness grafts do not contain adnexal structures, such as hair roots, and result in an epithelialized area without hair growth. Full-thickness grafts contain the

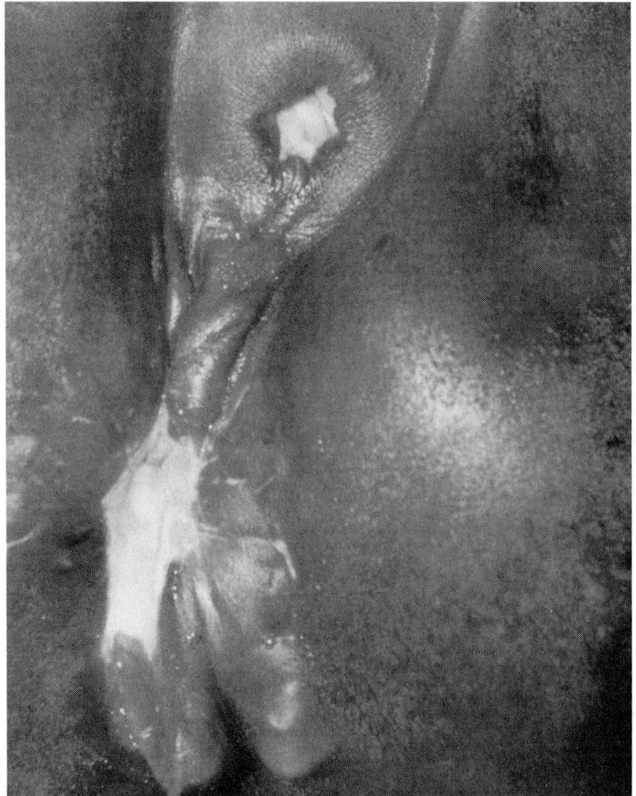

Fig. 2. A mare missing most of the left side of her vulva from a foaling accident.

epidermis and full thickness of the dermis but not the underlying subcutaneous tissue. Full-thickness grafts that take result in a more cosmetic final result because of hair regrowth. Hair growth reflects the normal growth at the donor site rather than at the recipient site (donor dominance). Composite grafts consist of the epidermis, dermis, and a variable depth of underlying tissue, possibly including fat, muscle, cartilage, or other structures.

Grafts can also be defined by the relation of the donor to the recipient. Autografts are taken from one site on a patient and transplanted to another site on the same patient. Isografts are grafts between identical twins or highly inbred strains. Allografts are transplanted from another individual of the same species, whereas xenografts are transplanted from another species. Autografts are the most common type of graft used in equine practice.

Physiology of grafting

The first critical process in the successful take of a graft is its adherence to the wound bed. Fibrin in the wound bed forms weak attachments of the

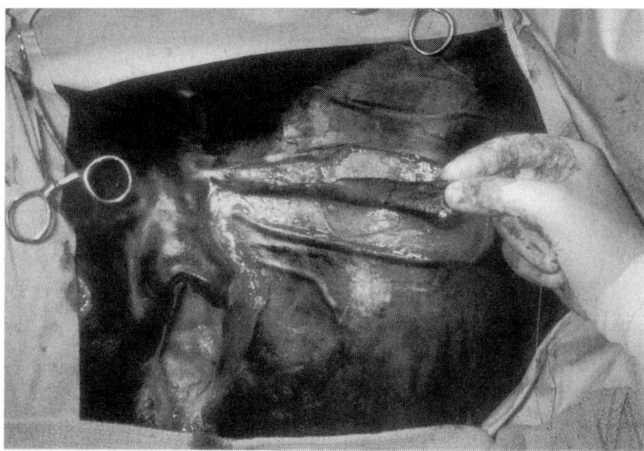

Fig. 3. Mare from Fig. 2 in dorsal recumbency. An axial pattern transpositional skin flap has been elevated to cover the vulvar defect.

graft to the wound. During this phase, it is easy to disrupt the fibrin attachments by motion or bacterial enzymatic destruction, leading to graft loss. Fibroblasts infiltrate the graft site and begin producing fibrous adhesions by 72 hours after transplantation [3]. A firm attachment should be present by 7 to 8 days [4].

Skin flaps receive nutrition and oxygen from their original vascular supply. This is the reason why random pattern flaps cannot have a length that far exceeds their width. Axial pattern flaps can be quite long and thin, because the vasculature supplying the flap is intact or is connected by anastomosis to the local vasculature. Grafts, conversely, must initially obtain their nutrition and oxygenation from the local environment at the recipient site until neovascularization occurs. Grafts obtain nutrients and oxygen initially through a process called osmotic or plasmatic imbibition. In this phase, the graft takes up nutrients from local fluids in the wound site. The graft metabolism becomes anaerobic, and the pH drops. This phase generally lasts 1 to 2 days. In intact dermis, the number of vessels increases in the more superficial portion of the dermis as a result of the normal arborizing pattern of dermal vessels. Thus, split-thickness grafts tend to survive better than full-thickness grafts because of their more numerous finer capillary network. This allows a shorter diffusion distance for nutrients during the phase of plasmatic imbibition and a greater chance of vessels at the recipient site healing to those of the graft.

Inosculation, the attachment of capillaries from the recipient site to the graft's vessels, follows. There is debate as to whether the budding vessels from the wound bed actually attach to the preexisting vessels in the graft or use the graft vessels as conduits as they grow into the graft. It has been shown that graft vessels become lined with endothelium of host origin [4].

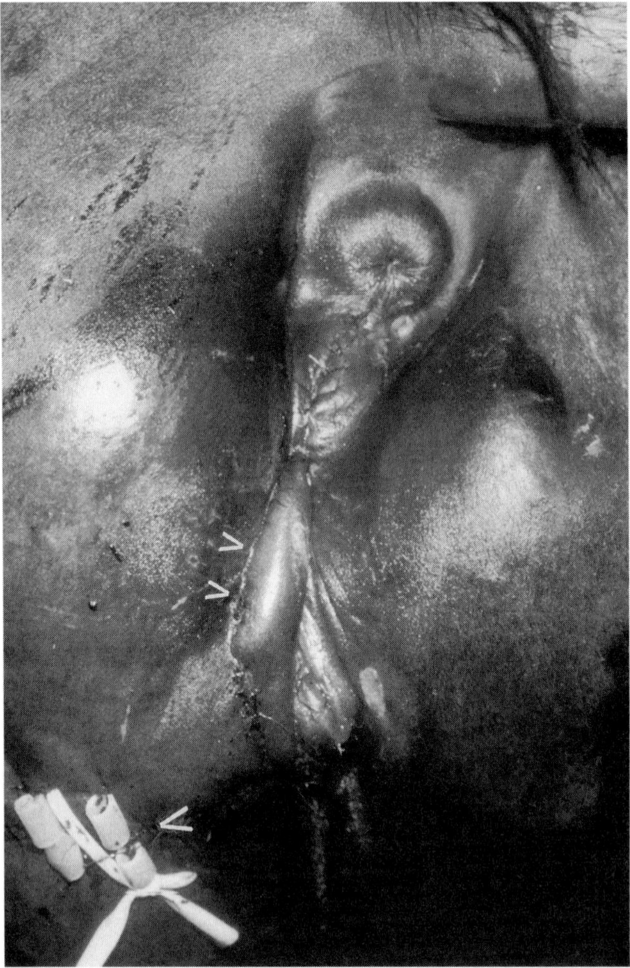

Fig. 4. Mare with rotational axial pattern flap in place (small arrowheads). Although the flap did not restore normal anatomy, it did provide coverage of the vaginal orifice so as to prevent fecal contamination. Vertical mattress sutures through stents have been used to relieve tension at the donor site (large arrowhead).

Blood flow can be re-established in the graft in as little as 2 days [3]. Neovascularization by direct ingrowth of capillaries into the graft also occurs. This is called secondary revascularization [4].

Application of grafts to wounds of the distal limbs of horses can decrease the contraction rate of those wounds. Although application of grafts 14 days after creating full-thickness circular wounds had no effect on contraction compared with nongrafted wounds, immediate grafting resulted in a lower rate constant of contraction compared with similar wounds grafted 10 days after they were created [6,7]. Thus, it seems that grafting had a negative effect on contraction only when performed before the onset of the latter. The clinical significance of this finding is that skin grafting can be delayed in areas in which contraction is helpful in closing large wounds (neck and trunk) but should be used early, during the lag period of contraction, to prevent contracture in other areas. An example of an indication for early grafting would be after removal of large masses near the ear, where contraction could result in a conformational deformity or inability of the horse to move the ear after second-intention healing.

After grafting, the elastin and collagen of the graft are progressively replaced by host elements. The graft is gradually reinnervated by nerve growth through preexisting neurolemmal sheaths or by direct invasion into the graft [4], which constitutes the organization phase of graft take.

Clinical approach to grafting

A number of conditions are prerequisite to optimal graft take. The recipient site must have a good vascular supply to nourish the graft. Wounds with exposed bone, ligaments, tendons, and other poorly perfused structures must granulate before skin grafting is attempted. Wounds should be cleaned and bandaged as fibroplasia progresses, until the granulation tissue almost reaches the level of the surrounding skin. Any wound with exposed bone that has lost its periosteum should be radiographed before grafting to check for the presence of a sequestrum. Draining tracts are further indications of sequestrate or foreign bodies and require a radiograph or ultrasound image to diagnose the source of the drainage so that it can be treated before grafting.

If excessive granulation tissue is present, it should be trimmed to slightly below the surrounding skin and bandaged to control bleeding, with grafting performed the next day. In extremely chronic wounds, resection of excess tissue may result in a graft bed that is fibrous in nature with a poor vascular supply. If this is the case, the surgeon should trim the tissue below the level of surrounding skin and wait for new granulation tissue to develop before grafting is attempted. Ideally, the recipient site should be aseptic (Fig. 5). Bacterial growth uses nutrients needed by the graft and can cause direct destruction of a graft, particularly through digestion of the fibrin required for adherence of the graft to the wound bed. There needs to be good contact between the recipient bed and the graft. If sheet grafts are to be placed over concave surfaces, they should be sutured at the depths of the wound or have a compression bandage applied that ensures good graft-wound contact. Finally, any hemorrhage at the recipient site must be controlled to prevent it from washing away or elevating the graft.

Once the recipient site is properly prepared, donor skin can be obtained. Four types of autografts are described: pinch grafts, punch grafts, strip grafts, and mesh grafts. Convenient areas from which to obtain donor skin from a horse are the ventral abdomen and ventral thorax. In addition, the

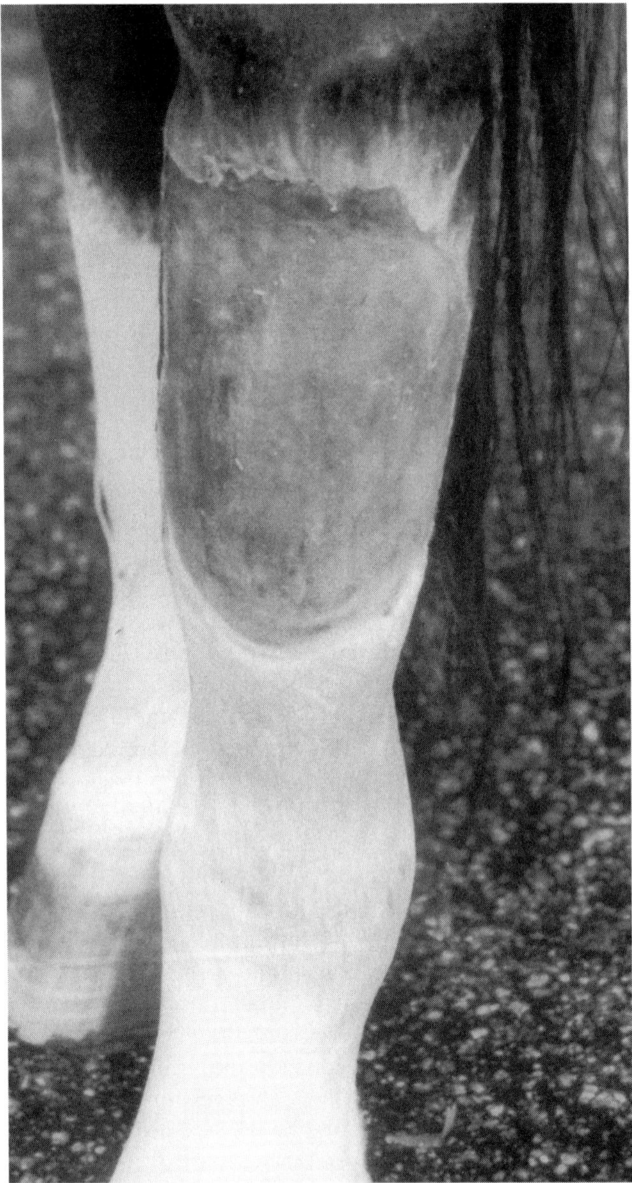

Fig. 5. Granulation bed on the metatarsus prepared for grafting. The bed is almost flush with the surrounding skin surface, has a healthy pink color, and has no evidence of infection. (Courtesy of Mat Gerard, PhD, Raleigh, NC.)

neck under the mane is a suitable site from which to harvest pinch and punch grafts. The mane is pulled to the opposite side of the neck from where it usually falls and is taped or tied in place. Regardless of the donor location, the skin is clipped and surgically scrubbed before obtaining grafts. The horse is sedated, and a local block is performed for pinch or punch grafts. The horse should be anesthetized if a dermatome is used to harvest sheets of skin.

Pinch grafts are created by "pinching" a small section of skin with forceps or elevating it with a fine-gauge needle and cutting it off with a scalpel. Because of the manner in which these grafts are obtained, they are thin split-thickness grafts at their periphery, gradually increasing in thickness toward their center, where they may approach full-thickness grafts. Because of this varying thickness, hair regrowth is variable. It has been the author's experience that hair growing from these grafts may not be normal in appearance and may grow to a longer length than the hair at the original donor site or the recipient site.

A large number of pinch grafts can be obtained and placed on gauze that has been moistened with physiologic saline solution or lactated Ringer's solution. A number 15 scalpel blade is used to create small pockets in the granulation bed to receive the grafts. Because the donor sites are usually not full thickness, they may be left open and require minimal postoperative care. Any that are full thickness can be closed with a single monofilament suture.

Punch grafts are obtained in a manner similar to pinch grafts, except that a biopsy punch is used to cut the skin at the donor site. The cut skin is elevated and freed from the underlying subcutaneous tissue. Any subcutaneous tissue still attached to the grafts should be removed before the grafts are placed at the recipient site because it may interfere with revascularization. A biopsy punch slightly smaller than the one used for obtaining the grafts is required to remove a plug of granulation tissue at the recipient site (Fig. 6), where the graft is placed. This ensures a tight fit for the grafts that undergo slight contraction after their harvest. The cosmetic outcome of punch grafts is improved if the surgeon considers the direction of hair growth within the graft. Each donor site should be closed with monofilament suture.

After pinch or punch grafting, the wound is bandaged with a sterile nonadherent pad or biologic dressing and a sterile soft wrap. Bandage conformation varies according to the location of the wound. Leg wraps are usually sufficient for metacarpal or metatarsal wounds. Immobilization of the limb is required in the case of wounds over joints to reduce excessive motion and subsequent graft loss. In these cases, a stiff splint or cast is used to protect the grafts until they heal to the graft bed. Although many authors recommend changing bandages daily after grafting, grafts are susceptible to mechanical dislodgement in the first few days after surgery. If a cast is used, it is usually left on for 10 to 14 days, at which time the attachments of the graft are fibrous as opposed to fibrinous and vascular attachments have occurred [4]. Although casting prevents observation of the graft site, the advantages of immobilization usually outweigh this disadvantage. The cast should be removed immediately if the horse shows any signs of additional pain in the limb or if the cast becomes warm, there is discharge seeping

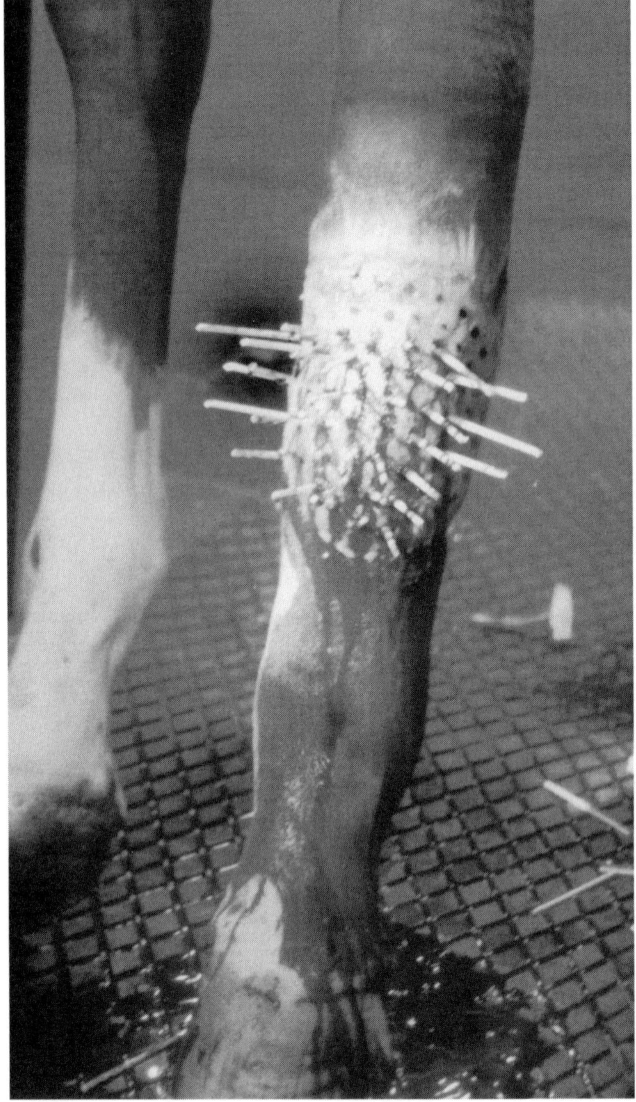

Fig. 6. A punch biopsy instrument 2 mm smaller than that used to obtain the skin grafts has been used to create the recipient sites in the granulation tissue. Cotton-tipped swabs control hemorrhage before graft placement. (Courtesy of Mat Gerard, PhD, Raleigh, NC.)

through it, or it becomes malodorous. Once the cast is removed, bandages should be changed daily and the wound gently cleaned until it has epithelialized (Fig. 7). Tie-over bandages can also be used to immobilize the wound dressing [4], depending on location. Tie-over bandages are applied by placing long-tailed sutures around the circumference of the wound. A

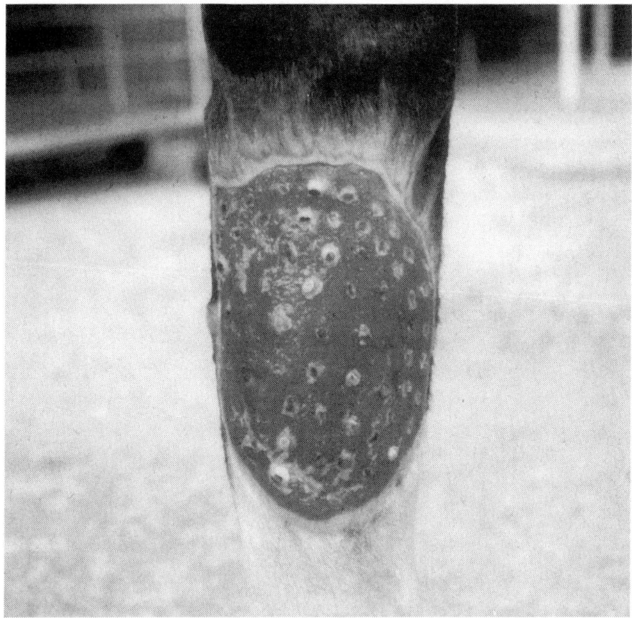

Fig. 7. The same limb 10 days after graft placement. Grafts have healed to the granulation tissue. Small circles of new epithelial tissue can be seen surrounding a number of the grafts. (Courtesy of Mat Gerard, PhD, Raleigh, NC.)

nonadherent pad is placed on the graft site, followed by bulky dressing material. The sutures are then tied over the dressing [4].

Strip or tunnel grafts [2,8] may be partial or full thickness. Partial-thickness grafts are obtained with a dermatome, whereas full-thickness grafts are harvested by making parallel incisions 2 mm apart and elevating the skin from the underlying subcutaneous tissue and excising it. The graft is then tunneled approximately 6 mm below the surface of the granulation tissue at the recipient site using a large-bore needle or alligator forceps, ensuring that the epidermal side of the graft faces the surface of the wound. The strips are placed parallel to one another 2 cm apart for the length of the wound. The cut ends of the skin strips are sutured to the skin on either side of the granulation bed (Fig. 8). When grafting is to take place on a limb, a tourniquet may be used to decrease hemorrhage and improve visualization of the strips. If placed sufficiently superficially, the granulation tissue overlying the graft should slough in 7 to 10 days [4]. If this does not occur, it should be excised at this time. The granulation tissue between grafts is removed down to the level of the grafts, and the area is bandaged once more. Bandages are changed daily and the wound gently cleaned until epithelialization is complete in 2 to 4 weeks [4].

Large split-thickness sheet grafts are usually obtained with a dermatome or freehand with a scalpel, according to the surgeon's skill and preference.

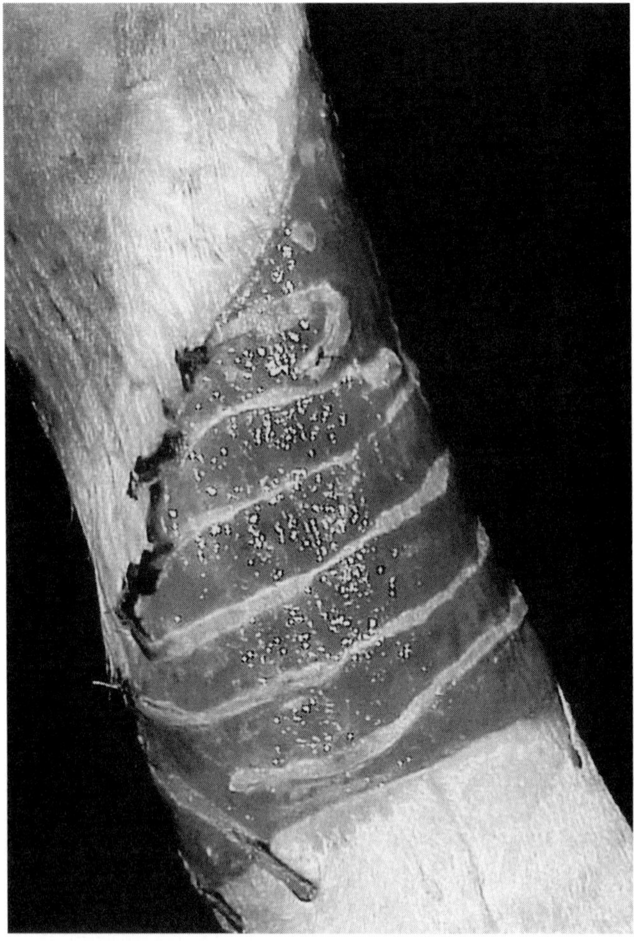

Fig. 8. Example of strip grafts on a metatarsal wound in a horse. The free ends of the strip grafts that were sutured over the skin adjacent to the wound have become necrotic, whereas most of the grafts have healed to the granulation bed. (Courtesy of Mat Gerard, PhD, Raleigh, NC.)

Harvesting split-thickness sheet grafts is painful, so general anesthesia is used. The sternal area is an optimum site from which to harvest skin, because the sternum provides a firm surface to push against and the resulting wound is fairly concealed. The skin is clipped and prepared for surgery. Sterile lubricant is applied to the dermatome and skin. An assistant is helpful in keeping the skin tense while the dermatome is pressed against the skin by the surgeon. Once an adequate length of skin is obtained, the dermatome is angled up from the skin to excise the graft. If the graft is not quickly and cleanly cut by the dermatome, it is better to turn the dermatome off and remove the graft with scissors than to put excessive tension on the graft with the dermatome. The graft is then placed on moistened gauze.

The graft may be placed directly on the recipient site and sutured in place. A disadvantage to this method is that any drainage from the recipient site can be trapped under the graft, lifting it from its nutrient source. In equine practice, the recipient sites are often much larger than the grafts obtained, so mesh grafting techniques are used to expand the grafts. The graft is cleaned of any underlying tissue and placed on a firm surface so that parallel alternating cuts can be made with a scalpel. Alternatively, the graft is placed on a specialized cutting block that has a series of parallel cutting blades. A dowel is rolled over the graft, pressing it against the blades. Once the graft has been meshed, it is sutured or glued over the recipient wound. The grafted site should be bandaged as mentioned previously for pinch and punch grafts.

Of the methods described in this article, a successful sheet graft yields the most cosmetic result. Mesh grafting is probably the best method for covering large defects. Conversely, pinch and punch grafting is technically simple and does not require any specialized equipment. The key to success with any of these methods is proper preparation of the wound site and meticulous aftercare.

Causes of graft failure

A poorly prepared recipient bed is an invitation for graft failure. A recipient bed that has poor perfusion (bare bone, mature granulation tissue, or fat) does not support a graft. An immediate cause of pinch or punch graft failure is simple displacement of the grafts from their recipient sites by hemorrhage. Full-thickness grafts fail if all underlying fat is not removed from the graft before it is placed on the wound bed, because fat prevents revascularization. Postoperative causes of failure are accumulation of material between the graft and the wound bed, motion that physically displaces the graft from the wound bed, and bacterial infection. Accumulation of material beneath the graft can be avoided by ensuring that hemorrhage is controlled before grafting and by meshing sheet grafts. Bacterial infection can result in direct destruction of grafted skin as well as displacement of the graft(s) from the recipient site by excessive wound exudate and enzymatic destruction of the fibrin that initially holds the graft in place. *Pseudomonas* spp and β-hemolytic *Streptococcus* spp are particularly prominent in equine wound infections. Infected wounds should be immediately treated with broad-spectrum antibiotics while awaiting culture results.

Skin graft storage

There are numerous reasons for storing grafts before their application. A horse may be anesthetized to clean and debride a wound that is not yet ready for grafting. For example, debriding excess granulation tissue results in significant hemorrhage, and grafting may need to be delayed for 1 to 2 days until hemorrhage is fully controlled. In this case, grafts can be harvested at the time of the initial surgery and stored to avoid subsequent anesthesia. Some grafts may be stored during an initial grafting procedure as a replacement source for grafts that do not take. Stored grafts may result in earlier vascularization as a result of the production of anaerobic metabolites [9]. Grafts may also be harvested from skin flaps that are expected to become necrotic when treating an acute traumatic wound and transplanted back to the same wound after it has begun to granulate.

In human medicine, grafts may be stored in gauze moistened with saline or nutrient media and refrigerated, frozen after cryopreservation, or stored at room temperature after freeze drying [10]. Skin that is stored in moistened gauze in a rolled configuration retains more of its normal histologic characteristics than skin that is stored flat (folded so that dermis is against dermis to prevent desiccation) [10]. Although there have been several studies on the effect of storage media and storage temperature on histologic changes or metabolic assays in skin grafts, the clinical consequences of observed changes are not always clear [10–12].

Excellent results have been achieved in horses with grafts stored up to 3 weeks in McCoy's 5A medium with 10% equine serum and gentamicin sulfate (80 mg/L). The grafts are stored at 4°C, with medium at a rate of 1 to 1.5 mL/cm^2 of skin surface area [9].

Application of skin flaps

Skin flaps differ from skin grafts in that they retain attachment to their original blood supply or their vascular pedicle is reconnected by microvascular anastomosis to vessels close to the defect the flap is intended to cover. Random pattern flaps are used most often in equine surgery [13]. Typically, a flap is elevated and advanced over a defect. Although an increased survival length has been correlated to increased width of the flap, a direct ratio between the two dimensions does not exist. For example, one study performed in horses showed that a 300% increase in width resulted in only a 34% increase in surviving length [5].

There is evidence in dogs that sharp dissection is superior to use of electrocautery and carbon dioxide and yttrium aluminum garnet lasers for elevating flaps. Although sharply dissected flaps take longer to elevate, there is less postoperative drainage and the grafts generate significantly higher wound bursting strengths. Sharply dissected flaps also have evidence of higher collagen content and fibroblast infiltration, with fewer polymorphonuclear leukocytes [14].

Axial pattern flaps are superior to random pattern flaps because of superior skin perfusion and the ability to maintain a greater percentage of baseline perfusion when submitted to tension [15]. Relatively few axial pattern flaps have been identified in horses compared with human beings, dogs, and cats [16–19]. A type of axial pattern flap called an Estlander flap has been used to repair a large chronic lip laceration in a colt [20]. This flap consisted of a full-thickness section of the colt's dorsal lip that was rotated to a ventral lip defect, preserving its vasculature and nerve supply.

Although there have been several attempts to use microvascular anastomosis to reconnect the vasculature of an excised axial pattern flap (free flap) to its original perfusing vessels (orthotopic flap) or to vessels at another location (heterotopic flap), a successful technique has not been reported for the horse [17,18]. Although it was assumed that the failure of equine free tissue transfer was caused by neutrophil-mediated injury associated with ischemia-reperfusion injury, a recent study does not support this hypothesis [21].

Skin expansion

Skin expansion has been used in human surgical practice for reconstructive and plastic procedures for many years; however, it has received relatively little attention in veterinary medicine. In 1989, Madison et al [22] described its use to repair cosmetic defects in three horses and a dog. Despite the success of those cases, little has been reported about this technique in the equine literature in the intervening years. This is surprising, because successful use of expanded skin to cover defects leads to more favorable cosmetic results than do grafting procedures. The primary disadvantage of tissue expansion compared with grafting techniques is the time it takes to achieve the desired expansion of skin and the necessity for two surgical procedures.

Skin has a tremendous capacity to expand over time, as evidenced by normal expansion during pregnancy, weight gain, or skin coverage over growing neoplasms. The epidermis of iatrogenically expanded skin remains of normal thickness, despite any increase in surface area. The dermis becomes thinner, with increasing numbers of fibroblasts. A capsule forms around implanted tissue expanders, with increased collagen synthesis in the dermis and capsule. There are minimal changes in skin appendages, such that the density of hair follicles only decreases slightly [23].

In planning tissue expansion, the surgeon must also consider the tissue that lies under the expander. Although not a major consideration in veterinary medicine, fat has low tolerance for the pressure of an expander, and any thinning of the fat layer is permanent. It is contraindicated to use tissue expanders over the skull until suture lines are mature, because a skull deformity can result [22].

Expansion devices are implanted adjacent to the defect to be covered, and the implantation incision is allowed to heal for approximately 12 to 14 days before initiation of expansion. Premature expansion, particularly in areas in which the skin is not particularly elastic, can result in incisional dehiscence and extrusion of the implant. A fine-gauge needle is used to fill the expander with saline. In human surgery, blanching of the skin or pain is an indication that too much saline has been injected, and some is removed. It is difficult to observe changes in skin color in many veterinary patients, however, and these patients also do not exhibit recognizable pain during normal expansion [22]. A potential solution is to measure transcutaneous oxygen tensions or use laser Doppler velocimetry to measure cutaneous blood flow during expansion, although this is rarely in the realm of equine practice.

Saline is added to the expander at regular intervals until the desired tissue expansion has occurred or the expander has reached its maximal limit. At that point, a second operation is performed to remove the expansion device and to create and advance the resulting skin flap over the defect. A capsule should have developed around the expander. This should not be removed, because its blood supply helps to support the overlying skin.

Complications of skin expanders include dehiscence of the initial incision for expander placement, infection of the initial surgical site, implant rupture, hematoma and skin ischemia, and subsequent necrosis over the expander.

The techniques described to this point are of classic or chronic tissue expansion. It is also possible to stretch skin more acutely. Presuturing takes advantage of a characteristic of skin known as stress relaxation [22–24]. If tension is applied by suturing across an area of skin and the length of the sutures remains constant, tension on the suture decreases with time. By presuturing a planned or existing wound 12 to 14 hours before surgery, it is possible to decrease the tension needed to close it significantly [24].

Acute or intraoperative tissue expansion is another technique to decrease tension on surgical wounds. In this method, a tissue expander is implanted and the surgical incision is temporarily closed. The tissue expander is filled until the overlying skin is under tension. The expander is drained 2 to 3 minutes later, and a 2- to 3-minute period of skin perfusion is allowed. The process is repeated for several cycles. Each time, it should be possible to inject more saline into the expander before similar resistance is felt [23]. The temporary sutures or towel clamps and the device are then removed, and the newly expanded skin is used to cover the defect.

Acute skin stretching can also be achieved using commercially available tensioning devices. A stretch-relaxation cycle similar to that described previously is also used with these devices. During periods of tension, blood flow decreases. The rest periods allow improved perfusion of skin between loads. Although skin that is not undermined returns to normal transcutaneous oxygen levels during the relaxation periods, skin that has been undermined does not, increasing the risk of necrosis of the skin edge [25].

An external skin-stretching device has been designed for use in small animal patients and may warrant further investigation in the horse [26]. Velcro squares are glued 5 to 10 cm away from the wound border with cyanoacrylate glue, and elastic bands are then attached to the latter in a shoelace pattern. The bands are placed under tension, which is gradually increased every 6 hours for a total of 72 to 96 hours. This technique may sufficiently attenuate tension so that extensive reconstructive procedures are avoided.

Skin substitutes

Numerous skin substitutes have been developed in the past 20 years, primarily for the human health care market. They can be divided into those with and without viable cells at the time of application.

Perhaps the most interesting of the acellular products are those derived from porcine small intestinal submucosa (PSIS). The PSIS is processed to lyse and remove all cellular components and is then sterilized. The PSIS has been shown to induce locally normal cell structure and to function when implanted in a number of different sites (vascular, urogenital, tendon, ligament, dura, and bone) [27]. The PSIS encourages rapid capillary ingrowth, increases resistance to infection, and does not induce adverse immunologic reactions. It has been used to treat a number of different wound types in people. Its effectiveness is thought to be a result, in part, of its content of glycosaminoglycans, proteoglycans, and growth factors, including fibroblast growth factor-1 and transforming growth factor-β [27].

Cellular skin substitute products were initially developed for application in human burn patients who do not have adequate skin for grafting; however, they are being applied much more frequently for chronic wounds (eg, venous leg ulcers, diabetic ulcers). It has been estimated that the cost of dressings alone to treat severe burns, diabetic ulcers, and venous leg ulcers is greater than $5 billion per year in the United States [28]. A number of different techniques have been reported for culturing autografts for application to patients with extensive skin loss. These consist of cultured keratinocytes, with or without a dermal component. Likewise, equine keratinocytes have been cultured successfully but not yet manufactured into grafts [29]. Although these procedures avoid the problem of rejection that occurs with allogenic skin substitutes, it can take weeks to produce a cultured sheet of autograft skin substitute.

Cultured allograft skin substitutes provide the advantage of an immediately available product. Because they are allografts, the patient does not undergo a procedure for harvesting the source material. There are a variety of products available. Most contain fibroblasts or keratinocytes that are derived from human neonatal foreskin and cultured in a collagen matrix. Bovine or porcine collagen is used in some products, whereas the cells are grown on a synthetic mesh in others, and they produce human collagen as well as other soluble mediators. Because collagen can be digested in wound fluid, some commercial products use cross-linked, partially protease-resistant, collagen in the matrix. Cocultured fibroblasts and keratinocytes produce cytokines and growth factors [28].

Use of allogenic skin substitutes can be thought of as application of biologically active bandages. Although the cells within the allogenic graft do not survive long term, they do provide a biologically superior wound environment compared with typical nonviable dressings and are thought to stimulate repair. The presence of dermal components also acts to prevent contraction, which can be important in select locations [28].

Skin substitutes take longer to vascularize than natural skin grafts because they do not contain any vascular structures when they are implanted. Genetic modification of keratinocytes used in synthetic products so that they overexpress growth factors, such as vascular endothelial growth factor, overcomes the delay in vascularization and improves survival of the transplanted keratinocytes [30,31].

Despite their successful applications in human medicine, there have been relatively few studies of skin substitutes in horses. When biologic materials have been applied to equine wounds, they have been used primarily as temporary bandages. Use of a bovine collagen membrane bandage showed no advantage when compared with traditional nonadherent dressings [32]. Similarly, a comparison of allogenic split-thickness skin, allogenic peritoneum, PSIS, and nonadherent dressings showed no advantage of the biologic dressings over traditional bandaging on equine limb wounds [33]. In contrast, when equine amnion was compared with nonadherent wound dressings in the postoperative management of pinch-grafted wounds, those bandaged with amnion had a significantly decreased mean healing time. There was no significant effect of the bandage on the percentage of grafts lost [34].

Certainly, the behavior of wounds on the limbs of horses differs from that of wounds elsewhere as well as differing in behavior from wounds in many other species. Further investigation is warranted to determine why skin substitutes do not seem to be as beneficial in horses as in people.

Summary

Although most equine wounds can be easily treated and heal without consequence, there are many that present special challenges. Skin grafts are a valuable part of the veterinarian's armamentarium for treatment of complicated wounds, particularly limb wounds. Attention to preparation of the recipient site and proper aftercare are critical to successful grafting. With better understanding of equine wound and graft physiology and the promise foretold by advances in human skin grafting, the outcome of treatments of difficult equine wounds should continue to improve in the future.

References

[1] Vacek JR, Honnas CM, Ford TS, et al. The principles of equine skin grafting. Vet Med 1992; 87:690–5.

[2] Vacek JR, Honnas CM, Ford TS, et al. Skin grafting techniques in horses. Vet Med 1992;87: 696–703.

[3] Lees MJ, Fretz PB, Bailey JV, et al. Principles of grafting. Compend Contin Educ Pract Vet 1989;1(8):954–61, 991.

[4] Caron JP. Skin grafting. In: Auer JA, Stick JA, editors. Equine surgery. 2nd edition. Philadelphia: WB Saunders; 1999. p. 152–66.

[5] Hinchcliff KW, MacDonald DR, Lindsay WA. Pedicle skin flaps in ponies: viable length is related to flap width. Equine Vet J 1992;24(1):26–9.

[6] Schumacher J, Brumbaugh GW, Honnas CM, et al. Kinetics of healing of grafted and non-grafted wounds on the distal portion of the forelimbs of horses. Am J Vet Res 1992;53(9): 1568–71.

[7] Ford TS, Schumacher J, Brumbaugh GW, et al. Effects of split-thickness and full-thickness grafts on secondary graft contraction in horses. Am J Vet Res 1992;53(9):1572–4.

[8] Lees MJ, Andrews GC, Bailey JV, et al. Tunnel grafting in equine wounds. Compend Contin Educ Pract Vet 1989;11(8):962–72.

[9] Schumacher J, Chambers M, Hanselka D, et al. Preservation of skin by refrigeration for autogenous grafting in the horse. Vet Surg 1987;16(5):358–61.

[10] Sterne GD, Titley OG, Christie JL. A qualitative histologic assessment of various storage conditions on short term preservation of human split skin grafts. Br J Plast Surg 2000;53(4): 331–6.

[11] Bravo D, Rigley TH, Gibran N, et al. Effect of storage and preservation methods on viability in transplantable human skin allografts. Burns 2000;26(4):367–78.

[12] Robb EC, Bechmann N, Plessinger RT, et al. Storage media and temperature maintain normal anatomy of cadaveric human skin for transplantation to full thickness skin wounds. J Burn Care Rehabil 2001;22(6):393–6.

[13] Peyton LC, Campbell ML, Wolf GA, et al. The use of random skin flaps in equine reconstructive surgery. Equine Vet Sci 1983;3(3):80–7.

[14] Gelman CL, Barroso EG, Britton CT, et al. The effects of lasers, electrocautery and sharp dissection on cutaneous flaps. Plast Reconstr Surg 1994;94:829–33.

[15] Bristol DG. The effect of tension on perfusion of axial and random pattern flaps in foals. Vet Surg 1992;21(3):223–7.

[16] Lees MJ, Bowen CV, Fretz PB, et al. Identification of a free skin flap from the region vascularized by the deep circumflex iliac artery of horses. Am J Vet Res 1990;51(5):796–9.

[17] Lees MJ, Bowen CV, Fretz PB, et al. Transfer of deep circumflex iliac flaps to the tarsus by microvascular anastomosis in the horse. Vet Surg 1989;18(4):292–9.

[18] Miller CW, Hurtig H. Identification and transfer of free cutaneous flaps by microvascular anastomosis in the pony. Vet Comp Orthop Traumatol 1989;1:21–4.

[19] Bristol DG, Hudson LC, Spaulding KA. The use of a barium/gelatin mixture to study equine vasculature with potential application to free flap transfer. Vet Radiol 1991;32:196–205.

[20] Smyth GB, Brown RG, Juzwiak JS, et al. Delayed repair of an extensive lip laceration in a colt using an Estlander flap. Vet Surg 1988;17(6):350–2.

[21] Scott WM, Fowler JD, Matte G, et al. Effect of ischemia and reperfusion on neutrophil accumulation in equine microvascular tissue flaps. Vet Surg 1999;28(3):180–7.

[22] Madison JB, Donawick WJ, Johnston DE, et al. The use of skin expansion to repair cosmetic defects in animals. Vet Surg 1989;18(1):15–21.

[23] Davis-Boute W, Taherpour SR, Moy RL, et al. Tissue expansion. In: Lask GP, Moy RL, editors. Principles and techniques of cutaneous surgery. New York: McGraw-Hill; 1996. p. 605–17.

[24] Liang MD. Presuturing: a new technique for closing large cutaneous defects: clinical and experimental studies. Plast Reconstr Surg 1988;81:694–702.

[25] Melis P, Noorlander ML, van der Kleig AJ, et al. Oxygenation and microcirculation during skin stretching in undermined and nonundermined skin. Plast Reconstr Surg 2003;112: 1295–301.

[26] Pavletic MM. Use of an external skin-stretching device for wound closure in dogs and cats. J Am Vet Med Assoc 2000;217:350–4.
[27] Brown-Etris M, Cutshall WD, Hiles MC. A new biomaterial derived from small intestinal submucosa and developed into a wound matrix device. Wounds 2002;14(4):150–66.
[28] Eisenbud D, Huang NF, Luke S, et al. Skin substitutes and wound healing: current status and challenges. Wounds 2004;16(1):2–17.
[29] Dahm AM, de Bruin A, Linat A, et al. Cultivation and characterization of primary and subcultured equine keratinocytes. Equine Vet J 2002;34(2):114–20.
[30] Supp DM, Supp AP, Bell SM, et al. Enhanced vascularization of cultured skin substitutes genetically modified to overexpress vascular endothelial growth factor. J Invest Dermatol 2000;114(1):5–13.
[31] Supp DM, Boyce ST. Overexpression of vascular endothelial growth factor accelerates early vascularization and improves healing of genetically modified cultured skin substitutes. J Burn Care Rehabil 2002;23(1):10–20.
[32] Yvorchuk-St. Jean K, Gauhan E, St. Jean G, et al. Evaluation of a porous bovine collagen membrane bandage for management of wounds in horses. Am J Vet Res 1995;56(12):1663–7.
[33] Gomez JH, Schumacher J, Lauten SD, et al. Effects of 3 biologic dressings on healing of cutaneous wounds on the limbs of horses. Can J Vet Res 2004;68:49–55.
[34] Goodrich LR, Moll HD, Crisman MV, et al. Comparison of equine amnion and a nonadherent wound dressing material for bandaging pinch grafted wounds in ponies. Am J Vet Res 2000;61(3):326–9.

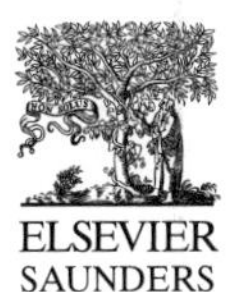
ELSEVIER
SAUNDERS

Vet Clin Equine 21 (2005) 145–165

VETERINARY
CLINICS
Equine Practice

Wounds of the Distal Limb Complicated by Involvement of Deep Structures

Henry Jann, DVM, MS[a,*], Chris Pasquini, DVM, MS[b]

[a]*Oklahoma State University, College of Veterinary Medicine, 002 Boren Veterinary Teaching Hospital, Stillwater, Oklahoma 74078, USA*
[b]*St. George's University, St. George, Grenada, West Indies*

Any wound of the lower limb has the potential of being career or even life threatening. This is because the musculoskeletal soft tissue structures (ie, tendons, ligaments, synovial cavities) that are so important to limb function and weight bearing are extremely susceptible to traumatic injury. When the speed and strength of the horse are considered, it is not unreasonable to assume that deeper structures may become involved on impact. Rapid and accurate recognition of damage to deep structures is mandatory for appropriate case management and a favorable prognosis for return to function. This article describes the location of critical musculoskeletal soft tissue components, the physiology of tendon and ligament healing, diagnostic techniques to verify deep structure involvement, current treatment options, and future perspectives that explore new treatment protocols.

Anatomy

To understand and treat wounds of the lower limb, the anatomy of the area must be understood. This section outlines the structures making up the distal limb, using the forelimb as the model. The distal hind limb is similar, except for the use of different terms (ie, metatarsal instead of metacarpal, plantar instead of palmar).

The superficial digital flexor (SDF) muscle flexes the carpus and the digital joints, except the distal interdigital (coffin) joint. The tendon of the SDF muscle passes through the carpal canal in a common synovial sheath with the deep digital flexor tendon (DDFT). In the metacarpal and/or metatarsal (cannon) region in all limbs, the superficial digital flexor

* Corresponding author.
E-mail address: jann@okstate.edu (H. Jann).

0749-0739/05/$ - see front matter
doi:10.1016/j.cveq.2004.11.008 ***vetequine.theclinics.com***

tendon (SDFT) flattens out, capping the DDFT superficially. At the metacarpophalangeal (MP) and/or metatarsophalangeal joint (fetlock), it widens and forms a ring (manica flexoria) through which the DDFT passes. In the digit, the SDFT divides into two branches that diverge to their insertions. The DDFT emerges between these two branches. Each branch inserts on either side of the pastern joint (the distal end of the proximal phalanx and the proximal end of the middle phalanx). These four insertions may prevent "dorsal buckling" (hyperflexion) of the proximal interphalangeal joint. The SDFT and DDFT share a common synovial sheath as they cross the palmar side of the proximal sesamoid bones (fetlock).

The deep digital flexor (DDF) muscle (flexor digitorum profundus) flexes the carpus and all the digital joints. Its tendon passes distally in the cannon region deep to the SDFT, receiving the accessory check ligament in the middle of the cannon region. The DDFT passes through the sleeve (manica flexoria) formed by the SDFT in the fetlock region. It then passes over the distal sesamoidean ligaments and the navicular bone before fanning out to insert on the semilunar line of the distal phalanx. The DDFT and SDFT share digital synovial sheathes through the carpal canal and over the fetlock and digit. The navicular bursa is situated between the DDFT and the navicular bone.

The proximal common tendon sheath (carpal flexor tendon sheath) encloses the SDFT and DDFT as they pass through the carpal canal deep to the flexor retinaculum. It extends 3 to 4 inches distal to the carpus to the middle of the metacarpus.

Other synovial sheaths of the carpus invest the tendons of the extensor carpi radialis, common digital extensor, lateral digital extensor, oblique carpal extensor, long tendon of the ulnaris lateralis, and flexor carpi radialis muscles (Fig. 1).

The digital synovial sheath (ie, distal common tendon sheath, fetlock flexor tendon sheath) is a combined synovial structure around the SDFT and DDFT as they pass over the MP and/or metatarsophalangeal joint (fetlock). It extends from the distal fourth of the cannon region to the middle of the middle phalanx. Lubricating the tendons over the fetlock, it facilitates their movement against each other.

The palmar annular ligament anchors the two flexor tendons as they pass over the fetlock. It is the thickening of the deep fascia over the flexor surface of the fetlock holding down the digital flexor tendons and their synovial sheaths in the groove of the sesamoid bones.

The common digital extensor muscle in the front limb or the long digital extensor muscle in the pelvic limb passes on the dorsal surface of the distal limb across the digital joints to insert on the extensor process of the distal phalanx (coffin bone; Fig. 2).

The suspensory ligament (SL) or interosseous (medius) muscle is the tendinous structure lying in the metacarpal groove that attaches to the

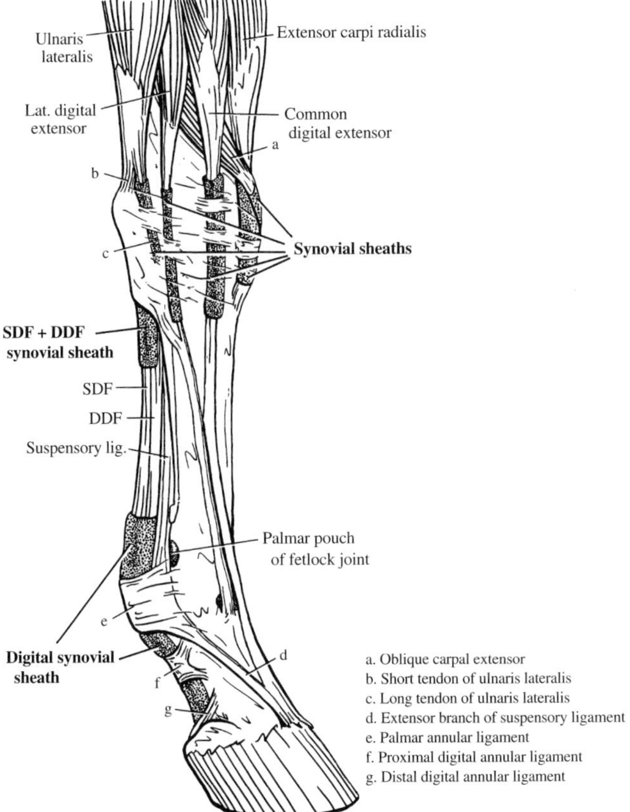

Fig. 1. Lateral view of synovial structures of the carpus and digit. (*Courtesy of* Chris Pasquini, DVM, MS, St. George's University, St. George, Grenada, West Indies.)

proximal sesamoid bones. Together with the sesamoid bones and the distal sesamoidean ligaments, it forms the suspensory apparatus that supports the fetlock. The origin of the SL is located at the proximal palmar end of the cannon bone and the distal row of the carpal bones. The body of the SL extends distally in the metacarpal groove and then splits into two branches in the distal fourth of the metacarpus. The branches of the SL attach on the abaxial side of the corresponding sesamoid bone and send two extensor branches to the common digital extensor tendon.

The suspensory apparatus consists of the SL, the proximal sesamoid bones, and the distal sesamoidean ligaments. Together, they act as a unit to support the fetlock joint (preventing excessive dorsal flexion). Disruption in any one of the three components results in the fetlock sinking. The distal sesamoidean ligaments of the proximal sesamoid bones, or "X, Y, and V" ligaments (the cruciate, the straight sesamoidean, and the oblique

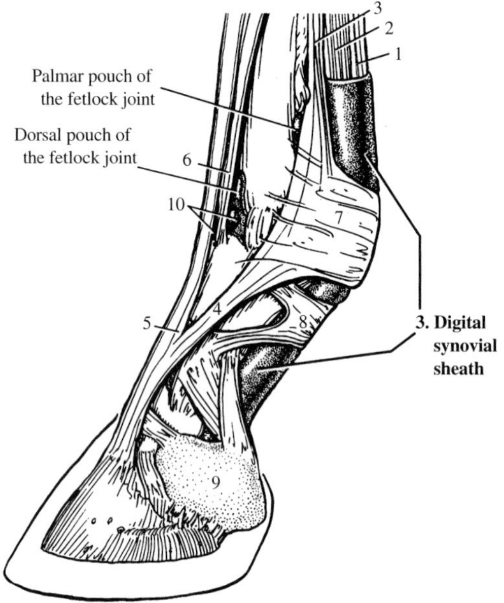

1. Superficial digital flexor (SDF) tendon
2. Deep digital flexor tendon (DDF) tendon
3. Suspensory ligament
4. Extensor branch of suspensory ligament
5. Common digital extensor tendon
6. Lateral digital extensor tendon
7. Palmar annular ligament
8. Proximal digital annular ligament
9. Cartilage of the hoof
10. Bursae for common & lateral digital extensor muscles

Fig. 2. Lateral view of the digit showing the digital tendon sheath and surrounding ligaments. (*Courtesy of* Chris Pasquini, DVM, MS, St. George's University, St. George, Grenada, West Indies.)

sesamoidean ligaments, respectively), are the three ligaments that anchor the sesamoid bones distally to the proximal and middle phalanges. They are part of the suspensory apparatus and the stay apparatus, counteracting the pull of the SL (Fig. 3).

Tendon and ligament healing

Our knowledge of how tendons and ligaments heal is constantly expanding and is still controversial at this juncture. The currently accepted models of tendon healing are based on intrinsic and extrinsic patterns of cellular response. The intrinsic pattern of tendon healing is characterized by an initial inflammatory phase, which initiates a proliferative phase in which a cellular response from the epitenon and endotenon results in migration of macrophage-like cells and fibroblasts. Cellular proliferation thus leads to bridging of tendon ends. This bridge is rapidly fortified during the remodeling phase when newly synthesized collagen is realigned in response

JOINTS - DIGITS

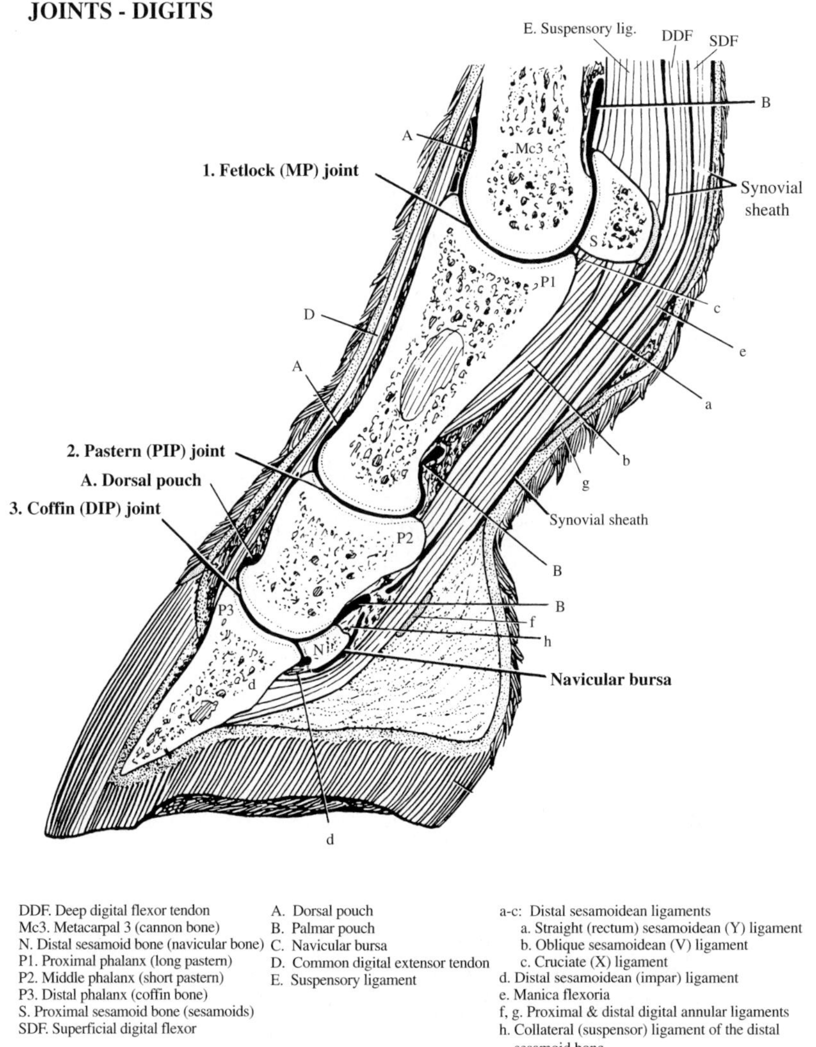

Fig. 3. Parasagittal section of the digit demonstrating tendons and ligaments. (*Courtesy of* Chris Pasquini, DVM, MS, St. George's University, St. George, Grenada, West Indies.)

to stress. The time frame for each of these processes is days, weeks, and months. The extrinsic pattern of healing occurs when tendons are injured within the confines of a synovial sheath and there is significant injury to the sheath itself. Under these conditions, the tendon sheath actually serves as the source of cells for the repair process. This is especially true when the tendon is immobilized within the sheath, such as during periods of external coaptation after tendon repair. This form of healing may lead to restrictive adhesions between the tendon sheath and injured tendon, which can be modulated by passive motion and minimizing damage to the sheath [1,2].

Ligament healing follows roughly the same pattern as tendon healing, although the extrinsic and intrinsic patterns have not been as clearly defined. Ligaments are responsive to exercise for maintenance of normal strength. This is clinically important in postoperative situations, where immobilized ligaments are significantly weaker than nonimmobilized ligaments [3–5].

Diagnosis

When examining a wound to the distal limb that has the potential of penetrating or compromising deep structures, it may be relatively easy to determine which structures are implicated, although this can be more challenging at other times. When tendons are compromised, there is an alteration in limb conformation during ambulation or on weight bearing. When flexor tendons have been compromised, there is always a certain degree of hyperextension of the digit. If the SDFT has been divided, the MP joint adopts a hyperextended attitude. In more simplistic terms, the fetlock drops when the limb is loaded (Fig. 4). If the SDFT and the DDFT have been compromised, the MP and the distal interphalangeal (DIP) joints hyperextend on weight bearing. This has the classic appearance of the dropped fetlock and the elevated toe (the toe comes off the ground when the limb is loaded; Fig. 5). When the SDFT, DDFT, and SL are involved, the MP joint is extremely hyperextended on weight bearing to the extent that its palmar (plantar) aspect actually makes contact with the ground surface. The toe is also raised off the ground because of hyperextension of the DIP joint [6,7]. When the common digital extensor tendon of the forelimb or the

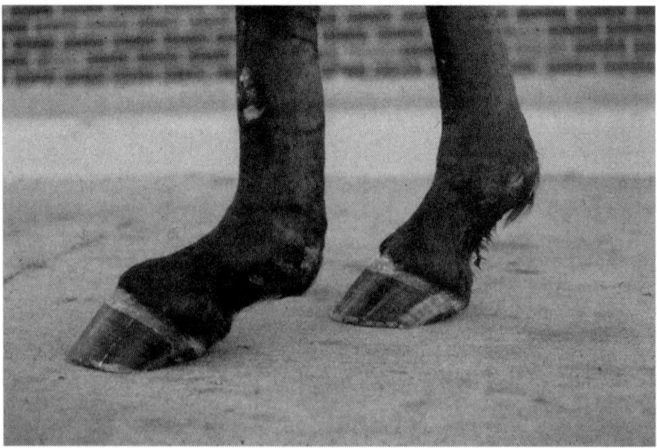

Fig. 4. Typical conformational change when the superficial digital flexor tendon is compromised. Note the hyperextended metacarpophalangeal joint (ie, dropped fetlock).

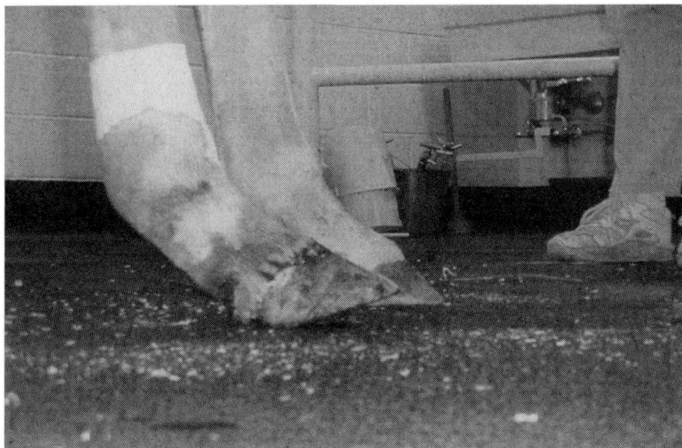

Fig. 5. Typical conformational change when the superficial digital flexor tendon and the deep digital flexor tendon are compromised. Note the hyperextension of the metacarpophalangeal and distal interphalangeal joints (ie, the fetlock is dropped and the toe is elevated on weight bearing).

long digital extensor tendon of the pelvic limb has been divided, the MP or metatarsophalangeal joint adopts an attitude of flexion when the limb is advanced. In more simplistic terms, the fetlock knuckles as the limb moves forward [8]. These changes in conformation are consistent, and they can be relied on for categorization of compromise to a specific tendon or tendon group. In cases in which tendons are only partially divided, a more accurate diagnosis can be obtained by exploring the wound in the conscious horse or after administering general anesthesia. In nonsheathed areas, the extent of damage and contamination can be determined during debridement of the wound (Fig. 6). In areas in which the tendons are surrounded by a sheath, the wound can be evaluated tenoscopically [9–12]. Distention of the tendon

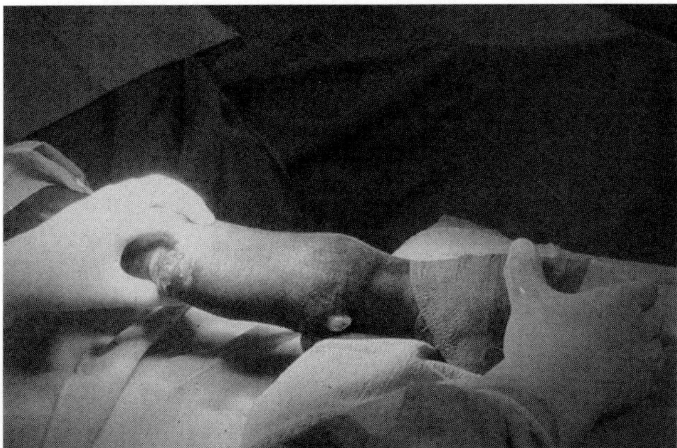

Fig. 6. Digital exploration of the wound before debridement. The digit is being flexed and extended to aid in evaluation of flexor tendon integrity.

sheath and insertion of the arthroscope are accomplished via the cul-de-sac region on the palmar or plantar surface of the tendon sheath 1 to 2 cm palmar or plantar to the digital neurovascular structures and between the annular ligament and proximal digital annular ligament. This technique provides excellent visualization of most surfaces of the digital flexor tendons and surrounding sheath while causing minimal trauma to the latter. Although tenoscopy is recommended in all wounds involving the digital sheath of the flexor tendons, it provides no information on deeper tendon architecture.

Treatment: nonsheathed flexor zones

Once an appropriate diagnosis has been established, the patient is best sent to a surgical referral facility for definitive treatment. The treatment of tendon lacerations is arguably one of the most challenging endeavors that a surgeon is confronted with. The importance of thorough case management cannot be overly emphasized. This is a multistep process with the ultimate goal of regaining maximal function; all steps are important and are thus discussed individually.

Immobilization of the limb

Immobilization of the limb is absolutely imperative to minimize further damage to the already dysfunctional limb and must be performed before transporting the horse. The Kimzey Leg Saver (Kimzey, Woodland, CA) is the most effective and quickest way to achieve immobilization of the distal limb (Fig. 7). If this device is not available, braces can be constructed with polyvinyl chloride (PVC) pipe (Fig. 8). This material is readily shaped with the application of heat from a butane torch so that it conforms to the limb.

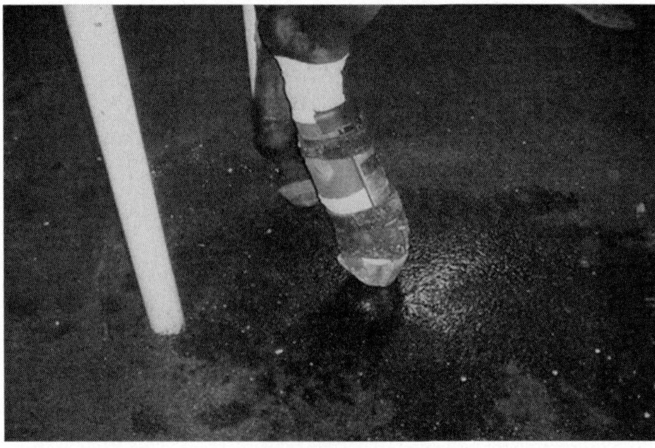

Fig. 7. Kimzey leg brace, which immobilizes the digit in an attitude of partial flexion.

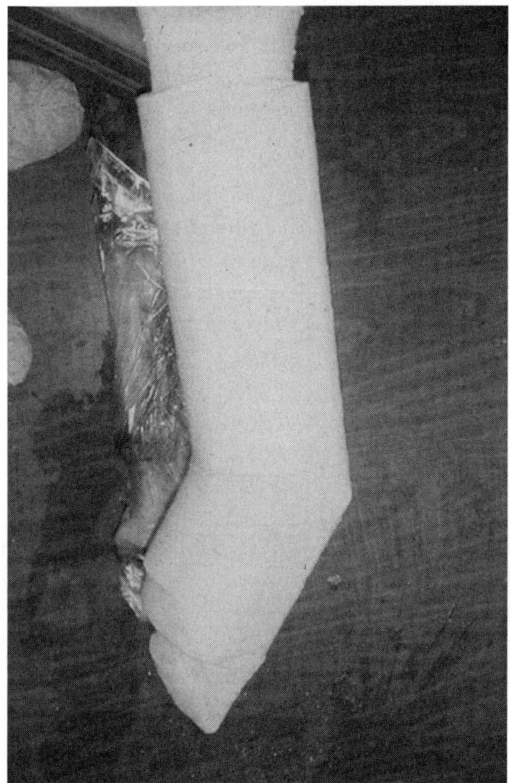

Fig. 8. Polyvinyl chloride pipe splint used to immobilize the digit in an attitude of partial flexion.

Typically, the limb is splinted in an attitude of partial flexion to decrease stress on the tendons.

Systemic treatment

With any tendon laceration, the potential for severe hemorrhage is always present. This is because of the proximity of major arteries to the flexor tendons and their relatively superficial location. Pale mucous membranes and a rapid pulse are indicative of hypovolemia, and intravenous fluids are indicated. Chemical restraint should also be kept to a minimum. Active hemorrhage can be controlled with pressure bandaging. It is not advisable to anesthetize these patients until they have been stabilized. Systemic antibiotics are indicated because of the typically contaminated nature of these wounds.

General anesthesia

Although initial treatment in the form of irrigation, rough wound debridement, and vessel ligation can be performed with regional anesthesia in the conscious horse, general anesthesia is required before definitive treatment of a tendon laceration. It is usually the authors' preference to initiate treatment using general anesthesia provided that the patient is stable. This expedites definitive treatment.

Wound debridement

This stage of tendon repair cannot be overemphasized. In fact, it would be appropriate to say that debridement is the *sine qua non* for successful repair of traumatic tendon lacerations. At this stage of treatment, the surgeon should focus not just on the tendon but on the entire wound. The typical presentation of these injuries is that of a highly contaminated wound with extensive devitalized tissue. The tissue that often seems grossly to be the most contaminated is the paratenon, and it must be debrided meticulously. The tendon ends themselves should also be debrided. The amount of tendon to be excised is determined by the gross appearance of the tendon ends. Any badly frayed, avascular, or contaminated areas must be removed. It is ideal for the ends of the tendon to demonstrate active hemorrhage before apposition with suture material. Any devitalized or compromised subcutaneous tissues and skin margins should also be debrided. When debridement is complete, all tissues should demonstrate active hemorrhage and be free of foreign contamination. Hemostasis is important to minimize postoperative hematoma formation.

Wound irrigation

No matter how meticulous the debridement process has been, there is still microscopic foreign debris remaining in the wound. Irrigation is thus essential to remove these remaining sources of infection. The irrigation solution shown to be bactericidal but minimally irritating to tissues and inhibitory to neutrophil migration is a 0.1% povidone-iodine and lactated Ringer's solution [12–15]. Large volumes of irrigation (2–3 L) are recommended along with active suction to mechanically remove gross and microscopic debris.

Tenorrhaphy

Primary repair of flexor tendons in the nonsheathed zone has been advocated for the past 2.5 decades [16–26]. The overall consensus is that suturing tendons is superior to a nonsutured treatment technique. The three goals of tendon repair are to minimize gap formation, minimize adhesion formation, and create minimal interference to the intrinsic vasculature of the tendon. In equine tendon repair, the compound locking loop and the three-loop pulley suture patterns have been shown to produce the strongest repair. The three-loop pulley pattern is the most resistant to gap formation. This is probably a result of its dynamic action of applying tension at the tenorrhaphy site as the ends of the tendon are being distracted. The other advantages of the three-loop pulley pattern include ease of placement, minimal amount of suture material in the wound, minimal crimping and distortion of tendon ends, and minimal disruption of the intrinsic vascularity of the tendon (Fig. 9) [27–29]. Nonabsorbable and absorbable suture material has been used for equine tendon repair. A study in chickens showed no statistical difference in breaking strength of tenorrhaphies that used absorbable or nonabsorbable suture material at 4 or 8 weeks [30]. Monofilament absorbable suture is probably the most desirable because it circumvents the possibility of suture sinus formation after implantation in a potentially contaminated wound [31]. Polydioxanone (PDS; Ethicon, Somerville, NJ) and polyglyconate (Maxon; Sherwood-Davis and Geck, St. Louis, MO) retain sufficient tensile strength for 4 weeks, which makes them appropriate for tenorrhaphy [32,33]. Four weeks is the time when tenorrhaphy scars begin to gain sufficient breaking strength to maintain apposition of tendon ends [22].

Wound closure

Every effort should be made to close the wound primarily. The tissue that is particularly important is the paratenon. This tissue layer should be meticulously closed over the actual tenorrhaphy site. This step is important because the paratenon provides the cells from which the tendon scar is formed. Closure of the paratenon also prevents the tendon ends from adhering to the subcutaneous tissues and the skin. The subcutaneous tissue and the skin should be closed in separate layers. This allows maximal covering of the tenorrhaphy site and maximizes the chances of primary wound healing. Primary wound healing is important to achieve whenever possible because it precludes the formation of excessive granulation tissue and maximizes the overall function of the limb.

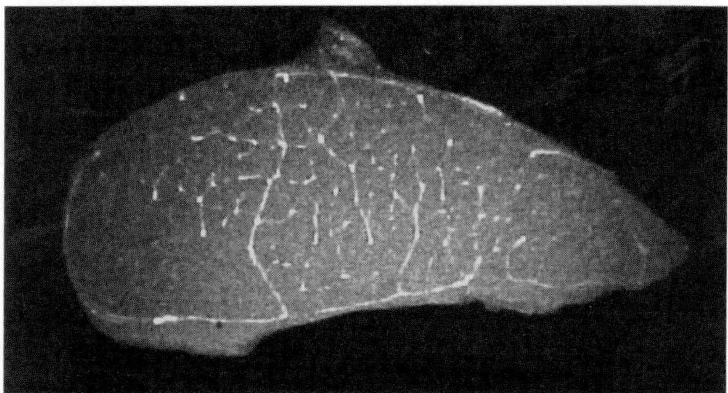

Fig. 9. Microangiogram of the superficial digital flexor tendon demonstrating the intrinsic vasculature, which the surgeon should try to maintain. (Courtesy of C. Crowson, DVM, Allison Park, PA.)

Post-tenorrhaphy immobilization of the limb

After surgery, the limb that was operated on should be immobilized for several weeks to allow the tenorrhaphy scar to gain sufficient strength before physiologic tensile forces are applied to it. Forelimb flexor tendon repairs can be immobilized in a fiberglass cast that extends from the proximal metacarpal region to and inclusive of the hoof. It is advisable to cast the limb in slight flexion (the long axis of the digit and metacarpus are parallel) to help maintain tendon apposition. Pelvic limb lacerations should be immobilized with the metatarsophalangeal joint in partial flexion. This is easily accomplished with the Kimzey leg brace or a PVC splint. This practice is important because tarsal flexion produces significant strain on the superficial flexor tendon, which can be extremely detrimental to a successful tenorrhaphy. The actual time required for external immobilization is somewhat controversial. Time requirements of 4, 6, and 12 weeks have been recommended. In the authors' opinion, the time of rigid immobilization should be kept to a minimum. This is because the overall process of external coaptation is not without complication (ie, cast sores, ligament laxity, cartilage degeneration). Also, early controlled stress results in more rapid scar remodeling and thus earlier restoration of function. Cases differ somewhat, but as a general rule, 4 weeks of external coaptation is considered a minimum. Periods of external immobilization exceeding 6 weeks are counterproductive. Scar remodeling requires several months; during this time, stall confinement is recommended. A heel extension shoe is required for several months after cast removal in cases involving the DDFT (Fig. 10) [26].

Post-tenorrhaphy ultrasonographic assessment of healing

Sequential ultrasonographic examination of a healing tendon provides objective information on the size of the tenorrhaphy gap and the degree of remodeling of scar tissue. The level of exercise must be regulated in the months after tendon repair, and ultrasound provides a means to recommend the advancement in the level of naturally occurring stress to which the repair site should be exposed [21,22,34]. Advancement from stall confinement, hand walking, small paddock turnout, and ponying to controlled ridden exercise comprises an appropriate rehabilitation protocol after tendon repair [26].

Prognosis

As a general rule, the overall prognosis for flexor tendon lacerations is favorable [35,36]. This statement is well substantiated in the literature; however, any discussion of prognosis is predicated on the quality of medical, surgical, and convalescent care. This, in turn, is dependent on the financial commitment of the owner and the temperament and intended use of the

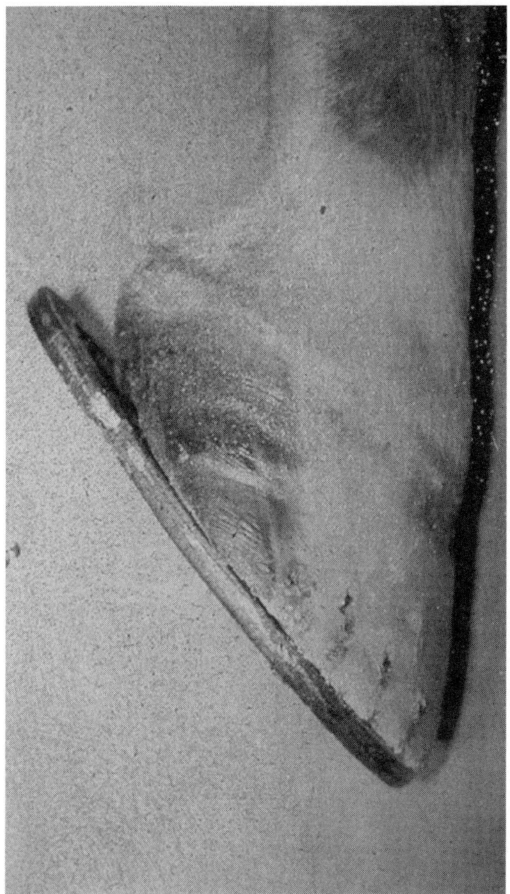

Fig. 10. Heel extension shoe required for 3 to 4 months after cast removal in cases of deep digital flexor tendon laceration.

injured animal. Owners must be informed of the cost of surgical treatment and the length of rehabilitation. They should also be informed that the overall prognosis can be favorable with appropriate patient management.

Treatment: sheathed flexor zones

Tendon lacerations that occur in the sheathed zones are more problematic than those that occur in the nonsheathed zones. The primary complicating factor in these regions is the potential development of septic tenosynovitis [37–39]. This is at best a career-threatening, and potentially a life-threatening, sequela to any traumatic wound involving a tendon sheath. In horses, any tendon laceration in the palmar and/or plantar aspect of the fetlock or pastern area automatically invades the tendon sheath, because the tendons are contained within sheaths in these anatomic zones. These areas are also the ones that are commonly traumatized. One recent report lists the digital sheath as the most commonly contaminated and infected synovial structure [12]. The primary goal of treatment is to prevent or treat septic tenosynovitis. This is an area where tenoscopy is useful not only to visualize the intrasynovial (intrathecal) portion of the tendon but to act as a conduit for lavage solutions. Tenoscopy allows excellent visualization of the sheath and is thus useful for locating any foreign material that may have been introduced into the tendon sheath at the time of injury [9–12]. After thorough tenoscopic lavage, it is important to place an ingress portal for postoperative lavage [26,37–39].

The most efficacious way to allow ingress of lavage fluids is via a fenestrated polyethylene tube inserted in the sheath from a proximal to distal direction using arthroscopic (tenoscopic) instrumentation (Fig. 11A). The tube is introduced at the most proximal portion of the digital sheath, allowing the entire sheath to be lavaged (see Fig. 11B). The initial wound should not be used as an ingress portal until complete debridement has been performed; however, it can be used as an effective egress portal, although other portals can also be created. Lavage is performed in the conscious horse for several consecutive days after the initial surgical debridement. The lavage system usually remains patent for several days and is removed when no longer functional [26].

Additional treatment steps for septic tenosynovitis are similar to those used for any other synovial cavity. These include systemic antibiotics, regional antibiotic perfusion, pre- and postoperative bacteriologic culture and/or sensitivity assays, synovial cytologic assessment, bandaging, external support (splinting), a heel extension shoe, and sequential radiographic and ultrasonographic evaluations [26,37–41].

A recent study has not been supportive of tenorrhaphy within the digital sheath. When tenorrhaphy was performed under ideal conditions, it was not possible to prevent a postoperative gap (5 cm) or adhesion formation between the DDFT and SDFT. The exact reason for this is not completely understood but possibly relates to biomechanical and physiologic influences unique to this anatomic region. All horses in this study were significantly lame at 6 months after surgery [42].

Prognosis

Wounds that involve the tendon sheaths can be successfully treated, and the prognosis can be favorable [37–40]. This has been clearly documented in the literature. What should be emphasized is the necessity of treating these injuries as being career and life threatening. This fact must be stressed from the onset of treatment, and a high level of compliance and financial commitment by the owner is essential for a favorable prognosis.

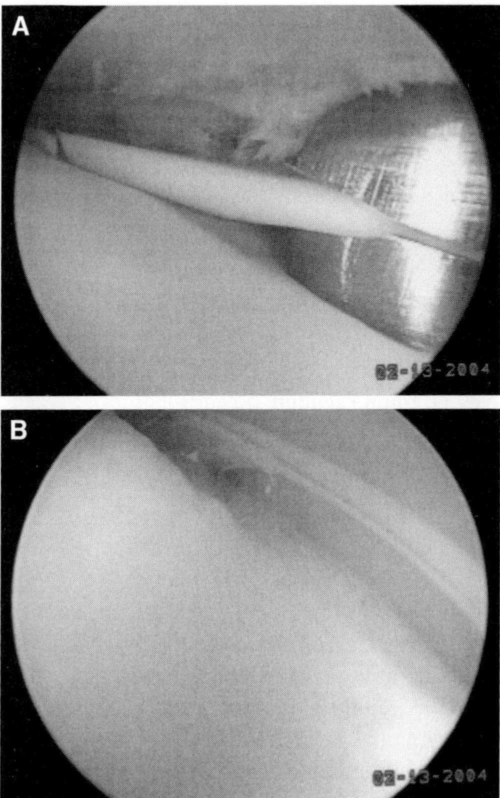

Fig. 11. (*A*) A polyethylene tube being placed in the digital sheath tenoscopically. The drain is being pulled into the sheath from a proximal to distal direction using an arthroscopic grasping instrument. (*B*) A polyethylene drain is placed in the digital sheath.

Treatment: extensor tendons

Nonsheathed zones

Lacerations that occur below the carpus or tarsus require little more than wound debridement and immobilization. Tenorrhaphy is recommended when feasible. Lacerated tendon ends are often separated to the extent that tenorrhaphy is not really possible. These injuries usually require external coaptation in the form of a cast or splint for 4 to 6 weeks. Scar tissue forms, which is gradually remodeled to function as a bridge between the tendon ends [24,26].

Sheathed zones

When injury occurs to the tendons over the dorsal aspect of the carpus or hock, there is the potential for development of septic tenosynovitis. This condition is treated in a similar manner to that of the flexor tendons (ie, debridement, lavage, possible postoperative drainage). In chronic cases, synovial resection has been used effectively [43]. If this latter approach fails and sepsis persists, removal of the intrathecal component of the common digital extensor tendon and ablation of the sheath lining has been shown to be effective and to allow a return to long-term soundness without gait abnormalities [44].

Prognosis

The prognosis for extensor tendon lacerations in the nonsheathed [8] and sheathed zones is generally favorable [43].

Future perspectives of equine tendon surgery

There are three major areas of research interest in equine tendon surgery: tendon grafting [45,46], bioabsorbable implants [47], and growth factors [48]. Tendon grafting in horses is technically feasible, and investigative reports have been encouraging with regard to the clinical efficacy of autologous grafts. The procedure affords a sixfold increase in strength early in the postoperative period [46]. Bioabsorbable implants represent an area that has not been investigated extensively but clearly shows promise according to one report in which the technique was used clinically [47]. This technique would be more simplistic from a technical aspect than autologous grafting, but biomechanical data have not yet been reported. The use of growth factors is another intriguing area that has some potential clinical application. A recent in vitro study has demonstrated increased migration of tenoblasts on absorbable suture material after exposure to epidermal growth factor [48]. The potentially beneficial effects of this are that increased migration could produce stronger repair at earlier postoperative times. This could circumvent prolonged periods of external coaptation and thus minimize the potential for adhesion formation.

Wounds involving the suspensory ligament

When a laceration is severe (deep) enough to compromise the SL, it also involves the SDFT and DDFT. In these situations, the neurovascular components of the metacarpal (metatarsal) region are almost always compromised. Even if the blood supply to the distal limb has not been totally compromised by the actual wound, it can be disrupted by overstretching because of loss of support to the fetlock joint. The digital arteries can also be compromised by blunt trauma to the palmar (plantar) aspect of the fetlock joint as a result of hyperextension. It is these neurovascular structures that must be carefully evaluated before treatment is initiated or a prognosis is given. In rare instances, there is sufficient blood supply to the distal limb to initiate treatment. All the principles of tendon repair that have been discussed apply to these situations, with the exception of a more prolonged period of external coaptation and external support devices. The Kimzey Leg Saver is particularly useful because it immobilizes the leg in partial flexion and can be removed easily to change bandages and padding, which is a necessary part of treatment. The time frame for external coaptation is 6 months to 1 year, and the prognosis is grave for any athletic purpose and guarded for breeding purposes [49].

Wounds involving the distal sesamoidean ligaments and the annular ligaments

Any wound severe enough to involve the distal sesamoidean ligaments also damages many of the structures mentioned previously. The most notable structures include the annular ligaments, digital tendon sheath, and flexor tendons themselves. Surgical repair of the distal sesamoidean ligaments has not been reported. The annular ligaments can be repaired, but the avoidance of septic tenosynovitis is clearly the factor that has the most impact on prognosis. To this end, it may be advisable not to be overzealous in the use of suture craft. What is important is to provide adequate drainage, because these wounds usually have extensive soft tissue damage and devitalized tissue. Primary closure may not be possible after debridement, and excess tension on the ligament could result in constriction of the flexor tendons and subsequent pain (ie, lameness). In fact, modified open desmotomy of the annular ligament has been advocated for treatment of septic tenosynovitis. In these cases, the annular ligament is not sutured after desmotomy and the wounds are left partially open distally to allow for drainage from the digital sheath [50].

Wounds involving the distal joints

Any significant traumatic wound of the distal limb that is in close proximity to a joint should be treated as if the joint were invaded until proven otherwise. There are several excellent descriptions of diagnostic techniques and treatment modalities for septic arthritis in horses [51–55]. Septic arthritis is a condition that should be avoided at all costs; the old adage "an ounce of prevention is worth a pound of cure" is perfectly applicable to the correlation of wounds of the distal limb to the potential for septic arthritis in one of the distal diarthrodial joints, particularly the fetlock, tarsus, and carpus. The severity of joint contamination and/or infection is primarily influenced by the rapidity and aggressiveness of treatment. To this end, these injuries are best approached in a stepwise fashion to ensure appropriate treatment:

1. Inspection: horses with acute injuries often show little or no lameness. This can give the owner and the attending veterinarian a false sense of

security regarding the potential for deep structure involvement. The wound must be thoroughly inspected visually and digitally; sedation may be required to this end. Before any digital inspection, the wound margins should be thoroughly cleansed and surgically prepared. This practice prevents further contamination of the deeper aspects of the wound and is particularly important if a synovial structure is thought to be involved. Digital exploration can be informative but is not always foolproof in detecting small perforations of the joint capsule. The simplest way to detect minor penetration of a joint is to assess its permeability. An area remote from the wound (ie, on the side of the joint opposite the wound) must be surgically prepared, through which sterile saline can then be injected intra-articularly with sufficient pressure to distend the joint fully. Any leakage in or around the wound confirms compromise of the integrity of the joint capsule. At this juncture, the problem changes from a simple laceration into a career- or life-threatening situation that must be conveyed to the client in no uncertain terms. The important aspect that must be conveyed is that the prognosis of wounds of this type is highly influenced by the rapidity of initiation of treatment. The prognosis has been documented at greater than 85% for survival and 50% for return to full function if appropriate treatment is initiated within 24 hours after the injury occurs [39,40]. A frustrating situation arises when the wound is several days old and an active cellulitis is present. In this situation, there is no safe place to penetrate the joint capsule without risking iatrogenic contamination. Systemic treatment (antibiotic therapy) of the cellulitis should precede any procedures that invade the joint. In these instances, arthrocentesis should be avoided until the cellulitis has been effectively treated. Plain radiography may be useful to check for gas accumulation in the joint space or a soft tissue deficit extending into an adjacent joint space.

2. Antimicrobial therapy: whenever joint involvement is suspected, broad-spectrum antibiotics should be started immediately. As with any rational antimicrobial therapeutic regimen, the choice of drugs should be predicated on serial culture and sensitivity results as well as on clinical response. The actual duration of therapy has been recommended to be 3 to 6 weeks and to be prolonged for 2 weeks after clinical signs have resolved [39]. Intravenous regional perfusion is advocated as an adjunct to systemic treatment in refractory cases [41]. Systemic analgesia is provided with phenylbutazone, which is administered in the smallest dose that keeps the patient comfortable. This usually requires a minimum of 2.2 mg/kg administered orally or intravenously every 12 hours.
3. Joint lavage: once joint involvement has been established, it is imperative to perform some form of joint lavage. Although joint lavage can be performed in the sedated horse under field conditions, the most efficacious way to achieve thorough joint lavage is via arthroscopy. General anesthesia is required, and the patient is referred to a surgical

facility. The same principles discussed for tendon sheath lavage apply to joint lavage. Copious fluids are used, and the wound is thoroughly debrided. At this juncture, the surgeon is faced with a decision. If the wound has been treated promptly and debridement has been adequate, the wound may be closed primarily. This should expedite healing and minimize aftercare. Alternatively, the wound can be left open to drain into a sterile bandage. From a practical standpoint, joint lavage can be performed daily until a positive clinical response is obtained. Drains can be placed to facilitate drainage and prevent premature closure of arthrotomy incisions. Ingress and/or egress drainage systems can be used for joint lavage and intra-articular antimicrobial administration. This practice allows for continual drainage of the synovial space and is probably the safest way to treat a wound involving a joint if the level of contamination is high or uncertain. This method of treatment is lengthy, costly, and labor-intensive because it requires daily bandage changes, which must be performed with the utmost sterility. These wounds usually heal with minimal complications if infection is avoided. Splints or casts are not usually necessary to obtain second-intention healing.

4. Clinical assessment of response to treatment: the most reliable way to assess the response to treatment is the way in which the patient uses the limb. What is desirable is a gradual improvement in weight bearing. Any increase in reluctance to bear weight in the face of analgesic and antibiotic therapy is a sign that a septic process is still ongoing. Serial synovial fluid analyses and bacterial culture and sensitivity procedures are then indicated. Once septic arthritis has become established, it is difficult to treat and intra-articular degenerative changes are inevitable. Therefore, aggressive therapy initiated early (within hours of the injury) is essential to a favorable prognosis.

References

[1] Gelberman R, Goldberg V, An K, et al. Tendon. In: Woo S, Buckwalter JA, editors. Injury and repair of the musculoskeletal soft tissues. Park Ridge, IL: American Academy of Orthopaedic Surgeons; 1988. p. 5–40.

[2] Gelberman RH, Vande Berg JS, Lundborg GN, et al. Flexor tendon healing and restoration of the gliding surface. J Bone Joint Surg Am 1983;65-A(1):70–80.

[3] Gelberman R, Goldberg V, An K, et al. Ligament: injury and repair. In: Woo S, Buckwalter JA, editors. Injury and repair of the musculoskeletal soft tissues. Park Ridge, IL: American Academy of Orthopaedic Surgeons; 1988. p. 103–66.

[4] Wright IM. Ligaments associated with joints. Vet Clin N Am Equine Pract 1995;11(2): 249–91.

[5] Amiel D, Frank C, Harwood F, et al. Tendons and ligaments: a morphological and biochemical comparison. J Orthop Res 1984;1(3):257–65.

[6] Stashak TS. Adam's lameness in horses. 4th edition. Philadelphia: Lea & Febiger; 1987. p. 472–5.

[7] Pasquini C, Jann HW, Pasquini S, et al. Guide to equine clinics lameness, vol. 2. Pilot Point (Texas): SUDZ Publishing; 1995. p. 160–1.

[8] Belknap JK, Baxter GM, Nickels FA. Extensor tendon lacerations in horses: 50 cases (1982–1988). J Am Vet Med Assoc 1993;203:428–31.
[9] Nixon AJ. Endoscopy of the digital flexor tendon sheath in horses. Vet Surg 1990;19(4):266–71.
[10] Frees KE, Lillich JD, Gaughan EM, et al. Tenoscopic-assisted treatment of open digital flexor tendon sheath injuries in horses: 20 cases (1992–2001). J Am Vet Med Assoc 2002;220(12):1823–7.
[11] Fortier LA. Tenoscopic surgery. In: Proceedings of the Equine 12th Annual American College of Veterinary Surgeons Symposium, Bethesda, MD, 2002. p. 177–9.
[12] Wright IM, Smith MRW, Humphrey DJ, et al. Endoscopic surgery in the treatment of contaminated and infected synovial cavities. Equine Vet J 2003;35(6):613–9.
[13] Bertone AL, McIlwraith CW, Powers BE, et al. Effect of four antimicrobial lavage solutions on the tarsocrural joint of horses. Vet Surg 1986;15(4):305–15.
[14] Bertone AL, McIlwraith CW, Jones RL, et al. Povidone-iodine lavage treatment of experimentally induced equine infectious arthritis. Am J Vet Res 1987;48(4):712–6.
[15] Watson ED. Effect of povidone-iodine on *in vitro* locomotion of equine neutrophils. Equine Vet J 1987;19(3):226–8.
[16] Jann HW, Alexander JW. Using a modified three-loop pulley tenorrhaphy to repair avulsion of the gastrocnemius tendon in dogs. Vet Med 1996;9:841–5.
[17] Pruitt DL, Manske PR, Fink B, et al. Cyclic stress analysis of flexor tendon repair. J Hand Surg 1991;16(4):701–7.
[18] Krackow KA, Thomas SC, Jones LC, et al. A new stitch for ligament-tendon fixation. J Bone Joint Surg Am 1986;68-A(5):764–6.
[19] Spurlock GH. Management of traumatic tendon lacerations. Vet Clin N Am Equine Pract 1989;5(3):575–90.
[20] DeKlerk AJ, Jonck LM. Tendon response to trauma and its possible clinical application. S Afr Med J 1991;80:444–9.
[21] Bertone AL, Stashak TS, Smith FW. A comparison of repair methods for gap healing in equine flexor tendon. Vet Surg 1990;19:254–65.
[22] Jann HW, Good JK, Morgan SJ, et al. Healing of transected equine superficial digital flexor tendons with and without tenorrhaphy. Vet Surg 1992;21(1):40–6.
[23] Nixon AJ, Stashak TS, Smith FW, et al. Comparison of carbon fiber and nylon suture for repair of transected flexor tendons in the horse. Equine Vet J 1984;16:93–102.
[24] Bertone AL. Tendon lacerations. Vet Clin North Am Equine Pract 1995;11(2):293–314.
[25] Watkins JP. Tendon and ligament disorders. In: Auer JA, Stick JA, editors. Equine surgery. 2nd edition. Philadelphia: WB Saunders; 1999. p. 711–21.
[26] Jann HW. Equine tendon lacerations. In: Tenth Annual American College of Veterinary Surgeons 2000 Symposium, Equine Proceedings, Bethesda, MD, 2000. p. 72–6.
[27] Jann HW, Stein LE, Good JK. Strength characteristics and failure modes of locking-loop and three-loop pulley suture patterns in equine tendons. Vet Surg 1990;19:28–33.
[28] Easley LK, Stashak TS, Smith FW, et al. Mechanical properties of four suture patterns for transected equine tendon repair. Vet Surg 1990;19:102–6.
[29] Crowson CL, Jann HW, Stein LE, et al. Quantitative effect of tenorrhaphy on the intrinsic vasculature of the equine superficial digital flexor tendon. Am J Vet Res 2004;65:279–82.
[30] Jann HW, Stein LE, Good JK. A comparison of nylon, polybutester, and polyglyconate suture materials to long digital flexor tenorrhaphy in chickens. Vet Surg 1992;21(3):234–7.
[31] Fackelman GE. Tendon surgery. Vet Clin North Am Large Anim Pract 1983;5:381–90.
[32] Bovane RB, Bitar H, Adreae PR, et al. In vivo comparison of four absorbable sutures: Vicryl, Dexon Plus, Maxon, and PDS. Can J Surg 1998;31:43–5.
[33] Sanz LE, Patterson JA, Kamath R, et al. Comparison of Maxon suture with Vicryl, chromic catgut, and PDS sutures in fascial closure in cats. Obstet Gynecol 1988;71:418–22.

[34] Micklethwaite L, Wood AKW, Andrew KW, et al. Use of quantitative analysis of sonographic brightness for detection of early healing of tendon injury in horses. Am J Vet Res 2001;62(8):1320–7.
[35] Foland JW, Trotter GW, Stashak TS, et al. Traumatic injuries involving tendons of the distal limbs in horses: a retrospective study of 55 cases. Equine Vet J 1991;23:422–5.
[36] Taylor DS, Pascoe JR, Meagher DM, et al. Digital flexor tendon lacerations in horses: 50 cases (1975–1990). J Am Vet Med Assoc 1995;206:342–6.
[37] Honnas CM, Schumacher J, Watkins JP, et al. Diagnosis and treatment of septic tenosynovitis in horses. Compend Contin Educ Pract Vet 1991;13(2):301–11.
[38] Honnas CM, Schumacher J, Cohen ND, et al. Septic tenosynovitis in horses: 25 cases (1983–1989). J Am Vet Med Assoc 1991;199(11):1616–22.
[39] Gaughan EM. Wounds of tendon sheaths and joints in horses. Equine Joint Dis 1994;16(4): 517–29.
[40] Schneider RK, Bramlage LR, Moore RM, et al. A retrospective study of 192 horses affected with septic arthritis/tenosynovitis. Equine Vet J 1992;24(6):436–42.
[41] Adams SB, Fessler JF. Regional antibiotic perfusion. In: Atlas of equine surgery. Philadelphia: WB Saunders; 2000. p. 393–6.
[42] Jann HW, Blaik MA, Emerson R, et al. Healing characteristics of deep digital flexor tenorrhaphy within the digital sheath of horses. Vet Surg 2003;32:421–30.
[43] Platt D, Wright IM. Chronic tenosynovitis of the carpal extensor tendon sheaths in 15 horses. Equine Vet J 1997;29(1):11–6.
[44] Booth TD, Abbot J, Clements A, et al. Treatment of septic common digital extensor tenosynovitis by complete resection in seven horses. Vet Surg 2004;33(2):107–11.
[45] Valdes-Valzquez MA, McClure JR, Oliver JL, et al. Evaluation of an autologous tendon graft repair method for gap healing of the deep digital flexor tendon in horses. Vet Surg 1996; 25(4):342–50.
[46] Reiners SR, Jann HW, Stein LE, et al. An evaluation of two autologous tendon grafting techniques in ponies. Vet Surg 2002;31:155–66.
[47] Eliashar E, Schramme MC, Schumacher Y, et al. Use of a bioabsorbable implant for the repair of severed digital flexor tendons in four horses. Vet Rec 2001;148:506–9.
[48] Jann HW, Stein LE, Slater DA. In vitro effects of epidermal growth factor or insulin-like growth factor on tenoblast migration on absorbable suture material. Vet Surg 1999;28: 268–78.
[49] Turner AS. Large animal orthopedics—lacerations of the suspensory ligament in the horse. In: Jennings PB, editor. The practice of large animal surgery. Philadelphia: WB Saunders; 1984. p. 925.
[50] Chan CC, Murphy H, Munroe GA. Treatment of chronic digital septic tenosynovitis in 12 horses by modified open annular ligament desmotomy and passive open drainage. Vet Rec 2000;147:388–92.
[51] Bertone AL. Infectious arthritis. In: McIlwraith CW, Trotter GW, editors. Joint disease in the horse. Philadelphia: WB Saunders; 1996. p. 397–409.
[52] Honnas CM, Trotter GW. The distal interphalangeal joint: septic arthritis of the distal interphalangeal joint. In: White NA, Moore JN, editors. Current techniques in equine surgery and lameness. 2nd edition. Philadelphia: WB Saunders; 1998. p. 394–7.
[53] Wagner von Matthiessen P, Orsini JA. Musculoskeletal. In: Orsini JA, Divers TJ, editors. Manual of equine emergencies treatment and procedures. 1st edition. Philadelphia: WB Saunders; 1998. p. 297–337.
[54] Crabill M. Wounds of joints. In: Tenth Annual American College of Veterinary Surgeons Equine Proceedings, Bethesda, MD, 2000. p. 67–71.
[55] Wright IM. Arthroscopic surgery in the management of contamination and infection of joints, tendon sheaths, and bursae. Clin Tech Equine Pract 2002;1(4):234–44.

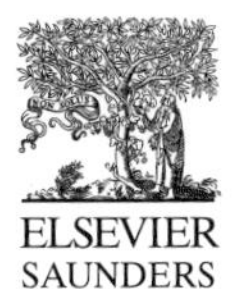

ELSEVIER
SAUNDERS

Vet Clin Equine 21 (2005) 167–190

VETERINARY
CLINICS
Equine Practice

Management of Equine Hoof Injuries

Christophe J. Céleste, DMV, IPSAV, DES[a,*],
Mihàly O. Szöke, DMV, DES, MSc[b]

[a]*Département des Sciences Cliniques, Faculté de Médecine Vétérinaire, Centre Hospitalier Universitaire Vétérinaire, Université de Montréal, CP 5000, Saint-Hyacinthe, Québec, Canada*
[b]*Hôpital Vétérinaire Lachute, 431, Rue Principale, Lachute, Québec, Canada*

Because of its distal position and constant contact with the environment, the horse's foot is frequently subjected to traumatic events. Although the hoof in itself is a hard structure, penetrating wounds are common. Some seemingly innocuous wounds might also involve deep structures and actually carry a poor prognosis for soundness, and they can even be life threatening. It is thus important to keep in mind the anatomy of the complex structures included in the hoof capsule. Particularities of the healing process are also relevant in establishing a treatment protocol.

Clinical anatomy

The bones contained in the equine foot are the second (middle) phalanx, the third (distal) phalanx, and the distal sesamoid (navicular) bone, forming the distal interphalangeal joint (DIJ). The stability of the latter is maintained by two short collateral ligaments, the collateral sesamoidean ligaments, a distal sesamoid impar ligament, and the joint capsule. Synovial pouches of the joint capsule are present on the palmar and/or plantar aspect of the joint dorsal and abaxial to the deep digital flexor tendon (DDFT) and axial to the collateral cartilages of the third phalanx. These pouches are in close contact with the podotrochlear (navicular) bursa on either side of the DDFT and, more proximally, with the digital flexor tendon synovial sheath (DFTSS) (Fig. 1) [1]. A penetrating wound just proximal and slightly axial to the cartilage of the third phalanx can involve any or all of these synovial structures.

* Corresponding author.
E-mail address: christophe.celeste@umontreal.ca

doi:10.1016/j.cveq.2004.11.009 ***vetequine.theclinics.com***

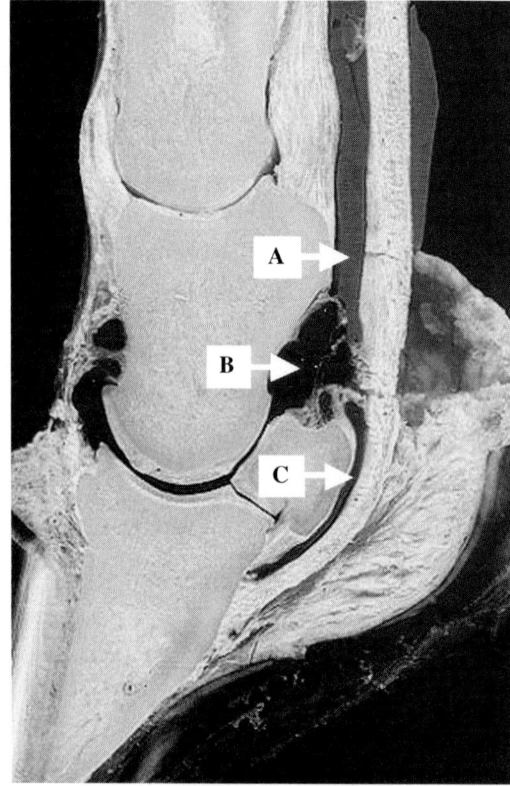

Fig. 1. Sagittal section of the distal part of the limb. As can be seen, the palmar/plantar pouches (*B*) of the interphalangeal joint are in close contact with the podotrochlear bursa (*C*) and, more proximally, with the digital flexor tendon synovial sheath (*A*), which is injected with latex. It is important to keep this closeness in mind when a penetrating injury involves the palmar/plantar area of the frog, the central or collateral sulci, and the cartilage of the third phalanx. Delayed recognition of the involvement of these synovial structures in a wound can worsen the prognosis dramatically. (Courtesy of S.M. Stover, DVM, PhD, Davis, CA).

The lamellar corium, of dermal origin, overlies the periosteum of the distal phalanx and is tightly interlocked with the epidermal laminae of the hoof. In cases of traumatic avulsion, the stratum germinativum of the epidermal laminae usually remains adherent to the lamellar corium. The spared living cells are responsible for the rapid epithelialization and keratinization often seen in the wound bed [2].

The hoof wall, or stratum corneum, is of epidermal origin and is usually divided into a stratum medium, which is thick and highly keratinized, and a softer stratum internum, of which the epidermal laminae were mentioned previously. The stratum medium is composed of horn tubules that grow from the stratum germinativum of the coronary epidermis. With the coronary corium and perioplic corium of dermal origin, the coronary epidermis constitutes the coronary band. Clinically, the underlying modified subcutis or coronary cushion is often considered a part of the coronary band, and it is included in surgical reconstruction of this structure.

The slow distad growth of the hoof wall (10 mm/mo) is a result of the differences between the primary and secondary epidermal laminae of the stratum internum. The cells of the primary epidermal laminae progressively keratinize while moving distally with the tubules of the stratum medium. The basal cells of the secondary lamellae, conversely, are adherent to the lamellar corium and do not keratinize. A continuous cycle of breaking and reforming links between the two cell populations is responsible for maintaining a strong attachment of the hoof wall to the parietal surface of the distal phalanx, allowing slow distal growth of the horn tubules [3]. On reaching the solar surface of the hoof, the keratinized cells of the epidermal laminae form the junction between the hoof wall and the sole. This zone of softer and whiter horn is commonly called the white line (Fig. 2). In avulsion injury, it is recommended to reconstruct the hoof wall with acrylic compounds as soon as sufficient keratinization has occurred in an attempt to limit excessive proliferation and keratinization of the lamellar epidermis, which would lead to widening of the white line.

Comparatively, growth of the sole and frog is much simpler and similar to that of normal skin. The high water content of the frog is responsible for its rubbery consistency. The digital cushion is a wedge-shaped structure of poorly vascularized elastic tissue placed between the frog and the DDFT, where it bends on the flexor surface of the distal sesamoid bone and reaches its insertion on the distal phalanx. The digital cushion provides the structural base for the bulbs of the heels between the cartilages of the distal phalanx.

Finally, it is important to remember that wounds in the pastern area often involve the medial or lateral digital arteries, veins, and nerves. Thanks to the terminal arch of the digital arteries, the blood supply to the foot is maintained if only one of the arteries is intact. Wounds in the bulbs of the heels often bleed profusely because of involvement of the venous plexus lining the axial and abaxial surfaces of the cartilages of the distal phalanx.

Healing characteristics of the equine foot

The anatomic structure and specific biomechanical properties of the foot affect the pattern of injury and healing. Any injury of sufficient force to invade the resistant stratum corneum usually results in a full-thickness wound. Full-thickness hoof wounds are rare, but when they occur, the rigidity of the stratum corneum usually prevents gaping of the wound margins, encourages fracture of the hoof capsule rather than tear, and causes the tissue to avulse completely from the underlying structures rather than just to lacerate [4]. Where the hoof wall is thinner and less rigid at the

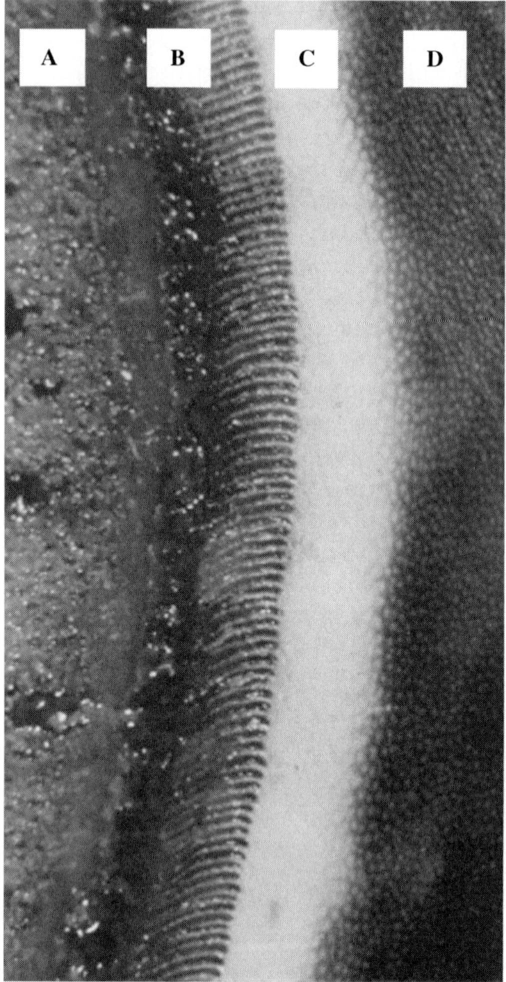

Fig. 2. Cross section of the hoof at the white line level. The distal phalanx (*A*), lamellae (*B*), white line (*C*), and hoof wall (*D*) are shown. The keratinized cells of the epidermal laminae usually form a junction between the hoof wall and the sole, which is made of softer and whiter horn, commonly called the white line.

coronary band and the heel area, lacerations, tears, and partial-thickness wounds occur more commonly.

Wound repair can be divided into three phases: inflammation, repair, and maturation. Wounds affecting tissue below the coronary band are contained within the rigid stratum corneum, such that swelling is impossible during the inflammatory phase. Furthermore, the rigid nature of the hoof may prevent adequate drainage of exudate and spontaneous elimination of foreign bodies and necrotic tissue, leading to subsolar abscess formation or infection of deeper underlying structures. In skin wounds, the repair phase involves contraction, fibroplasia, and epithelialization. Contraction does not occur in hoof wounds [5], and epithelialization differs. A full-thickness hoof wound involving the frog or sole usually evolves similar to a full-thickness skin wound, with homogeneous epithelial coverage coming from surrounding epithelium and re-establishment of epithelial strata by local epithelial proliferation. In a full-thickness wound involving the hoof wall, epithelium is re-established by progressive hoof wall growth from the coronary band downward rather than by local epithelial proliferation. In some hoof wounds, especially those involving the coronary band region, the epithelial margins may be of one or more origins, however. In these cases, the final appearance and structure of the healed wound reflect the nature and source of epithelium that filled the defect [4]. Thus, full-thickness wounds involving the skin and the coronary band often cause the formation of horny spurs or persistent defects in the hoof wall.

Principles of hoof injury management

Hoof wounds need special consideration because of structural particularities and usually heavy contamination. Lacerations occurring in the field may also go unrecognized for hours or even days, allowing infection to be well established at the time of diagnosis. If the wound is fresh and contamination is minor, a sterile water-based gel should be used to protect the exposed tissue while the skin is clipped and scrubbed with an antiseptic-soaked sponge. Lavage of the wound should be performed in the same manner as for other wounds.

Because of the rigidity and thickness of the hoof capsule, wound closure is rarely possible. Exceptions are wounds to the coronary band or heel bulbs, which should be reconstructed whenever feasible in an effort to retain the structural and functional properties of the foot (see the section on avulsion injury). In these cases, primary or delayed primary closure may be used.

Topical treatments used to treat other wounds on the body may be applied with similar considerations. Caution must be taken with the use of full-strength povidone-iodine solution, iodine tincture, Lugol solution, and topical astringents. Overzealous application of caustic agents can destroy granulation tissue and may further damage the deeper underlying structures and worsen the prognosis.

Dressing the horse's foot follows the same principles as for the rest of the distal limb, except that the middle layer is frequently omitted. Modified wet-to-dry dressings are commonly used and a waterproof layer usually completes the bandage (Fig. 3). In selected cases with sole injury or perforation, a special shoe with a treatment plate can also be used (see the section on deep puncture injury) to provide better solar protection (Fig. 4). A treatment plate does not provide adequate protection against moisture

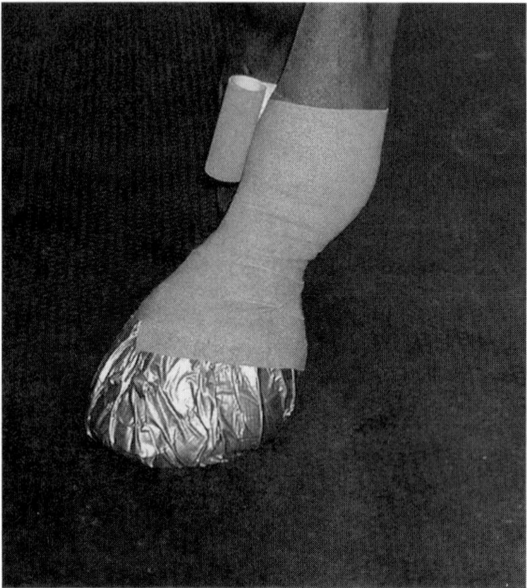

Fig. 3. Regular foot dressing with a waterproof layer (duct tape).

and contamination from the environment, however [6–8]. Because dressings seldom impart sufficient stability to the hoof for wounds involving the coronary band or heel bulbs, casting is recommended and improves healing as well as functional and cosmetic results as well as preventing the likelihood of persistent hoof wall defects (see the section on avulsion injury) [9–11]. In

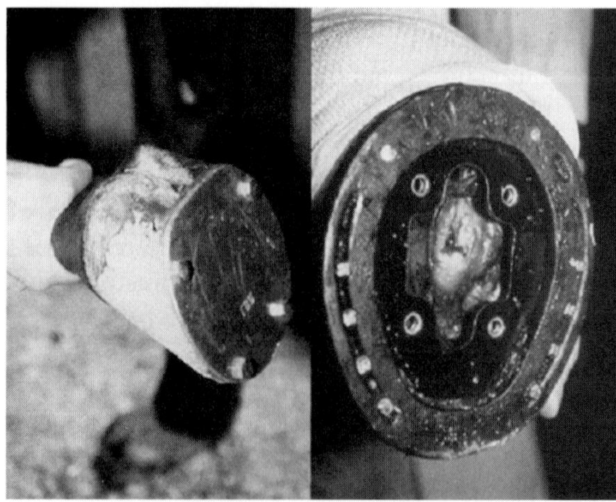

Fig. 4. Different models of treatment plates. To the left is an aluminium treatment plate bolted to the shoe. To the right is a commercialized plastic hospital plate with the insert removed. (Courtesy of M. Marcoux, DVM, MSc, Saint-Hyacinthe, Québec, Canada).

many cases, therapeutic trimming and shoeing with bars, clips, a plate, a pad, extensions, or elevations may be used to promote healing.

Most healing complications afflicting hoof injuries resemble those occurring in skin injuries, although excessive granulation tissue is rarely a problem. A hoof injury usually heals slowly and sometimes seems to be idle for no apparent reason. Light surface debridement of the granulation tissue, irritating ointment, and wet-to-dry dressings usually boost the deficient healing.

Superficial puncture injuries

Superficial puncture wounds are among the most common causes of acute lameness in horses. Subsolar abscesses may originate from a penetrating wound in the white line, a nail hole, a deep subsolar bruise, or a contaminated subsolar hemorrhage. Lameness is usually acute and severe; the horse may not bear full weight on the affected limb. Distal limb swelling and systemic signs of infection, such as fever and lethargy, may be present. The digital pulse in the affected limb is usually increased, as is the heat of the hoof when compared with the other feet. Hoof tester examination often reveals a focal painful region. Careful and gentle paring and trimming of the sole and frog may help to locate the abscess. Foot poultices applied overnight and foot baths with Epsom salts several times a day can be used to soften the horn and to help localize the affected region in a foot with diffuse pain.

Treatment of superficial puncture wounds that do not involve underlying vital structures is usually straightforward and is aimed at establishing adequate drainage, removing infected and necrotic tissue, and protecting the site from subsequent contamination. This can be performed in a standing horse, although sedation and perineural anesthesia at the level of the proximal sesamoid bones may be required in some uncooperative horses. If the draining tract is open at the solar surface, it should be enlarged just enough with a sharp hoof knife to ensure good irrigation and drainage. The edges of the horn defect must be thinned in a gentle slope to avoid pinching of exposed tissue. Underlying necrotic or infected tissue should be removed with curettes. As soon as pink tissue or blood is encountered, debridement should be discontinued to limit disruption of the solar corium and subsequent prolonged healing and painful sequelae [12,13]. If the draining tract is open at the coronary band, debridement should be done carefully to prevent iatrogenic DIJ contamination and further damage to the coronary band itself [12,13]. Once drainage is established and necrotic tissue is removed, the foot must be protected from the environment with a clean bandage, including a waterproof layer (polythene bag and adhesive or duct tape). Foot baths (warm water with povidone-iodine, Javel solution, or Epsom salt solution) should be continued until resolution of infection and inflammation. When the affected area is healed and dry and the epithelium is sufficiently keratinized, the shoe can be replaced. In some selected cases, a treatment plate or a plastic pad may be applied under the shoe to provide better solar protection. Antibiotics and nonsteroidal anti-inflammatory drugs (NSAIDs) are not usually indicated, unless infection is severe or spreads to deeper or more proximal structures (eg, coronary band, pastern region). Tetanus prophylaxis is mandatory. The prognosis is excellent unless deeper structure involvement has not been recognized in a timely manner [12,13].

Deep puncture wounds: penetrating injury of the sole or hoof wall

Infectious osteitis of the distal phalanx

Infectious osteitis of the distal phalanx commonly results from deep puncture wounds of the sole as well as from dissection by subsolar abscesses, hoof wall avulsions, soft tissue infections, solar margin fractures, or chronic laminitis with recurrent abscessation and ischemia [6,13,14]. Deep puncture wounds through the hoof wall are rare. Clinical signs are variable and include moderate to severe intermittent and recurrent lameness, a unilaterally increased digital pulse, increased heat in the affected foot, and soft tissue swelling. A chronic recurrent dark draining tract is usually noted at the solar surface or coronary band. Gentle paring of the hoof and poultice bandages applied to the sole for 24 to 48 hours are sometimes required to soften the horn and help find the tract. In rare cases, a tract may not be identified. The final diagnosis is usually made by radiographic assessment. Lateromedial, dorsopalmar and/or plantar, and dorsal proximopalmar and/or plantar distal oblique views at 60° to 65° are used (Fig. 5) [6,14]. Whenever a draining tract is identified, radiology is recommended, using a sterile metal probe or the injection of contrast medium into the tract to determine the direction and depth as well as possible communications with adjacent synovial structures. Radiographic signs of infectious osteitis, although not immediately apparent, include osteolysis, gas shadows in contact with the bone, decreased bone radiodensity, and widening of the vascular channels of the distal phalanx [6,14]. With the progression of bone infection, blood supply to the affected area of the distal phalanx may be compromised, leading to sequestration of avascular fragments [13].

Surgical treatment of infectious osteitis is recommended. Debridement and curettage of all infected soft tissue and necrotic bone can be performed in a sedated standing horse; however, better aseptic conditions, visualization of the lesion, and hemostasis are achieved under general anesthesia. Twenty-four hours before surgery, the affected foot is carefully pared and rasped to remove the superficial layer of the hoof capsule; it is then scrubbed with povidone-iodine soap, and a povidone-iodine solution–soaked sterile dressing is applied [15]. After induction of sedation or general anesthesia,

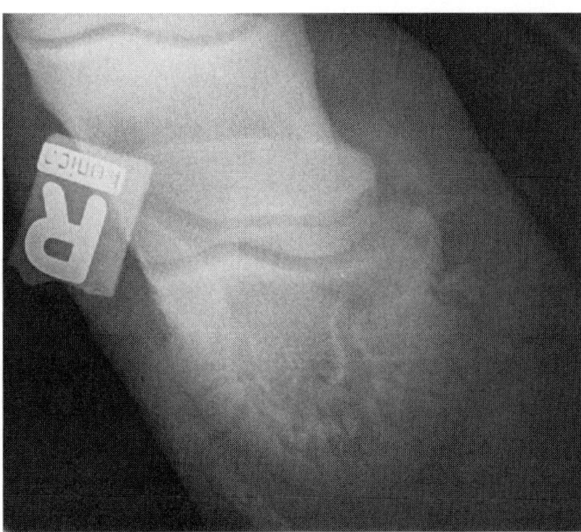

Fig. 5. Radiographic assessment of the foot of a horse with a recurrent subsolar abscess. A 60° oblique radiographic view is shown. A bone sequestrum can be seen on the solar margin of the distal phalanx.

the foot is desensitized using perineural analgesia at the level of the proximal sesamoid bones and is prepared aseptically for surgery. Hemostasis may be achieved by wrapping an Esmarch bandage firmly around the fetlock joint to compress the palmar and/or plantar digital arteries. Good hemostasis is helpful when performing surgery on a standing horse. Under general anesthesia, the use of an Esmarch bandage may be omitted to allow better visualization of healthy tissue and bone margins and to maintain better local diffusion of antibiotics. The approach chosen then depends on the location of the bony lesion and the extent of soft tissue infection. An approach through the hoof wall is used for lesions involving the parietal surface of the distal phalanx, whereas lesions on the solar margin or surface are approached through the sole. The horn and soft tissue surrounding the tract over the affected area are excised sharply, using a sterile hoof knife and scalpel. The edges of the horn defect must then be thinned as previously described (Fig. 6). The infected soft tissue, bone (usually discolored and softer than normal bone and fails to bleed when curetted), and all identifiable loose bony fragments are removed using bone curettes or motorized devices (eg, Dremel tool, Galt trephine). The infected bone should be aggressively curetted down to healthy bone margins (ie, until bleeding bone is exposed). If the coronary band is involved, care must be taken during debridement to preserve the overlying coronary corium. Culture of the infected bone and microbial sensitivity testing should be performed. Bacterial cultures usually reveal contamination by gram-positive and gram-negative organisms. Anaerobes are often suspected. A post-operative radiograph should be obtained to ensure complete debridement. The wound is then lavaged with sterile physiologic solution and packed with

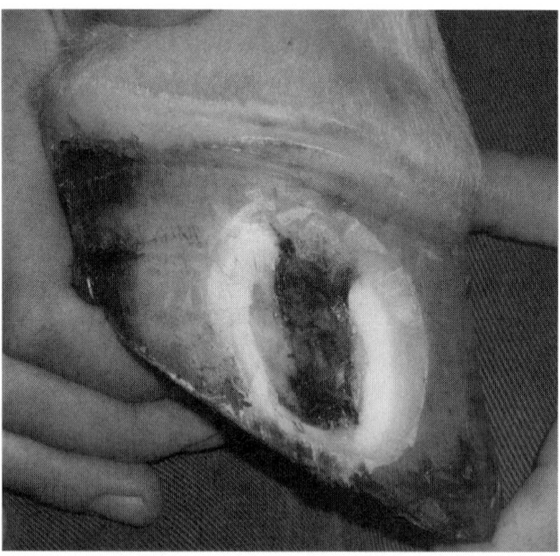

Fig. 6. Deep puncture of the lateral surface of the hoof wall with bone sequestration. The abscess was approached through the hoof wall. The coronary band and the solar margin were preserved. After removal of necrotic tissue and bone sequestrum, the edges of the horn defect were thinned to prevent pinching of the granulation tissue.

sterile gauze sponges soaked in an antiseptic or antimicrobial solution. A sterile pressure bandage is applied, and the digit is further covered with a waterproof layer.

After surgery, horses are given broad-spectrum antibiotics until sensitivity results are available. Subsequently, antimicrobial therapy is adjusted. Local antibiotic delivery systems, including regional limb perfusion and antibiotic impregnated beads of polymethylmethacrylate (AIB-PMMA), can be of interest in selected cases. Antimicrobial therapy is usually continued for 2 to 3 weeks after resolution of clinical signs of infection. NSAIDs are administered during and after surgery to minimize inflammation and pain. As usual, tetanus prophylaxis is mandatory.

After surgery, the frequency of bandage changes depends on the amount of exudate. When infected tissue is adequately removed, healthy granulation tissue usually covers the bone in approximately 10 days and the wound drains minimally. At this point, in case of sole penetration, a shoe or bar shoe with a bolted removable treatment plate can be applied [6–8]. In the case of a hoof wall defect, granulation tissue is covered by keratinized epithelium only 4 to 6 weeks after surgery. Only then can acrylic resin be applied in the defect to protect the wound; if it is applied earlier, the exothermic reaction results in necrosis of the underlying laminae and recurrence of infection. The convalescence period is long (2–4 months) [14] and requires extensive postoperative care and limited exercise.

The prognosis is excellent for return to soundness (80%–95%) and good for return to previous use (70%–80%) if the cause of infection is not laminitis. Up to 24% of the distal phalanx can be removed with a successful outcome [6,14,16,17]. The main complications are recurrence of infection, pathologic fracture of the distal phalanx, and contamination of the podotrochlear bursa or DIJ.

Infection of the collateral cartilage of the distal phalanx

Infection of the collateral cartilage usually results from injuries to the cartilage itself or to the soft tissue surrounding it. These injuries include puncture of the hoof wall, coronary band or heel bulb; subsolar abscesses draining at the coronary band; heel bulb lacerations; and deep hoof cracks. Septic chondritis induces moderate to non–weight- bearing lameness according to the patency of draining tracts. Diagnosis is mainly based on moderate to severe swelling and pain over the affected cartilage, the presence of fistulous tracts draining proximal to the coronary band over the affected collateral cartilage, and intermittent recurrent lameness. Radiographic assessment with insertion of a flexible metal probe or contrast medium is recommended to determine the depth and direction of the draining tracts and to rule out bone or DIJ involvement.

Because of the limited blood supply to the cartilage, medical treatment is often ineffective and surgical treatment is strongly recommended. Excision of all necrotic and infected tissue (eg, cartilage, surrounding soft tissue, draining tracts) is performed under general anesthesia. The affected foot is carefully prepared as previously described. A slightly curved incision is made over the infected cartilage and draining tracts (methylene blue dye can be injected in fistulous tracts to facilitate their identification), and all involved tissue, including necrotic blue or reddish cartilage, is removed by sharp dissection and curettage. If necrotic and infected tissue extends distally below the coronary band and is inaccessible through the proximal skin incision, a hole can be made in the hoof wall with a trephine (19 mm) at the distal border of affected cartilage. This hole allows better access and provides better drainage after surgery. Caution must be taken to avoid further damage to the coronary band. Culture of the infected cartilage and microbial sensitivity testing should be performed. After all the necrotic and infected tissue has been removed, arthrocentesis of the DIJ should be performed and the joint distended with sterile physiologic solution to assess its integrity. The skin incision is then closed, and the trephine hole is packed with sterile gauze sponges soaked in an antiseptic or antimicrobial solution.

After surgery, the bandage is changed daily to remove exudate and evaluate drainage and growth of granulation tissue. When primary healing is the objective, a short-limb cast is usually applied to the affected limb for 2 to 3 weeks to minimize movement at the skin suture line. Postoperative management is similar to that previously described for infectious osteitis of the distal phalanx. Exercise can usually be resumed 2.5 to 3 months after surgery.

The prognosis for acute and subacute cases with early complete surgical removal of diseased tissue is good. The most frequent complications are dehiscence of the skin wound, infectious osteitis of the distal phalanx, and sepsis of the DIJ, which worsen the prognosis considerably [12,18].

Deep punctures wounds: penetrating injury of the frog and sulci

Sepsis of the deep digital flexor tendon, podotrochlear bursa, distal interphalangeal joint, and digital flexor tendon synovial sheath

All puncture wounds should be considered as potentially serious, but those in the palmar and/or plantar region of the frog and in the central or collateral sulci (Fig. 7) require special attention because of the consequences associated with infection of underlying structures. Sepsis of the DDFT, podotrochlear bursa, navicular bone, DFTSS, or DIJ is common and may be career ending or even life threatening if aggressive treatment is not promptly initiated. Septic navicular bursitis with septic deep digital flexor

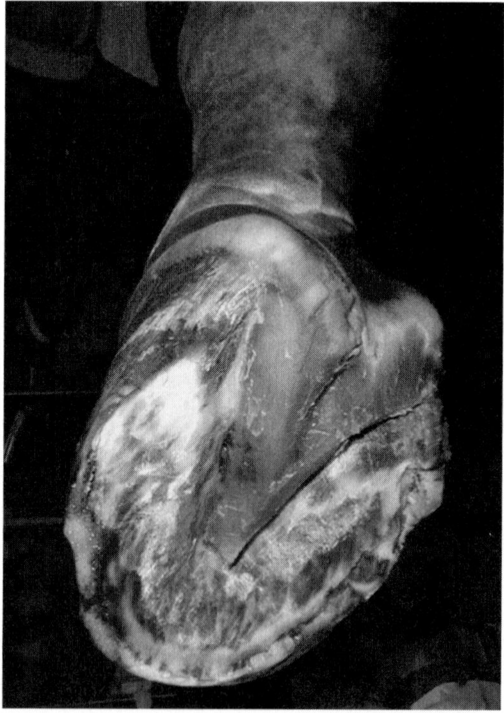

Fig. 7. Solar surface of the foot. A puncture wound in the lateral sulcus of the frog of 2 weeks' duration is shown. A small dark spot with moderate drainage can be seen. Surgical treatment revealed podotrochlear bursa sepsis with navicular bone osteomyelitis.

tendonitis and osteomyelitis of the navicular bone are the most common complications and the most frequent reasons for euthanasia of horses with deep puncture wounds of the hoof in the region of the frog [19].

The clinical signs vary with the structure involved and duration of the injury. Lameness may be mild at the time of injury and then moderate to severe once inflammation and infection occur. Careful examination of the foot must be performed. If the horse is presented with the foreign body in place, radiographic assessment should be performed immediately to determine the depth and orientation of the wound. If the foreign body has been removed, which is often the case, light paring of the sole and frog with a hoof knife and hoof tester examination to determine focal pain may help to find the puncture site, although the entire surface of the hoof is often reactive and the horse may not be cooperative. The horse can be sedated and the foot desensitized with proximal perineural analgesia to facilitate further examination. Because of the collapse of hoof structures around the puncture site after removal of the foreign body, it may be difficult to locate the hole. Whenever a hole is identified, radiographic assessment using a sterile flexible metal probe or injection of contrast medium to determine affected underlying structures is recommended (Fig. 8). Caution must be taken to avoid penetration of unaffected structures with the metal probe. Distention of the navicular bursa, DIJ, and DFTSS with contrast medium through a needle inserted percutaneously at a distant location may also allow detection of a fistulous tract and contamination of these structures. This technique is preferred over direct injection of contrast medium through the puncture site because it minimizes further contamination. Lateromedial, dorsopalmar (plantar), and oblique radiographic views are useful to

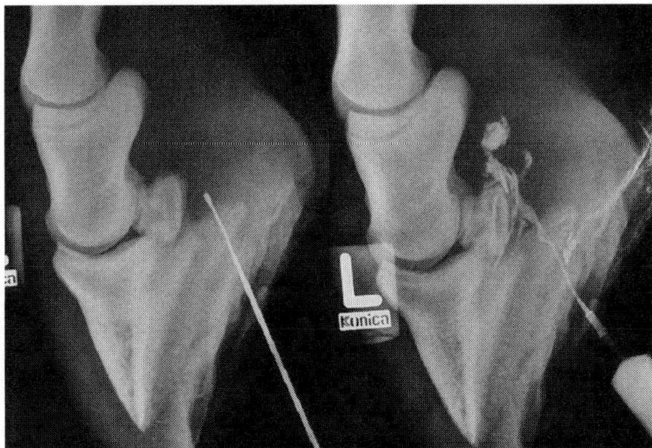

Fig. 8. Radiographic assessment of a foot after a deep puncture injury in the medial sulcus of the frog 2 weeks previously, using a sterile metal probe (left side) and contrast medium injected through the solar hole (right side). Lateromedial radiographic views are shown. The contrast medium extends proximally into the podotrochlear bursa and reveals contamination of this synovial cavity, which is not obvious with the probe examination.

determine the spread of contrast medium and to assess the distal phalanx and navicular bone. If involvement of the navicular bursa, DIJ, or DFTSS is suspected, synovial fluid should be collected from these cavities and cytologic evaluation and bacterial culture and microbial sensitivity tests should be conducted.

To maximize the prognosis, medical treatment should not be used alone but rather combined with surgical interventions unless economic considerations dictate otherwise. In this case, medical treatment alone might still be successful in some patients. Systemic broad-spectrum antibiotics, NSAIDs, and tetanus prophylaxis should be administered immediately after synovial fluid sampling. Systemic antibiotic therapy is usually modified according to microbial sensitivity and should be continued for at least 3 weeks after resolution of all clinical signs of infection. Debridement of all necrotic tissue and copious percutaneous lavage with sterile physiologic solution is then indicated. Administration of antibiotics intrasynovially or by regional perfusion should be performed [20,21]. Lavage and local administration of antibiotics should be undertaken at least every other day and continued until significant improvement of cytologic synovial fluid parameters is noted.

Surgical treatment under general anesthesia remains the gold standard. Preparation of the foot is performed as previously described. If only the DDFT is involved, surgical debridement of the infected tendon is carefully performed to prevent penetration of the navicular bursa. Postoperative care resembles that for deep puncture wounds of the sole. Use of a 4° to 8° wedge pad is useful because it may decrease forces on the DDFT and provide some pain relief. The wedge pad is then gradually lowered over several months as the DDFT heals and strengthens [13].

If the podotrochlear bursa or navicular bone is involved, prompt surgical exploration, lavage, and debridement are strongly recommended. Two surgical techniques (endoscopy of the podotrochlear bursa and the "streetnail" procedure) have been described to access the podotrochlear bursa and navicular bone. Both are performed under general anesthesia.

Surgical opening of the puncture site down to the podotrochlear bursa by creating a window in the DDFT is referred to as the streetnail procedure. If the puncture site can be identified and is still patent, a sterile flexible metal probe is inserted in the hole to facilitate visualization and removal of the sinus tract and surrounding necrotic tissue in successive layers (frog, digital cushion, and deep digital flexor tendon). Care must be taken to ensure that the DDFT is incised over the flexor surface of the navicular bone caudal to the distal sesamoid impar ligament. This ligament is intimately associated with the DDFT and, if incised, results in penetration of the DIJ. Once the navicular bursa is open, debridement of necrotic tissue and bone is performed using curettes. This surgical procedure allows limited visualization of the synovium of the bursa and the flexor surface of the navicular bone (Fig. 9). Communications between the DIJ or DFTSS and the

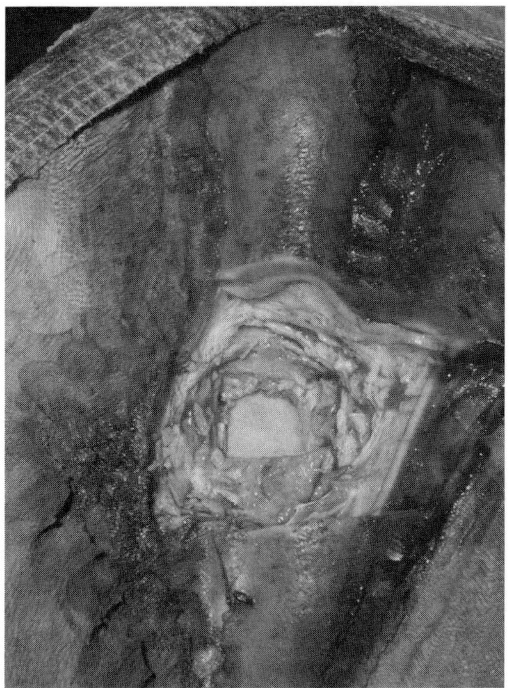

Fig. 9. Surgical treatment of podotrochlear bursa sepsis by a streetnail procedure. The flexor surface of the navicular bone is apparent. There is evidence of cartilage degradation and osteomyelitis.

podotrochlear bursa can be identified at this point by injecting sterile physiologic solution in each of these synovial structures from a proximal percutaneous site. If the DIJ or DFTSS is involved, fluid should be seen coming through the surgical opening into the navicular bursa. After abundant lavage, the surgical wound can be left open to heal by second intention or packed with autogenous cancellous bone graft [19] or AIB-PMMA (Fig. 10) [12], which fills in the dead space, reduces the opportunity of ascending contamination, and may help to prevent desiccation of underlying tissue. Bone grafts also provide a scaffold for subsequent formation of granulation tissue [19], enhance the local immune system's chances of resolving the infection [22], and significantly decrease the convalescent period [19], whereas AIB-PMMA provides a high concentration of antibiotic locally [12]. The surgical wound is then covered with a sterile bandage and a waterproof layer. Drainage is often abundant in the first days after surgery. Once the wound has granulated enough and drainage has decreased, a shoe or bar shoe with a treatment plate can be used. Drainage must be minimal before this step; otherwise, it may soak through the dressing and allow ascending infection from the contaminated

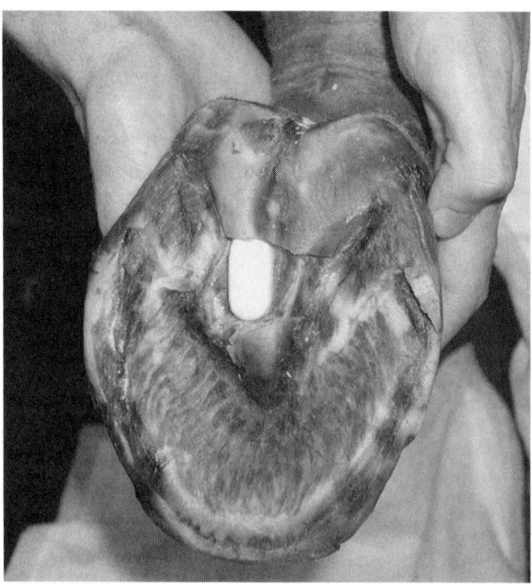

Fig. 10. Solar surface of the foot. Surgical treatment of podotrochlear bursa sepsis was performed by means of a streetnail procedure 10 days after surgery. The horn defect is nearly filled with granulation tissue. An antibiotic-impregnated bead of polymethylmethacrylate was used as a local antibiotic delivery system and can be seen in the horn defect.

plate [8]. AIB-PMMA is usually used until a healthy bed of granulation tissue develops and all signs of infection are gone [12].

Endoscopy of the podotrochlear bursa has been described [23]. This surgical procedure allows visualization of the synovium of the bursa, the suspensory ligaments of the navicular bone, the flexor surface of the navicular bone, and the dorsal surface of the DDFT. A combination of hand and/or motorized instrumentation and high-pressure lavage systems can be used to debride infected and inflamed synovium, subchondral bone defects, fibrin, foreign material, and the puncture site if present. When the original penetrating wound is still open, other surgical instruments can be passed through the wound into the navicular bursa. Only the skin portals are closed, and the distal part of the limb is dressed with a sterile bandage [23]. If a puncture site is present and draining, management of the wound is similar to that previously described for the streetnail procedure.

The DIJ or DFTSS can also be involved. They should be promptly and aggressively lavaged with sterile polyionic solution. Lavage can be performed percutaneously or more aggressively by means of endoscopy of the DFTSS [24–26] and arthroscopy of the DIJ [27]. Convalescence depends on the structures involved and the surgical procedure used and varies from 2 to 6 months.

According to a retrospective study of 50 cases with deep puncture wounds of the foot, only 50% of horses with a puncture in the frog region fully recovered from the injury [17]. Nevertheless, 80% of the horses operated on within a few days after such an injury returned to full function [17]. The return to athletic soundness after endoscopy of the navicular bursa was 63%, but it was only 31.5% after the streetnail procedure [23,28]. Horses treated by endoscopy seem to have a shorter hospitalization period, a shorter convalescence, less intensive postoperative care, and fewer complications, especially necrosis of the DDFT [23,28]. The prognosis for a forelimb is worse than for a hind limb and is significantly improved by early therapeutic intervention (surgery within 1 week of injury). Based on these results, it is strongly recommended to treat puncture injuries involving the frog region promptly and to favor endoscopic treatment whenever the navicular bursa is involved. Failure is most often attributed to osteomyelitis of the navicular bone, necrosis and rupture of the DDFT, and sepsis of the DIJ or DFTSS.

Lacerations involving the coronary band

Lacerations in the pastern region are common in horses. They may be caused by wires, ropes, or any kind of sharp object. The tendency to panic, get entangled in fence wire, or kick puts a horse at risk for such injuries. Often, the laceration involves the heel bulbs from somewhere between the bulbs at the palmar or plantar aspect of the pastern, curving dorsally and then distally to reach the coronary band at the level of the quarter. A cut by a sharp object is often limited by the hoof wall, whereas wire entanglement or entrapment of the foot often results in an avulsion similar to degloving injuries of the skin.

As for any other wound, integrity of major blood vessel should be verified as soon as possible. Wounds in the pastern area frequently result in transection of one or both digital arteries and veins and can bleed profusely. Owners or handlers in a stressful situation do not always think of applying a pressure bandage, and a horse is occasionally presented in hemorrhagic shock. The bleeding is controlled most efficiently with a pressure bandage. An Esmarch bandage can also be used as a tourniquet for a short time. Eventually, ligation of a major vessel may be necessary. Before any sedation is used to help evaluate the wound in a nervous horse, the cardiovascular status of the patient should be closely monitored and vascular volume re-established if necessary. In some cases, examination and cleansing of the wound must be delayed until all bleeding is effectively stopped and the cardiovascular status is stable enough to allow the safe use of tranquilizers and perineural blocks.

After the procedures common to most types of hoof wounds have been followed, a more thorough exploration can be carried out. Sterile gloves are mandatory. With smaller tracts, the use of a sterile probe might be necessary, but great care must be taken to avoid driving contamination deeper or involving structures (ie, synovial compartments) that were not contaminated initially. Radiographs can be taken with the probe inserted in the wound. The same care is taken with contrast studies, where gentle insertion of a catheter and low-pressure injection of the medium should be used. In the field, invasion of the DIJ or the DFTSS can be more easily assessed by distending these structures with sterile saline injected through a needle inserted in a distant site. Once again, gentle pressure and careful monitoring of distention should be used, because in the absence of counter-pressure provided by the subcutis and skin, an intact synovial pouch might easily burst. A more complete description of these techniques has been provided in the section reviewing deep penetrating wounds.

Contrast radiographic studies are important to assess soft tissue structures involved in a wound. In the case of any traumatic event, however, the importance of a complete radiographic examination, including bones and joints, can never be stressed enough. There are cases where type I and type II fractures of the distal phalanx, fractures of the navicular bone, proximal phalanx sagittal fractures, or plantar and palmar eminence fractures have been diagnosed incidentally during routine radiographic examination of patients with moderate to severe wounds.

Depending on the age of the wound, level of contamination, involvement of deep structures, and necessity to control hemorrhage, treatment options are primary closure, delayed primary closure, or secondary closure. If the coronary band is involved, reconstructive surgery should always be recommended, because treatment with bandages alone often leads to poor functional results, including horn spurs, permanent cracks, or deformation of the hoof wall, as well as costs that are much higher than anticipated.

Although in horses kept outside, secondary closure may be the norm, the authors generally undertake primary closure. Closure is most often delayed because of hemorrhage originating from the venous plexus of the heel bulbs, and that must be controlled by pressure wraps rather than because of heavy contamination. This must be accomplished before granulation tissue appears in the wound bed around the fourth day after injury.

In the case of a recent, sharp, and minimally contaminated wound, primary closure is advocated. Wound debridement is performed by means of sharp dissection and kept superficial. The scalpel blade is often changed in an attempt to limit trauma to exposed tissue. One must be particularly conservative when approaching the coronary band, because any deficit may lead to a permanent defect in the hoof wall. Undermining under the coronary cushion and aggressive thinning of the hoof wall distal to the laceration are sometimes required to allow sufficient apposition of the lacerated ends of the coronary band. A combination of vertical and horizontal mattress sutures with number 0 or 1 nonabsorbable monofilament material and simple interrupted sutures on the edges of the wound with number 2-0 similar material is appropriate. Like others, we have had no problems placing number 2-0 simple interrupted sutures in the coronary band itself

(Fig. 11), including the coronary cushion, and have even sutured full-depth incisions parallel to the axis of the coronary band in a similar fashion with good success [29]. Delayed primary closure is performed in exactly the same way.

Repair of any wound deep and extensive enough to induce increased movement or instability in a portion of the hoof wall or a gap while weight bearing, as is most likely the case with wounds involving the heel bulbs, should be protected by a cast. In the case of a wound with moderate proximal extension, a slipper cast can be used with good results (Fig. 12). It should be applied to just below the fetlock or just proximal to the coronary band but should never end at the level of the midpastern, where deep horizontal skin erosions are likely to appear at the dorsoproximal and caudoproximal borders of the cast. The cast must be kept in place for 2 to 3 weeks, depending on wound configuration. After removal, it is often helpful to use some kind of bar shoe with side clips to stabilize the hoof wall just distal to the wound. At the beginning, the wall at this level can be shortened so that it is not bearing on the shoe surface. The weight can be transferred to the frog, and the bar can be left long enough to contact the surface of a wide flat bar welded between the branches of the shoe.

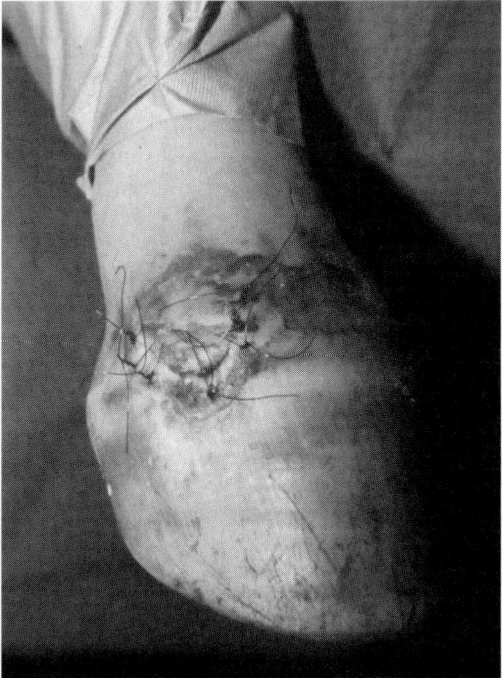

Fig. 11. Laceration of the coronary band on a weanling after surgical debridement and suture (simple interrupted) under general anesthesia. A slipper cast was applied immediately after surgery and left in place for 3 weeks.

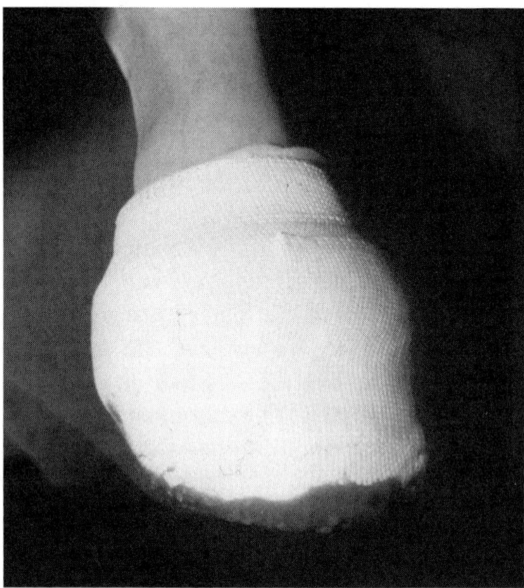

Fig. 12. Regular slipper cast. Caution must be taken to avoid ending the cast at the level of the midpastern. Otherwise, deep skin erosions appear in a few days, and the cast has to be removed earlier.

In cases of chronic infected wounds, extensive tissue trauma, or involvement of deep structures, secondary closure is usually the treatment of choice. The wound is lavaged and debrided in the manner described previously, but closure is delayed. The wound is medicated with an antiseptic or antibiotic ointment and kept under a sterile bandage. Systemic antibiotic therapy is indicated in most cases. Debulking of the wound is performed as soon as a sound granulation bed is obtained so as to decrease the bacterial population and to provide enough space to allow good apposition of the wound edges without excessive tension. The rest of the procedure is identical to delayed primary closure.

Involvement of synovial structures even in a clean acute wound was formerly considered an indication for secondary closure. It is now known that not all synovial invasions result in synovial sepsis, however. Endoscopic techniques using a rigid arthroscope to explore and copiously lavage the synovial structures of the equine foot have been reported. The efficiency of intrasynovial antibiotic injections and other means of regional antibiotic delivery has also been demonstrated, and these techniques are now widely used in association with primary closure of a clean wound.

Avulsion injuries

Partial or complete avulsion injuries of the hoof may involve any of the structures contained in the foot. Although the hoof has the capacity to heal completely, this occurs much more slowly, because contraction does not contribute to repair. The treatment is often protracted and extremely costly, and the outcome is uncertain. Luckily, injuries with extensive deep structure involvement are rare, and most have a partial avulsion of only a portion of the hoof wall, often in the quarter or heel area.

Initial assessment resembles that described for lacerations in the pastern area. Depending on the extent of the lesion, the horse is moderately to severely (non–weight-bearing) lame. Deep structures are evaluated after the foot region has been properly clipped, scrubbed, and rinsed.

Treatment of an incomplete partial avulsion is generally straightforward and can often be conducted in a standing horse after regional perineural anesthesia. The loose portion of the hoof wall is simply excised. Any part still attached to the lamellar corium is left in place in an attempt to maintain stability. In some cases, however, the traumatized and swollen coronary band bulges above the hoof wall still attached to the lamellar corium distally. Thinning or removal of the horn just distal to the coronary band is then important to avoid compression and necrosis of this delicate structure. No section of the hoof wall should be left square angled but should be thinned in a gentle slope around the exposed lamellar epidermis. The wound is then bandaged until sufficiently healed. Once a dry keratinized epithelium is obtained, iodine tincture may be used to speed up hardening of the surface, although the authors prefer to wait until 0.5 inch of new horn growth is visible at the coronary band and a fully keratinized surface is present in the defect, at which time the deficit is filled with hoof acrylic. Subsequently, a bar shoe with side clips and acrylic repair not fully bearing on the shoe surface is recommended.

Incomplete avulsions with a piece of hoof wall attached to the coronary band present a special challenge. The coronary band is often separated from the underlying subcutis and elevated proximally. If left untreated, a wedge of granulation tissue forms in the defect and a horny spur appears from the elevated portion of the coronary band. If it is clean and acute, the coronary band is best sutured back in place, with the detached wall partially removed and thinned to allow suturing. In more chronic cases, debulking of the underlying granulation tissue is necessary before good apposition and reconstruction of the coronary band is possible. In cases with more extensive avulsions, it might be necessary to protect the repaired area and exposed tissue using a half-limb or slipper cast. The cast is left in place for 2 to 3 weeks as previously described.

Horny spurs are not only unsightly but are subject to trauma and often painful (Fig. 13). They cannot simply be excised without risking the creation of a permanent hoof wall defect. Surgical reconstruction has been described, where the spur is contoured to fit in the hoof wall defect after the scar tissue has been removed from under the elevated coronary band and skin flap and is sutured in place (Fig. 14) [29].

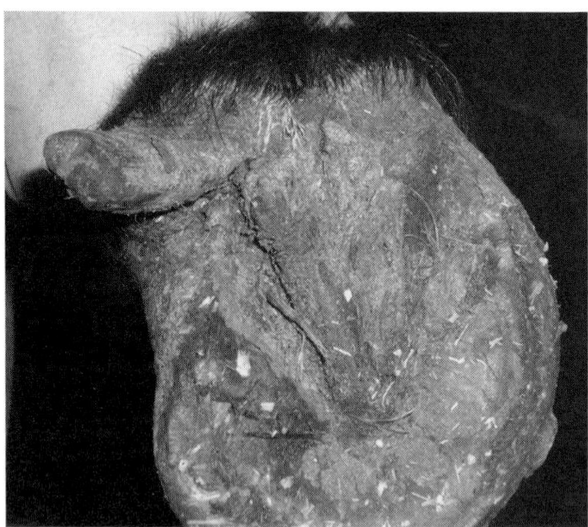

Fig. 13. Solar surface of the foot. A horny spur on the left heel bulb is visible.

Treatment of a complete avulsion involving deep structures of the foot varies according to which structures are injured. In general, treatment requires thorough debridement, drainage, and lavage of invaded synovial compartments, bandaging until all infectious complications are resolved, and, finally, casting for successive periods of 2 to 3 weeks, with periodic debridement until sufficient horn growth is obtained. This treatment is a life-saving procedure that takes months of effort in most cases, and the prognosis can only be fully assessed after several weeks.

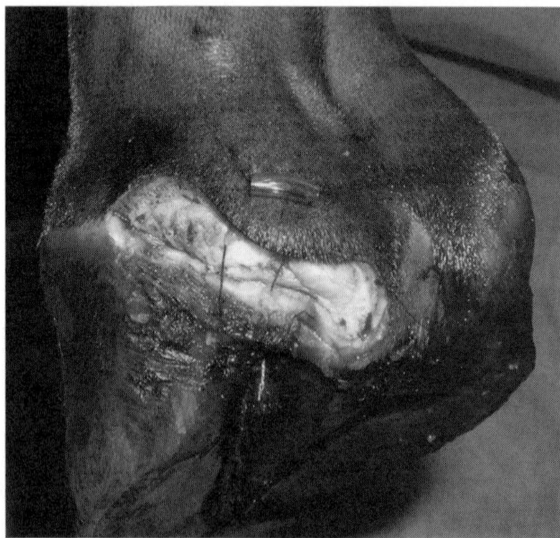

Fig. 14. Same horse as in Fig. 13 after horny spur removal. Caution was taken to preserve the normal underlying coronary band. The skin flap was sutured in place, and a slipper cast was applied for 3 weeks. The healing was perfect.

Acknowledgments

The authors thank Dr. Sarah Despatie for her contribution in the preparation of this article.

References

[1] Barone R. Anatomie comparée des mammifères domestiques. In: Vigot E, editor. Anatomie comparée des mammifères domestiques. Paris: Vigot Frères; 1980. p. 211–31.
[2] Kainer RA. Clinical anatomy of the equine foot. Vet Clin N Am Equine Pract 1989;5:1–27.
[3] Leach DH, Oliphant LW. Ultrastructure of the equine hoof wall secondary epidermal lamellae. Am J Vet Res 1983;44:1561–70.
[4] Parks AH. Equine foot wounds: general principles of healing and treatment. Proc Am Assoc Equine Pract 1999;45:180–7.
[5] Fessler JF. Hoof injuries. Vet Clin N Am Equine Pract 1989;5:643–64.
[6] Linford S, Embertson R, Bramlage L. Septic osteitis of the third phalanx: a review of 63 cases. Proc Am Assoc Equine Pract 1994;40:103.
[7] Moyer WA. Subsolar abscesses and foot infections. In: Colahan PT, Mayhew IG, Merritt AM, et al, editors. Equine medicine and surgery. 4th edition. Goleta: American Veterinary Publications; 1991. p. 1343–4.
[8] Ragle CA. Treatment plate applications. In: White NA, Moore JN, editors. Current techniques in equine surgery and lameness. 2nd edition. Philadelphia: WB Saunders; 1998. p. 521–3.
[9] Blackford JT, Latimer FG, Wan PY. Treating pastern and foot lacerations with a phalangeal cast. Proc Am Assoc Equine Pract 1994;40:97–8.
[10] Booth TM, Knottenbelt DC. Distal limb casts in equine wound management. Equine Vet Educ 1999;11:273–80.
[11] Booth TM, Dart AJ, Watkins JP. Equine limb casts: classification and indications. Compend Contin Educ Pract Vet 2003;25:701–6.
[12] Stashak TA. The foot. In: Adam's lameness in horses. 5th edition. Philadelphia: Lippincott Williams & Wilkins; 2002. p. 645–733.
[13] Dabareiner RM, Moyer WA, Carter GK. Trauma to the sole and wall. In: Ross MW, Dyson SJ, editors. Diagnosis and management of lameness in the horse. 1st edition. St. Louis: WB Saunders; 2003. p. 275–82.
[14] Cauvin ER, Munroe GA. Septic osteitis of the distal phalanx: findings and surgical treatment in 18 cases. Equine Vet J 1998;30:512–9.
[15] Hennig GE, Kraus BH, Fister R, et al. Comparison of two methods for presurgical disinfection of the equine hoof. Vet Surg 2001;30:366–73.
[16] Gaughan EM, Rendano VT, Ducharme NG. Surgical treatment of septic pedal osteitis in horses: nine cases (1980–1987). J Am Vet Med Assoc 1989;195:1131–4.
[17] Steckel RR, Fessler JF, Huston LC. Deep puncture of the equine hoof: a review of 50 cases. Proc Am Assoc Equine Pract 1989;35:167–76.
[18] Honnas C. The foot. In: Auer J, Stick J, editors. Equine surgery. 2nd edition. Philadelphia: WB Saunders; 1999. p. 779–91.
[19] Honnas CM, Crabill MR, Mackie JT, et al. Use of autogenous cancellous bone grafting in the treatment of septic navicular bursitis and distal sesamoid osteomyelitis in horses. J Am Vet Med Assoc 1995;206:1191–4.
[20] Murphey ED, Santschi EM, Papich MG. Local antibiotic perfusion of the distal limb of horses. Proc Am Assoc Equine Pract 1994;40:141–2.
[21] Santschi EM, Adam SB, Murphey ED. How to perform equine intravenous digital perfusion. Proc Am Assoc Equine Pract 1998;44:198–201.

[22] Richardson GL. Surgical management of penetrating wounds to the equine foot. Proc Am Assoc Equine Pract 1999;45:198–9.
[23] Wright IM, Phillips TJ, Walmsley JP. Endoscopy of the navicular bursa: a new technique for the treatment of contaminated and septic bursae. Equine Vet J 1999;31:5–11.
[24] Nixon AJ. Endoscopy of the digital flexor tendon sheath in horses. Vet Surg 1990;19:266–71.
[25] Fortier LA, Nixon AJ, Ducharme NG, et al. Tenoscopic examination and proximal annular ligament desmotomy for treatment of equine "complex" digital sheath tenosynovitis. Vet Surg 1999;28:429–35.
[26] Frees KE, Lillich JD, Gaughan EM, et al. Tenoscopic-assisted treatment of open digital flexor tendon sheath injuries in horses: 20 cases (1992–2001). J Am Vet Med Assoc 2002;220: 1823–7.
[27] Vacek JR, Welch RD, Honnas CM. Arthroscopic approach and intra-articular anatomy of the palmaroproximal or plantaroproximal aspect of distal interphalangeal joints. Vet Surg 1992;21:257–60.
[28] Richardson GL, O'Brien TR, Pascoe JR, et al. Puncture wounds of the navicular bursa in 38 horses: a retrospective study. Vet Surg 1986;15:156–60.
[29] Stashak TS. Management of lacerations and avulsion injuries of the foot and pastern region and hoof wall cracks. Vet Clin N Am Equine Pract 1989;5:195–220.

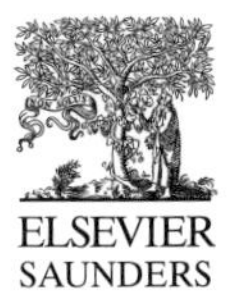

ELSEVIER
SAUNDERS

Vet Clin Equine 21 (2005) 191–215

VETERINARY
CLINICS
Equine Practice

Management of Neck and Head Injuries

Spencer M. Barber, DVM

Department of Large Animal Clinical Sciences, Western College of Veterinary Medicine, University of Saskatchewan, 52 Campus Drive, Saskatoon, Saskatchewan, Canada S7N 5B4

Injuries of the neck

Neck lacerations

Lacerations of the neck occur commonly in horses kept in cattle pastures fenced with barbed wire. The wounds are usually horizontal, located at the base of the neck, and often involve only the skin and subcutaneous tissue; however, arbitrary amounts of the brachiocephalicus, sternocephalicus, and sternothyrohyoidius muscles may be transected. There usually is no loss of function, but the skin edges may retract a variable amount as a result of tension, which is increased by movement of the head and neck (Fig. 1A). Treatment options consist of primary closure, delayed closure, and healing by second intention [1,2].

Narrow lacerations (2–3-cm wide gap) can be debrided and sutured in the standing horse without excessive tension. With intermediate-sized wounds (10–15-cm wide gap), dehiscence is more likely because of greater tension, and tension sutures or stents are needed. In our practice, many clients allow these wounds to heal by second intention with excellent results unless early return of the horse to normal activities is necessary. Large wounds (greater than 15-cm wide gap) or those that cause complete transection of the neck muscles are rather uncommon (see Fig. 1B). Because second-intention healing is protracted and labor-intensive and may result in loss of function, primary or delayed repair is recommended and is best performed under general anesthesia. Fractious, head shy, or uncooperative horses do not make good candidates for repair. If possible, the horse should be conditioned to a rope "martingale" to restrict elevation of its head before surgical repair (see Fig. 1D). A successful outcome can be expected when skin edges are closely approximated without excessive tension before induction of anesthesia. Thorough debridement and the use of Penrose drains as well as suture material

E-mail address: spence.barber@usask.ca

doi:10.1016/j.cveq.2004.11.010 **vetequine.theclinics.com**

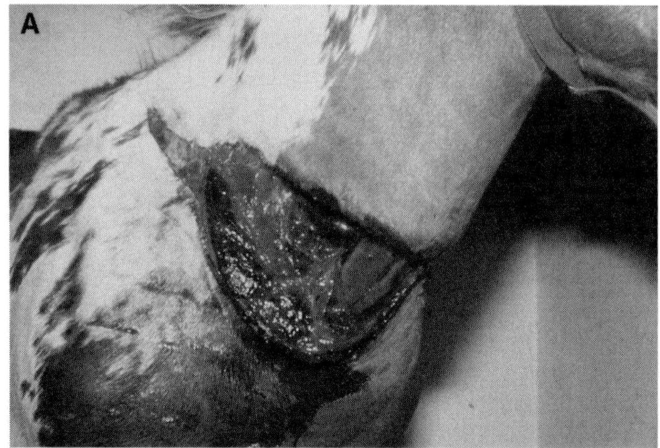

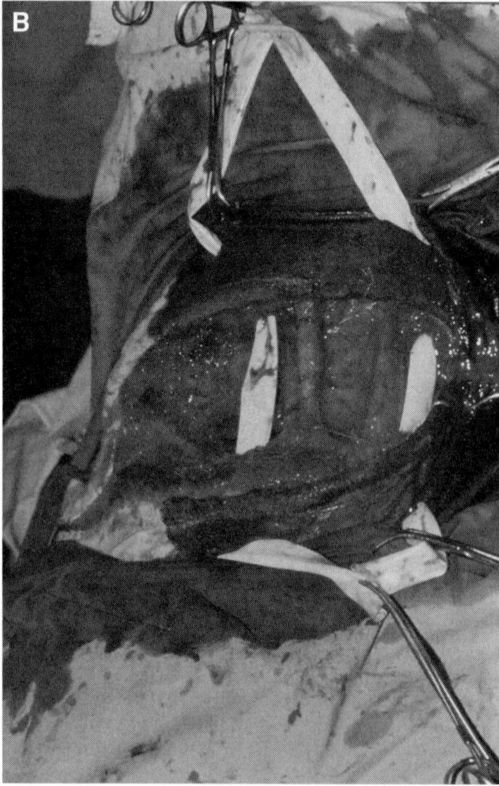

Fig. 1. (*A*) Acute laceration to the base of the neck with complete transection of the brachiocephalicus and sternocephalicus muscles. Skin edges could be apposed with minimal tension. (*B*) After aggressive debridement, Penrose drains were placed. The muscle layers were apposed with tension sutures without excessive tension but are not shown in this photograph. Note the exposed jugular vein that is stripped of much of its adventitia. (*C*) A stent bandage was placed over the wound and tightened to relieve pressure on the primary suture line and to discourage neck movement. (*D*) Three weeks after the repair, the stent bandage was removed; however, the rope "martingale," which was applied immediately after surgery, remained in use to prevent excessive movement of the neck. The wound healed by primary intention.

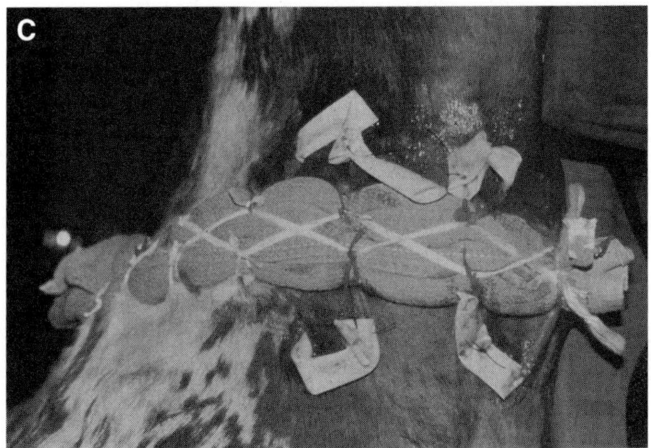

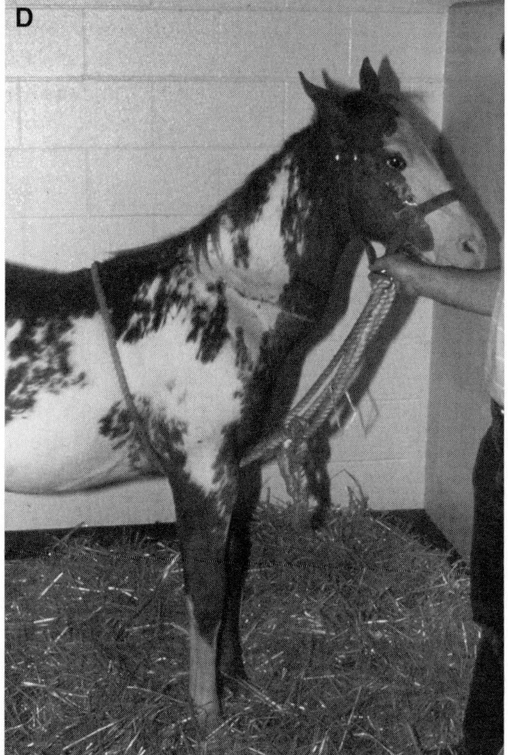

Fig. 1 (*continued*)

strong enough to withstand considerable forces and applied in a tension pattern, such as a vertical mattress or near-far-far-near pattern, are crucial to success. A stent bandage not only prevents contamination and trauma to the repair but may take pressure off the primary suture line. The stent bandage is maintained for 10 to 14 days, and the martingale is maintained for 2 to 3 weeks (see Fig. 1C). Judicious use of nonsteroidal anti-inflammatory drugs is recommended; some tenderness at the wound site is desirable because it prevents the horse from using the neck too much.

With second-intention wound healing, treatment is aimed at stimulating granulation tissue formation. Moist wound management helps to achieve this objective as well as to enhance wound contraction and epithelialization rates. Hydrotherapy twice daily for 15 to 20 minutes is initially helpful in physically debriding the wound and later increases circulation and subsequent granulation tissue formation. Although bandaging would be desirable in keeping the wound moist, it is often not possible. To help prevent desiccation and promote enhanced wound contraction, the author applies an ointment to the wound after hydrotherapy. In experimental leg wounds, live yeast cell derivative (Preparation H; Whitehall Laboratories, New York, NY) may cause excessive development of granulation tissue [3]; however, it can be used to enhance healing in body wounds that are not predisposed to the formation of proud flesh. Another product used by the author to promote moisture retention is scarlet red contained in an oil base (Red Kote or Vetoquinol; H.W. Naylor Co., Morris, NY) [1]. Treatment with hydrotherapy and topical ointment is continued until the wound is completely healed.

Neurovascular injuries

The vagosympathetic trunk, recurrent laryngeal nerve, common carotid artery, and jugular vein can all be injured after laceration to the cranial aspect of the neck. The jugular vein is the most susceptible because of its superficial location just beneath the external musculature of the neck.

Although the jugular vein and common carotid artery are rarely severed, they may be exposed and have their perivascular tissue stripped away by injury, predisposing them to desiccation and subsequent rupture. Exposed intact vessels should be covered with viable soft tissue whenever possible to provide protection and a source of nourishment for the vessels (see Fig. 1B). Complete rupture of the jugular vein or common carotid artery is life threatening. If the vessels appear devitalized or are torn, they can safely be ligated at both ends to prevent fatal hemorrhage [4].

Injury to the recurrent laryngeal nerve results in laryngeal hemiplegia. Clinical signs associated with this may not be noticed at rest, but laryngeal paralysis can be identified by endoscopic examination. Injury to the vagosympathetic trunk may result in a multitude of clinical signs, including alterations in heart rate or esophageal function, abnormal gastrointestinal motility and/or colic, and possible sweating or changes in skin temperature. Thus, care must be taken during the aforementioned vessel ligatures to prevent injuries to the vagosympathetic trunk and the recurrent laryngeal nerve.

Tracheal injuries

Anatomy

The trachea is a flexible air-carrying tube extending from the cricoid cartilage to the left and right mainstem bronchi. The trachea lies on midline, with the common carotid artery, laryngeal nerve, and vagosympathetic trunk approximating its dorsolateral surface and the esophagus to its left in the cervical area. The trachea is composed of hyaline cartilaginous rings that are incomplete dorsally [5], where they are bridged by the tracheal membrane. The rings are flattened dorsoventrally, with an average dorsoventral diameter of 5 cm and a transverse diameter of up to 7 cm [5]. The stiffness of the cartilaginous rings prevents collapse during inhalation, whereas the dorsal area not spanned by cartilage allows for tracheal expansion when large volumes of air are required, such as during exercise. The rings are connected to one another by fibroelastic tissue, the annular tracheal ligament, which ensures flexibility during neck movement.

Tracheal trauma

Injuries to the trachea are not common but can be serious. The thoracic portion of the trachea is well protected within the thorax and is rarely injured, whereas the cervical portion, despite being covered by substantial musculature, is often the site of injury. Damage may result from external blows such as a kick, rope, or impact with a solid or sharp object [6–8]. Injury can also result from puncture by a foreign body or by excessive pressure created by an endotracheal tube [9].

Clinical signs depend on the patency and integrity of the trachea and whether the skin and subcutaneous tissues are intact. Any full-thickness defect to the tracheal wall allows air to escape subcutaneously. If the skin and subcutaneous tissues are open, the amount of subcutaneous emphysema is minimal; however, if they are closed, the emphysema can be extensive and affect large portions of the body [7,8]. Horses do not experience respiratory distress as long as the tracheal lumen remains patent. If structures of the tracheal wall are ruptured and invaginate into the lumen, they may compromise breathing and can lead to elevations in heart rate and respiratory rate, inspiratory and expiratory noise, and possible respiratory distress. In large open wounds, tracheal integrity may be assessed visually and by palpation, whereas in smaller skin wounds and injuries without skin penetration, this is more difficult. Occasionally, a small swelling of the cervical area may be the only indication of external trauma [6], and any swelling may make palpation of the trachea difficult. Radiographs are useful to evaluate the diameter of the tracheal lumen, to check for the presence of an intraluminal mass, and to detect peritracheal gas in full-thickness tracheal defects in which the surrounding skin remains intact. Endoscopic examination of the trachea is well tolerated by most standing horses and allows identification of full-thickness defects of the tracheal wall as well as injuries that result in prolapse of tracheal rings or the invagination of the tracheal membrane or peritracheal tissue into the lumen.

Management depends on the structures involved and the insult to the respiratory system. Small full-thickness defects of the tracheal wall that result in only minimal subcutaneous emphysema usually heal spontaneously by second intention [7]. If a larger perforation is present in the trachea but the skin and subcutaneous tissues are open, a similar approach is adequate. In the presence of a large perforation and intact skin, however, the creation of a full-thickness defect at the site of injury, or a tracheostomy adjacent to it, prevents air from being forced subcutaneously and allows the injured site to heal by second intention. If there is prolapse of the tracheal membrane or pieces of extraluminal connective tissue present in the lumen, these must be excised before reconstruction of the tracheal defect [6,7]. Complete disruption of the trachea occurs uncommonly but represents a surgical emergency [8]. The trachea must be closed with small-gauge stainless steel wire or, preferably, absorbable suture material [8] without penetrating the mucosa or the cartilage. Broken tracheal rings can cause instability or collapse of the tracheal wall, may project into the lumen and interfere with air flow, or may act as a stimulus to granulation tissue formation that subsequently causes partial obstruction of the lumen. Any structures causing collapse of the tracheal wall must be stabilized, and any intraluminal masses must be removed to prevent subsequent respiratory difficulties. If a small portion of a ring is broken and projects into the lumen, it should be surgically excised as long as the trachea is stable. Conversely, when tracheal ring rupture results in collapse of the trachea, application of an external polypropylene splint may be required [10,11]. An alternative treatment for broken tracheal rings that cause respiratory difficulty is resection and anastomosis of the injured area, with removal of four to five rings allowing a fair to good prognosis [12]. Removal of a larger number of rings is not advised, because excessive tension on the suture line may cause disruption of the trachea that usually requires euthanasia of the patient. When damage to a tracheal ring is limited to its ventral aspect, this portion can be removed to create a permanent tracheostomy, with a fair prognosis [13,14].

Esophageal injuries

Anatomy

The esophagus, a musculomembranous tube that extends from the pharynx to the stomach, is approximately 125 to 200 cm long, with its cervical portion representing greater than 50% of its length [15,16]. It is located dorsal to the trachea in the cranial third of the neck, on the left side in the midcervical area, and ventral to the trachea near the thoracic inlet. The common carotid artery, vagosympathetic trunk, and recurrent laryngeal nerve are all located adjacent to the esophagus. The esophageal wall is composed of four layers. The mucosa and submucosa, easily distinguishable from the underlying muscularis, form longitudinal folds in the esophageal lumen and provide the greatest tensile strength during closure. The third layer is composed of two helically oriented striated muscles in the cranial two thirds that blend into a smooth muscle layer at the base of the heart. The thickness of the muscular layers increases caudally, whereas the size of the lumen decreases correspondingly. A tunica adventitia covers the outer surface of the esophagus, except in the short abdominal segment, where it has a serosal covering [15,16].

Clinical signs

The clinical signs depend on the type of esophageal injury. A tubular shaped nonpainful swelling may be palpated proximal to an obstruction in the cervical portion of the esophagus in the area of the jugular groove. In the case of a pulsion diverticulum, the swelling is more discrete and fluctuates in size in association with the intake of food and water. A cervical swelling that is diffuse, hot, and painful to digital pressure and has crepitus suggests a full-thickness rupture of the esophageal wall with discharge of saliva, food, air, and bacteria into the fascial planes. The resulting infection may lead to necrosis of the overlying skin [17,18] or may gravitate toward the thoracic inlet and cause mediastinitis or pleuritis [19]. Injury to the adjacent carotid artery can cause profuse fatal hemorrhage [18], whereas damage to the recurrent laryngeal nerve causes laryngeal hemiplegia [17] and injury to the vagosympathetic trunk causes Horner's syndrome. If a skin wound is present, saliva and food may be seen discharging; however, ventral drainage may be inadequate and lead to seepage along fascial planes with resulting cellulitis.

Esophageal healing

The stratified squamous epithelium of the mucosa has an excellent regenerative power that enables partial- and full-thickness defects to heal without stricture [20]. Wounds that extend into the submucosal and muscular layers heal by means of granulation and wound contraction [20]. Circumferential wounds, which are common in horses after esophageal impactions, can produce a stricture that causes recurrent obstruction [15]. The maximal reduction in lumen size occurs 30 days after the injury, but luminal diameter may thereafter spontaneously increase to normal by day 60 [21–23], possibly as a result of scar remodeling and dilation from normal eating. If surgical correction is contemplated, it should thus be delayed until at least 60 days after the trauma.

Surgery of the esophagus often results in complications [15] and is associated with a low long-term survival rate [24]. Constant tension, motion, and expansion; lack of a serosal surface, and thus limited tissue holding strength; need for a watertight seal; and a less than abundant blood supply [25,26] are all factors that contribute to dehiscence, stricture, and other complications [22,24].

Esophageal diverticulum

A traction diverticulum results when periesophageal scar tissue contracts, pulling the esophageal wall outward [15]. This may occur after surgical penetration or wounding of the esophagus but rarely causes clinical signs or requires surgical treatment [15,16]. A pulsion diverticulum results from rupture of the muscular wall with mucosal protrusion through the defect [15,16]. It causes intermittent swelling and signs of esophageal obstruction and may continue to enlarge to cause complete obstruction and rupture eventually [15,27,28]. Surgical repair of a pulsion diverticulum is indicated and has a reasonable prognosis. Inversion of the prolapsed mucosa and closure of the mural defect decrease the likelihood of postoperative leakage, infection, or fistula formation [16,28]. If the mucosal sac is large and may cause obstruction of the esophageal lumen on inversion, however, a diverticulectomy is recommended [16,27].

Esophageal rupture

Rupture of the esophageal wall can result from an external blow, penetration by a foreign body, or extension of a necrotic or infectious process, or it may be secondary to stomach tubing or a chronic obstructive lesion [15,29–31]. It is most common in the cervical area, with 2- to 5-cm longitudinal traumatic ruptures being frequent [29–31]. Clinical signs are variable, depending on the duration of injury and whether the skin is intact. Rupture of the esophageal wall allows the escape of saliva, food, and water into the periesophageal tissue. If the skin is open, this material is visible; however, if the skin is intact, the material is trapped in the fascial planes, resulting in an enlarging hot, tender, and diffuse cervical swelling and a horse that is febrile, dehydrated, and depressed [16,17,29,31]. Signs of cellulitis are exacerbated with chronicity, and rupture of the overlying skin can occur by extension of the infectious and necrotic process [16], or the infection may gravitate to the thoracic inlet, resulting in mediastinitis and pleuritis [16,19]. An esophageal defect may be seen on endoscopic examination [17], but small lesions may be hard to locate if they are located adjacent to the cranial esophageal sphincter [15]. Gas is noted in the periesophageal tissue on plain radiographic films, whereas contrast material confirms leakage through a defect in the esophageal wall.

If the wounds are fresh and minimally contaminated, primary closure is indicated and has been used successfully [29,30,32]. Placement of a nasogastric tube after primary repair is not recommended [25]; rather, placement of a cervical esophagostomy tube into a normal segment of esophagus distal to the perforation enables nutritional support and allows the damaged area to heal with fewer complications [16]. Wall defects can also heal successfully by second intention [17,29], and although a traction diverticulum develops at the site of injury, this is not usually of clinical importance [16]. If food material has collected in the fascial planes, aggressive wound debridement, the establishment of ventral drainage, and systemic antibiotic therapy are paramount to successful treatment [15–17]. Considerable fluid, electrolyte, and nutritional losses can occur and must be addressed in the treatment plan [16,17]. Although the outcome of esophageal rupture is improved by surgery, the long-term survival rate is still poor [24]. Notable complications include laryngeal hemiplegia and rupture of the common carotid artery [18,24].

Injuries of the head

Injuries of the head occur commonly in horses, which are flight animals that respond to situations in which they detect danger by running, pulling back, and throwing their head. Furthermore, the head is frequently handled for leading and transporting, and the horse is used for activities that have inherent risks and employ equipment that can lead to injury if used inappropriately. Finally, the horse is sometimes kept in unsafe facilities presenting dangerous objects, such as nails, wire, and tin.

The head is a complex region, containing portions of several body systems with important physiologic functions. Damage to various structures of the head can result in abnormalities that not only threaten the horse's health and well-being but can have a dramatic impact on its athletic performance or appearance and consequent value to its owner.

Lacerations

Lacerations are a common head injury, and the principles of wound management resemble those for wounds in other locations. Head lacerations are usually presented early and with little contamination and tension, but there can be considerable mobility of certain tissues (eg, lips). An abundant blood supply leads to rapid and strong healing [33]; however, when debriding, care should be taken to preserve all viable tissue to allow more accurate reconstruction, which ensures normal function and appearance [34]. Primary or delayed closure is often chosen over second-intention healing to maximize the restoration of function and to minimize blemish. Even chronic and contaminated wounds can often be repaired.

Scalping lacerations

These occur commonly and often are associated with the horse throwing its head while being loaded into a trailer or going through a low gateway. An inverted V-shaped skin flap exposes the temporalis muscle and frontal bone (Fig. 2). The skin flap usually has a wide base and is viable and minimally contaminated but is retracted and curled at the tip. Second-intention healing would be slow because of the minimal tissue available for wound contraction and not cosmetic, because the flap is retracted and curled; thus, primary closure is advocated. An extremely thin slice should be trimmed to freshen

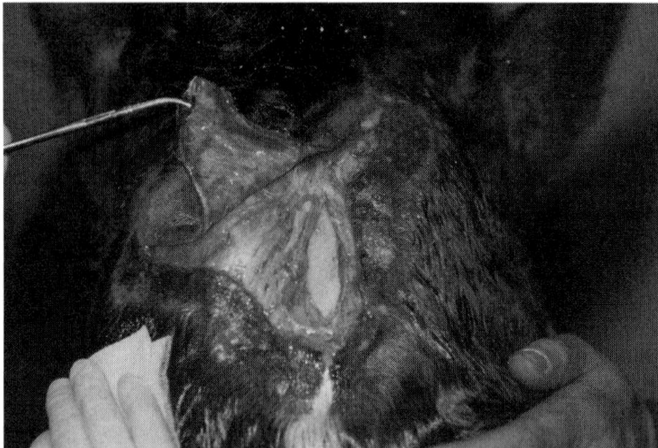

Fig. 2. A typical scalping injury with production of a triangular skin flap and exposure of the temporalis muscle and the frontal bone.

the edge of the flap before closure. If the periosteum was damaged by injury, aggressive debridement of the bone surface is important to reduce bacterial contamination and decrease the risk of sequestrum formation. This can be accomplished by scraping the bone with the edge of a scalpel or curette, high-pressure lavage, or use of a rotary burr. Subsequently, the bone must be protected by viable muscle, subcutaneous tissue, or skin. Separate closure of subcutaneous tissue and skin is desirable when possible. The skin is closed with a combination of mattress and appositional interrupted sutures, which leads to a good cosmetic result.

Lip lacerations

The integrity of the upper lip is critical to facial symmetry and cosmetic appearance but also plays a major role in prehension and the horse's ability to whinny [35]. The lower lip retains food and saliva within the oral cavity [35], whereas the commissure serves as a seat for the bit. The lips are areas of high motion; thus, dehiscence is a common problem after suturing [36]. Although lip lacerations are highly contaminated, infection is prevented by an abundant blood supply [36]. Horses usually can eat well despite a lip laceration unless it is severe and interferes physically with prehension or is extremely painful.

Partial-thickness lip defects can be treated conservatively but heal more rapidly and more cosmetically after primary or delayed closure. Full-thickness defects should always be reconstructed. After debridement, the skin and mucosa are separated from the musculature over approximately 1 to 1.5 cm, creating three separate layers. Mucosal edges are apposed with absorbable suture in a continuous or interrupted pattern with buried knots.

The muscle layer is apposed with preplaced quill sutures, with the knots external to the skin or buried within the musculature. The skin is closed with a combination of tension and appositional sutures. Penrose stents are useful to reinforce the suture line [34,36].

Lacerations involving the lip commissure are at greater risk of dehiscence because of high tension in this area, which ultimately leads to drooling and a poor seat for the bit. Accurate reconstruction and placement of tension or quill sutures and stents help to decrease the incidence of dehiscence [35].

Degloving injuries of the lower lip, although uncommon, present a serious problem because they interfere significantly with eating and there is little tissue remaining on the mandible for repair. The mucosal edges on the mandible and lips are undermined to create flaps for suturing. The lip is then held in position by drilling holes through the rostral mandible for the placement of mattress sutures between it and the skin; the sutures are tied externally over stents. Because there can be considerable dead space, Penrose drains are placed for a few days to prevent accumulation of exudate [36].

If a major portion of the lip is lost (more than 30%), simple closure and reconstruction may not be possible, which may result in disfigurement and loss of function. In these cases, additional reconstructive techniques, such as the Estlander flap, may be required [35].

It is recommended to cross-tie or muzzle the horse to prevent disruption of the repair from rubbing. Horses eat after surgery, but soft feed and analgesics are indicated.

Tongue lacerations

Tongue lacerations can result from the inappropriate use of bits, the placement of foreign objects in the mouth, or self-inflicted bites. The first two causes usually injure the dorsum of the tongue at its midbody, whereas bites occur at the tip of the tongue. Horses can eat well despite the laceration, but blood and saliva may be seen coming from the mouth [37]. Severe lacerations, especially those that lead to avascularity or loss of control of the tongue tip, interfere with eating.

Most lacerations heal well by second intention, and surgical repair is not needed [37]. Deep lacerations heal with a scar and a defect in the dorsum of the tongue that is not cosmetic and may trap the bit and cause abnormalities in performance or reinjury to the tongue (Fig. 3). Surgical closure of the defect results in a more rapid return of the horse to normal riding activities, with less chance of altered performance or repeat injury. If the laceration to the muscle is so severe that the horse has lost control of the tip, surgical repair is definitely indicated.

Although significant contamination with bacteria and feed is common, these factors do not seem to be detrimental to repair. Conversely, continued

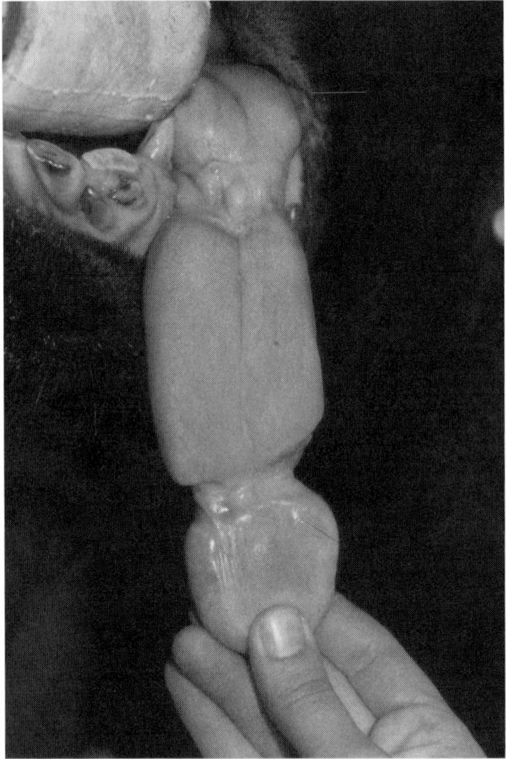

Fig. 3. Two healed lacerations of the tongue caused by the bit.

movement of the tongue and the creation of dead space within the closure are thought to be significant deterrents. Small lacerations at the tip can be repaired in a standing sedated horse; however, general anesthesia is preferred for more extensive injuries or those that are located more caudally on the tongue (Fig. 4). In the latter case, the tongue is exteriorized by traction with a towel clamp placed in the dorsum or by a gauze loop placed caudal to the laceration. The surface of the wound should be sharply debrided with a scalpel to produce a fresh edge; however, this must be done without excessive removal of viable tissue so as to prevent further deformity. The lacerations normally run transversally across the tongue and extend from the dorsal surface into the depths of the musculature. The laceration is closed from the bottom of the defect upward using multiple layers to close all dead space [36,37]. Knots can be buried in the muscle or tied on the external surface [36,37]. Absorbable suture is preferred because it obviates removal. The dorsal surface of the tongue has the greatest strength and holds tension sutures well. The external surface is closed with a combination of tension and appositional interrupted sutures, with accurate anatomic approximation to prevent bacteria, food material, or saliva from entering the repair site.

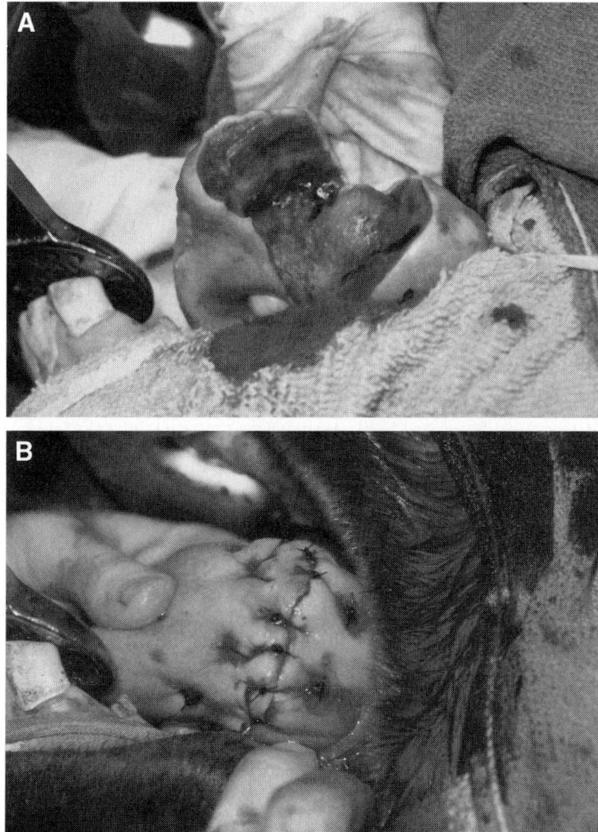

Fig. 4. (*A*) Severe laceration of the caudal aspect of the tongue extending from the dorsal surface obliquely through most of the musculature. (*B*) After wound debridement, the tongue was closed in multiple layers with a combination of simple interrupted and interrupted mattress sutures of absorbable material.

Although the tongue has an excellent blood supply, a severe injury could result in avascularity [34,36,37]. In this case, amputation at the level of the frenulum is well tolerated [34]. A wedge-shaped piece of tissue is removed from the remaining viable tip to create dorsal and ventral edges that are closed over the end of the tongue, usually in layers, without excessive tension [37].

Nostril lacerations

Lacerations of this area occur periodically from the horse catching or impaling the tissue on sharp protruding objects. The significance of the injury depends on the extent of the laceration. Normal function of the nostril is required for whinnying [35] and for efficient inspiration during exercise [36]. Furthermore, nostrils are readily apparent, and a defect to them can depreciate the horse's value.

Lacerations are usually minimally contaminated, can be closed without excessive tension or postoperative motion, and are well vascularized. Thorough debridement is needed, but it is important to save all viable tissue for reconstruction so as to avoid a deformity. A figure-of-eight suture has been advocated in lacerations of the arch of the nostril at the entry into the false nostril [36], but the author prefers multilayered closure at all locations. The edges are sharply freshened and slightly undermined, and the deep layer is closed first with at least a three-layer closure. The surface of the wound is closed with accurate anatomic positioning of the edges by interrupted tension and appositional sutures. Chronic wounds that have healed with a large flap are repaired in a similar manner after debridement that creates a raw surface and slightly undermines the edges to produce multiple layers (Fig. 5) [36]. If a scar restricts the ability of the nostril to dilate, surgical procedures, such as Z-plasties, have been reported to increase the diameter of the nostrils [36]. The surgical site must be protected from mutilation by muzzling or cross-tying the horse.

Ear lacerations

Because of its great mobility, the ear is uncommonly lacerated; it is damaged more frequently by being bitten or frozen. Most injuries occur to the tip of the ear and can be cosmetically unacceptable to owners.

Surgical repair is highly recommended, because untreated lacerations result in an ear that is thickened, curled, or has a forked tip. The skin and cartilage are sharply debrided by removing a narrow strip of tissue with a scalpel or scissors. To prevent deformities, all possible tissue is preserved for reconstruction. Only the skin is sutured in the closure to prevent thickening of the cartilage and subsequent deformity of the ear [36]. If the ear tends to curl after repair, a splint made of a portion of radiographic film can be attached to it by placing sutures through the film and the cartilage well back from the defect. Bandaging is not recommended and often leads to self mutilation; however, cross-tying is useful to prevent dehiscence and deformity of the ears after reconstruction.

Eyelid lacerations

Eyelids are commonly injured by blunt or sharp projecting objects. The eyelid has an important role in protecting the eye and bathing it with lacrimal fluid. The upper eyelid is larger and more mobile and is important in blinking. Loss of eyelid function can lead to numerous complications, including epiphora, conjunctivitis, exposure keratitis, and corneal ulcers. For this reason, eyelid repair is always indicated. Some lacerations create small

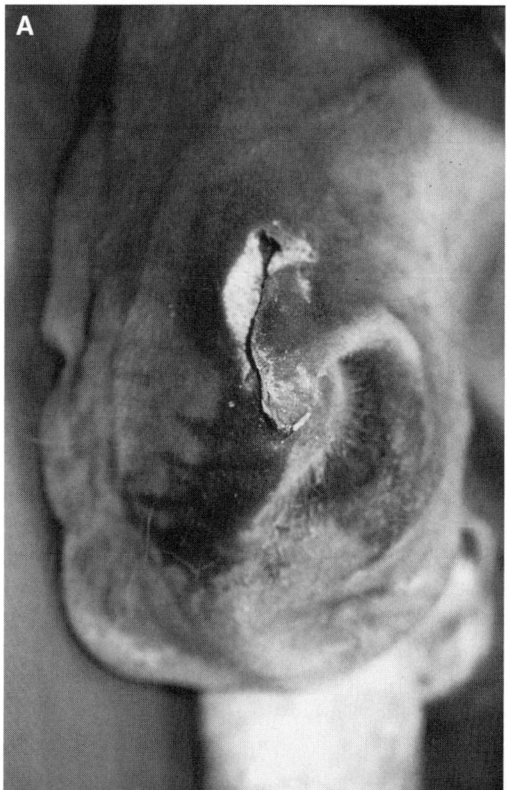

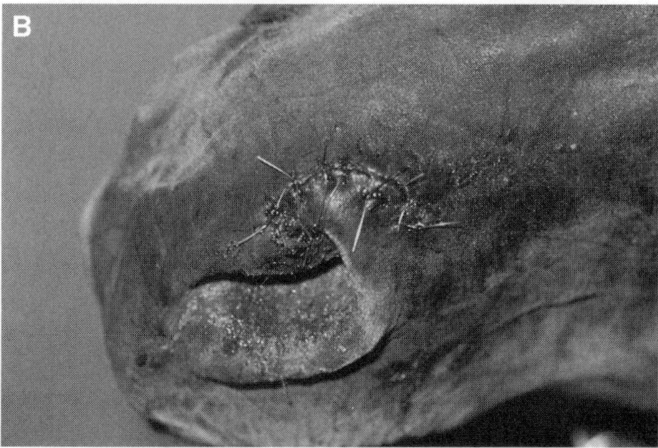

Fig. 5. (*A*) Chronic laceration of the arch of the nostril producing a skin flap that interfered with function, decreased performance, caused a noise, and was cosmetically unacceptable. (*B*) Appearance after the chronic wound was debrided to produce viable edges that were sutured in a three-layer closure. The sutured wound healed, and the horse returned to normal activities.

pieces of tissue with a precarious blood supply; however, reconstruction is still recommended in an attempt to salvage a normal and functional eyelid margin [36]. Luckily, blood supply to the eyelid is excellent, and lacerations are often minimally contaminated.

Occasionally, lacerations are partial thickness and do not involve the lid margin. When the margin is intact, the chance of deformity and complications is greatly reduced. These wounds are debrided, preserving a maximum amount of tissue, and sutured in a one- or two-layer closure. They usually heal uneventfully and with return to full function. When scar contracture results in retraction of the eyelid margin from the globe, blepharoplasty techniques are required to restore normal function (Fig. 6).

Full-thickness lid defects with disruption of the margin are more commonly encountered. Surgical repair is best performed with the horse under general anesthesia. Debridement should be gentle and conservative; only obviously dead and highly devascularized tissue is removed. The conjunctiva is closed first with a simple interrupted or simple continuous suture pattern [36,38,39]. It is paramount that the knots be buried within tissue to avoid rubbing on the cornea. When closing the skin layer, it is important to place the first suture at the lid margin to realign the edges accurately and restore function. A figure-of-eight suture has been recommended in this location, once again ensuring that the knot is placed externally to avoid rubbing on the cornea. The next skin suture is placed adjacent to the one at the lid margin and penetrates deeply into the eyelid and the tarsal plate, such that it takes up much of the tension of the repair. Fine suture material (4-0 or 5-0) is used for the conjunctival layer and for sutures placed at the lid margin, but simple interrupted sutures of larger caliber can be used for the rest of the skin closure.

Lacerations that result in defects greater than 30% or 40% of the lid margin may require special blepharoplasty techniques to restore function [38,39]. One of the simplest methods of reconstructing the margin is the sliding skin flap (single pedicle advancement flap) [38]. Rhomboid graft flaps have been used to repair defects involving more than 50% of the eyelid, and defects of the lateral upper eyelid can be closed with a sliding Z flap [38]. If a scar results in ectropion, a Z-plasty is useful (see Fig. 6) [39]. The reader is referred elsewhere [36,38,39] for a detailed description of these procedures and their applications.

Lacerations of the medial canthus can disrupt the nasal puncta or canaliculus [40]. To reduce the likelihood of developing chronic epiphora from obstruction of a damaged nasolacrimal system, surgical repair is indicated. A probe can been used to place suture material through the severed ends of the canaliculus. Stents made of silicone or silastic tubing are then drawn through the canaliculus down the nasolacrimal duct and secured to the skin for several weeks to allow repair of the canaliculus around them [40]. Cross-tying the horse is indicated for several days to prevent rubbing and premature stent removal.

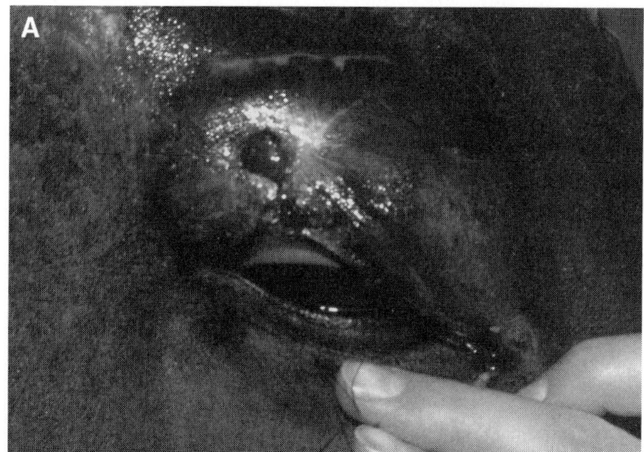

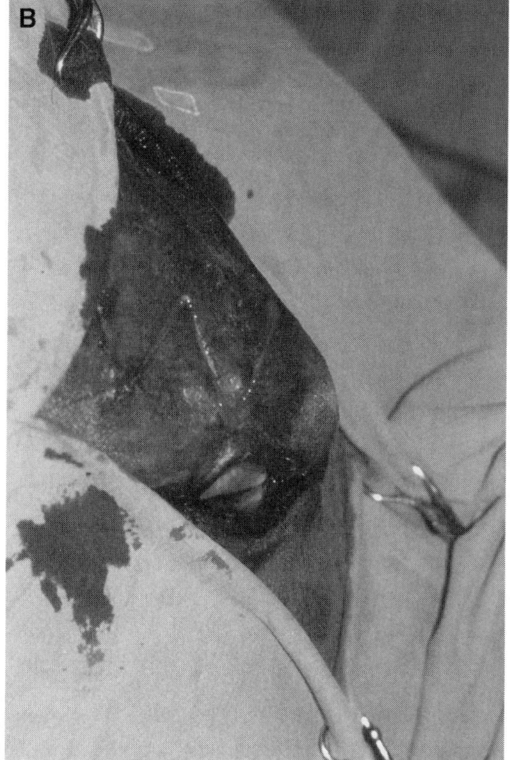

Fig. 6. (*A*) Ectropion of the upper eyelid with exposure keratitis caused by scar contracture after trauma to the eyelid and bony sequestration of the zygomatic arch. (*B*) A Z-plasty with 3.5-cm bar was performed to relieve the scar contracture. (*C*) Normal function and minimal blemish of the eyelid were attained after Z-plasty reconstruction.

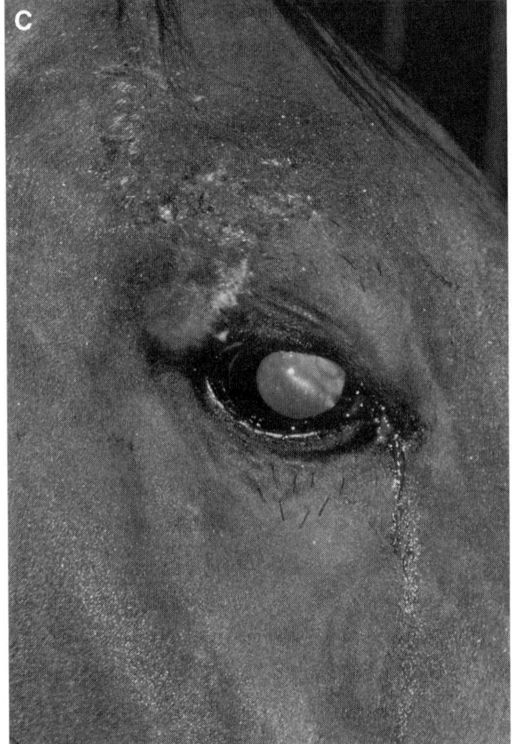

Fig. 6 (*continued*)

Fractures of the facial bones, sinuses, and orbit

Clinical signs and diagnosis

Clinical signs depend on the severity of injury and whether the nasal passage, paranasal sinuses, or orbital rim is involved. Fractures of the rostral nasal bones can be associated with degloving injuries of the overlying soft tissue (Fig. 7) [41]. Most fractures occur more caudally, however, and usually involve the maxilla and nasal, frontal, and lacrimal bones with or without disruption of the overlying skin [42].

When the skin is open, the presence of bony fragments and penetration of the nasal passage or sinus are usually obvious; however, a precise diagnosis is more difficult if the skin is closed. Injury frequently generates facial asymmetry [43,44], although this may be difficult to detect because of local edema and hemorrhage at the impact site [42]. Digital palpation is painful and may preclude a detailed examination. Crepitus is present if there are comminuted mobile fragments, but many fractures are incomplete, impacted, and nonmobile. If the injury is chronic, crepitus is not present because of fibrosis and callus formation. Epistaxis indicates that the fractures have penetrated the

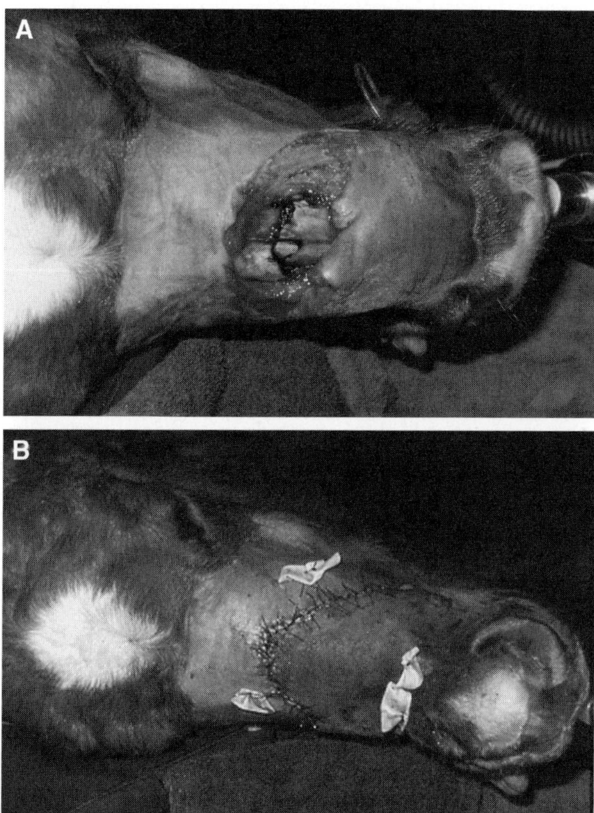

Fig. 7. (*A*) Laceration of the rostral portion of the face, with slight degloving of the soft tissue and fracture of the nasal bones in a foal. (*B*) After thorough debridement of the bone and soft tissues, the unstable fragments were stabilized with interfragmentary wires, Penrose drains were placed for ventral drainage, and the wound was closed.

mucosal lining of the nasal passage or paranasal sinus [42,43]. In this case, the fractures should be considered compound because of bacterial contamination from the nasal passage or sinus [42]. Penetration of the airway can occasionally lead to subcutaneous emphysema [45]. Dyspnea may occur if there is a large blood clot in the nasal passage or if there is a major narrowing of the nasal passage secondary to fractures of the nasal bones or nasal septum [45,46]. Epiphora results from obstruction of the nasolacrimal duct; however, if the fracture severs the duct, secretions drain into the wound and epiphora is not evident [47]. Fractures of the orbital rim can result in fragments impinging on the globe, preventing normal movements of the eye within the orbit [47,48]. Corneal edema and photophobia can accompany corneal ulceration and uveitis [47].

Diagnosis is often obvious if facial asymmetry, crepitus, or an open skin wound is present. Radiographs should always be taken to document and delineate the extent of the fractures; however, because of the complex anatomy and shape of the head, it is often difficult to "profile" the area of concern. Hence, the extent of bony injury is often found at surgery to be greater than was visible on the radiographs [47,48]. The presence of a fluid line in the maxillary sinus indicates penetration of the mucosa and collection of blood in the sinus. Clotting may prevent drainage of blood through the normal slit-like openings of the sinus into the nasal passage.

Treatment

Systemic antibiotics are indicated, because the fractures are usually compound and contaminated. Blood retained in an occluded sinus is an excellent nidus for bacterial infection and may result in a sinus infection. A lavage system for the sinus should be installed and can be performed with the patient standing or can be placed while the horse is under general anesthesia for fracture repair. An intramedullary pin just slightly larger than a silastic drain is used to create a percutaneous hole in the maxilla, nasal, or frontal bone adjacent to the fracture site. A silastic drain is then inserted into the frontal or maxillary sinus and secured by suturing butterfly tape to the skin. An extension set allows lavage from a remote distance from the head. The sinus is lavaged twice daily with physiologic saline or dilute antiseptic solution for several days, and hay is fed on the ground to encourage natural drainage.

Surgical treatment is not necessary if the skin and nasolacrimal duct are intact, eye movement is not impeded, nasal passage is not narrowed, and cosmetic appearance is not a priority. Even in these cases, however, the author encourages reconstruction to diminish the risk of complications.

Reconstruction should be performed with the horse under general anesthesia for optimal debridement and accurate repair. Access to the fractures for reconstruction can be through extension of an existing open skin wound [47] or, if the fracture is closed, via a curved skin incision adjacent to the site of injury [44]. Skin wounds on the face heal well despite contamination; however, aggressive debridement of the soft and hard tissues is important. The fractures are complete with mobile unstable fragments, sometimes with a tenuous blood supply, or incomplete with depressed but stable fragments [47]. Any small mobile fragments with minimal blood supply should be discarded to decrease the possibility of sequestrum formation. If these pieces are small, their removal should not lead to deformity of the face, because the defect is filled with fibrous tissue and new bone. When the sinus is open, any bone fragments, debris, and blood clots should be removed and a lavage system installed.

Surgical repair is much easier and cosmetically successful if performed in acute fractures, because fibrosis and callus formation hinder reduction and reconstruction in chronic cases. If a small piece of avascular bone was discarded, elevators, retractors, or a bone hook can be introduced through the newly created opening and used to pry, lever, or retract the depressed fragments back into position. If a hole is not present, one can be made with rongeurs along the edge of the fracture [47] or holes can be drilled in contiguous stable bones [44]. Bone screws can also be inserted into the depressed fragments and traction used to elevate them [49]. If the fracture is chronic, orthopedic wire or an orthopedic bone saw may be needed to cut areas where the fragments have started to heal in an abnormal position [47]. Incomplete fragments usually interdigitate enough that further stabilization after reduction is not needed. Complete fractures sometimes remain unstable after reduction and require stabilization with stainless steel wires placed between the fragments and solid surrounding bone [44,47]. Holes can be drilled in the edge of the fragments before or after reduction, but if the holes are made before reduction, the wires can be preplaced. The wire should not be overtightened, because this can break the soft bone; an alternative is to use absorbable suture material. Suturing the periosteum often is all that is required for stability; however, this covering may be stripped from the fragments, necessitating the placement of wire or suture through the bone. If stability cannot be achieved with wiring or suturing alone, bone plates can be used but may lead to drainage, screw loosening, and eventual removal of the implants [45,46]. Alternatively, stability can be achieved by drilling holes in unstable fragments and preplacing wires or sutures that exit the skin and are tied over an external splint that rests on the stable bone adjacent to the fracture and therefore prevents collapse. The splint, wire, and sutures can be removed in a few weeks when healing has provided stability.

A large bony defect may yield a concavity from lack of support of the overlying skin. In these cases, the opening may be bridged with synthetic mesh that is then covered with skin [50]. Aggressive debridement and use of antibiotics are necessary to help prevent infection of the implant.

Closure of the skin is important to prevent continued contamination of the repair site and, possibly, the sinus and to provide vascularity to fragments whose blood supply is impaired by comminution and periosteal elevation. Undermining of the skin or relief incisions made a few centimeters from the skin edge may be required to close the defect without excessive tension. The openings created by the relieving incisions can be closed with other plastic procedures or left to heal by second intention.

Fractures of the orbital rim

Impingement of bone fragments against the eye can injure it or prevent its normal movement [47,48]. This is evident by means of proptosis and/or "entrapment" of the eye in one position when the head is moved. Entrapment of the globe occurs after fractures of the lacrimal bone at the medial canthus of the orbit or of the zygomatic process of the frontal or temporal bone. Fractures of the zygomatic process can usually be elevated into position by lifting the fragment with a bone hook inserted into the conjunctival fornix [48]. Further stabilization often is not needed, although insertion of wires or suture between the fragments may improve stability. Fracture fragments from the medial canthus of the orbit are often difficult to reduce, but pressure on the globe can be relieved by removing the portion of bone pressing on the globe with rongeurs placed subconjunctivally or by simply breaking it off [47]. A careful examination of both eyes is recommended, because corneal ulceration and uveitis of the ipsilateral eye [47] and retinal detachment in the contralateral eye [51] have been reported after facial fractures.

Nasolacrimal duct injury

Although the proximal portion of the nasolacrimal duct is enclosed in a bony canal within the lacrimal bone and maxilla and seems to be fairly resistant to trauma [47], its integrity can be lost when facial bones fracture [51–53]. Epiphora may not occur initially, because the tears may drain into the wound, but it may be seen later when scarring and callus obstruct the duct. Patency of the duct should always be checked by catheterization or flushing with fluorescein dye. If the severed ends of the duct can be identified, it may heal over silicone tubing used as an internal splint [40]. Otherwise, a permanent communication with the maxillary sinus can be created by placing a polyethylene catheter through the proximal puncta and proximal segment of the duct into the sinus through a bony hole created by the fracture or the surgeon [51–53]. The catheter is left in place for 2 to 3 weeks until a permanent fistula forms.

Antibiotics, nonsteroidal inflammatory drugs, and sinus lavage are continued for several days after surgical repair. Care should be taken to prevent reinjury to the face during recovery from anesthesia. Bandages and cross-tying may be necessary to protect the incision, and especially the nasolacrimal catheters, from rubbing. If a concavity is still present after healing has occurred, the defect can be cosmetically corrected by implanting a prosthetic device subperiosteally [54].

Summary

The horse, a flight animal that is used extensively by man, frequently receives injuries to its neck or head that result mostly from its management and handling. Better facilities, training of the horse, and horsemanship skills of the handler could prevent many of these injuries. Because many body systems can be involved, with potentially major consequences regarding health, performance, and appearance, early recognition of trauma and competent treatment are crucial.

Progress has been made in the treatment of some tracheal and esophageal injuries. Severe tracheal trauma and rupture of the esophagus still represent major challenges for the attending veterinarian, however. Lacerations of the head generally heal well, likely because of an abundant blood supply. Thorough yet conservative debridement is necessary, as is accurate reconstruction of the tissues to maintain normal function and an acceptable cosmetic appearance. Fractures of the facial bones can result in complications, such as sequestrum formation, sinusitis, nasolacrimal duct injury, facial deformity, and injury to or entrapment of the globe. An awareness of the treatment methods available can help to diminish the complication rate and to restore a normal or acceptable appearance.

References

[1] Stashak TS. Wound closure. In: Equine wound management. Philadelphia: Lea & Febiger; 1991. p. 40–8.
[2] Baxter GM. Wounds and wound healing. In: Colahan PT, Merritt AM, Moore JN, et al, editors. Equine medicine and surgery. 5th edition. Philadelphia: Mosby; 1999. p. 1801–41.
[3] Bigbie RB, Schumacher J, Swaim SF, et al. Effects of amnion and live yeast cell derivative on second-intention healing in horses. Am J Vet Res 1991;52(8):1376–81.
[4] Barber SM. Diseases of the guttural pouches. In: Colahan PT, Merritt AM, Moore JN, et al, editors. Equine medicine and surgery. 5th edition. Philadelphia: Mosby; 1999. p. 502–12.
[5] Shappell KK. Trachea. In: Auer JA, Stick JA, editors. Equine surgery. 2nd edition. Philadelphia: WB Saunders; 1999. p. 376–81.
[6] Caron JP, Townsend HGG. Tracheal perforation and widespread subcutaneous emphysema in a horse. Can Vet J 1984;25:339–41.
[7] Fubini SL, Todhunter RJ, Vivrette SL, et al. Tracheal rupture in two horses. J Am Vet Med Assoc 1990;187(1):69–70.
[8] Kirker-Head CA, Jakob TP. Surgical repair of ruptured trachea in a horse. J Am Vet Med Assoc 1990;196(10):1635–8.
[9] Freeman DE. Trachea. In: Beech J, editor. Equine respiratory disorders. Malvern: Lea & Febiger; 1991. p. 389–402.
[10] Robertson JT, Spurlock GH. Tracheal reconstruction in a foal. J Am Vet Med Assoc 1986; 189(3):313–4.
[11] Yovich JV, Stashak TS. Surgical repair of a collapsed trachea caused by a lipoma in a horse. Vet Surg 1984;13:217–21.
[12] Tate LP, Koch DB, Sembrat RF, et al. Tracheal reconstruction by resection and end-to-end anastomosis in the horse. J Am Vet Med Assoc 1981;178(3):253–8.
[13] Shappell KK, Stick JA, Derksen FJ, et al. Permanent tracheostomy in Equidae: 47 cases (1981–1986). J Am Vet Med Assoc 1988;192(2):939–42.
[14] McClure SR, Taylor TS, Honnas CM, et al. Permanent tracheostomy in standing horses: technique and results. Vet Surg 1995;24:231–4.
[15] Fubini SL, Starrak GS, Freeman DE. Esophagus. In: Auer JA, Stick JA, editors. Equine surgery. 2nd edition. Philadelphia: WB Saunders; 1999. p. 199–209.
[16] Stick JA. Diseases of the esophagus. In: Colahan PT, Merritt AM, Moore JN, et al, editors. Equine medicine and surgery. 5th edition. Philadelpha: Mosby; 1999. p. 677–98.
[17] Read EK, Barber SM, Wilson DG, et al. Oesphageal rupture in a Quarter Horse mare: unique features of liquid enteral hyperalimentation and fistula management. Equine Vet Educ 2002;14(3):126–31.
[18] Risnes I, Mair TS. Traumatic oesophageal rupture in a horse complicated by subsequent rupture of the common carotid artery. Equine Vet Educ 2003;15(3):120–4.
[19] Dechant JE, MacDonald DG, Crawford WH, et al. Pleuritis associated with perforation of an isolated oesophageal ulcer in a horse. Equine Vet J 1998;30:170–2.

[20] Peacock EE. Esophagus. In: Wound repair. 3rd edition. Philadelphia: WB Saunders; 1984. p. 451–5.
[21] Todhunter RJ, Stick JA, Trotter GW, et al. Medical management of esophageal stricture in seven horses. J Am Vet Med Assoc 1984;185(7):93–9.
[22] Todhunter RJ, Stick JA, Slocombe RF. Comparison of three feeding techniques after esophageal mucosal reaction and anastomosis in the horse. Cornell Vet 1986;76:16–29.
[23] Knottenbelt DC, Harrison LJ, Peacock PJ. Conservative treatment of oesophageal stricture in 5 foals. Vet Rec 1992;131:27–30.
[24] Craig DR, Shivy DR, Pankowski RL, et al. Esophageal disorders in 61 horses: results of non surgical and surgical management. Vet Surg 1989;18(6):432–8.
[25] Suann CJ. Oesophageal resection and anastomosis as a treatment for oesophageal stricture in the horse. Equine Vet J 1982;14(2):163–4.
[26] Wagner PC, Rantanen NW. Myotomy as a treatment for esophageal stricture in a horse. Equine Pract 1980;2(6):40–5.
[27] Murray RC, Gaughan EM. Pulsion diverticulum of the cranial cervical esophagus in a horse. Can Vet J 1993;34:365–7.
[28] Hackett RP, Dyer RM, Hoffer RE. Surgical correction of esophageal diverticulum in a horse. J Am Vet Med Assoc 1978;173(8):998–1000.
[29] De Moor A, Wouters L, Mouens Y, et al. Surgical treatment of a traumatic oesophageal rupture in a foal. Equine Vet J 1979;11(4):265–6.
[30] Wingfield Digby NJ, Burguez PN. Traumatic oesophageal rupture in the horse. Equine Vet J 1982;14(2):169–70.
[31] Lunn DP, Peel JE. Successful treatment of traumatic oesophageal rupture with severe cellulitis in a mare. Vet Rec 1985;116:544–5.
[32] Stick JA, Krehbiel JD, Kunze DJ, et al. Esophageal healing in the pony: comparison of sutured vs non sutured esophagotomy. Am J Vet Res 1981;42(9):1506–13.
[33] Colahan PT. Diseases of the lips, mouth, tongue, and oropharynx. In: Colahan PT, Merritt AM, Moore JN, et al, editors. Equine medicine and surgery. 5th edition. Philadelphia: Mosby; 1999. p. 652–8.
[34] Howard RD, Stashak TS. Reconstructive surgery of selected injuries of the head. Vet Clin N Am Equine Pract 1993;9(1):185–98.
[35] Smyth GB, Brown RG, Juzwiak JS, et al. Delayed repair of an extensive lip laceration in a colt using an Estlander flap. Vet Surg 1988;17(6):350–2.
[36] Stashak TS. Wound management and reconstructive surgery of the head region. In: Equine wound management. Philadelphia: Lea & Febiger; 1991. p. 89–144.
[37] White NA, Hoffman PE. Surgical repair of equine lingual lacerations. Equine Pract 1980; 2(2):37–42.
[38] Miller TR. Eyelids. In: Auer JA, Stick JA, editors. Equine surgery. 2nd edition. Philadelphia: WB Saunders; 1999. p. 450–64.
[39] Hamilton HL, Whitley RD, McLaughlin SA, et al. Basic blepharoplasty techniques. Compend Contin Educ Pract Vet 1999;21(10):946–53.
[40] Dziezyc J. Nasolacrimal system. In: Auer JA, Stick JA, editors. Equine surgery. 2nd edition. Philadelphia: WB Saunders; 1999. p. 476–80.
[41] Debowes RM. Fractures of the mandible and maxilla. In: Nixon AJ, editor. Equine fracture repair. Philadelphia: WB Saunders; 1996. p. 323–35.
[42] Easter JL, Watkins JP. Diseases of the head and neck. In: Colahan PT, Merritt AM, Moore JN, et al, editors. Equine medicine and surgery. 5th edition. Philadelphia: Mosby; 1999. p. 1669–76.
[43] Levine SB. Depression fractures of the nasal and frontal bones of the horse. J Equine Med Surg 1997;3:186–90.
[44] Turner AS. Surgical management of depression fractures of the equine skull. Vet Surg 1979; 8(2):29–33.

[45] Dowling BA, Dart AJ, Trope G. Surgical repair of skull fractures in four horses using cuttable bone plates. Aust Vet J 2001;79:324–7.
[46] Burba DJ, Collier MA. T-plate repair of fractures of the nasal bones in horses. J Am Vet Med Assoc 1991;199(7):909–12.
[47] Caron JP, Barber SM, Bailey JV, et al. Periorbital skull fractures in five horses. J Am Vet Med Assoc 1986;188(3):280–4.
[48] Blackford JT, Hanselka DV, Heitmann JM, et al. Noninvasive techniques for reduction of zygomatic process fractures in the horse. Vet Surg 1985;14(1):21–6.
[49] Haynes PF. Surgery of the equine respiratory tract. In: Jennings PB, editor. Practice of large animal surgery. Philadelphia: WB Saunders; 1984. p. 388–487.
[50] Martin GS, McIlwraith CW. Repair of a frontal sinus eversion in a horse. Vet Surg 1981;10: 149–52.
[51] Wilson DG, Levine SA. Surgical reconstruction of the nasolacrimal system in the horse. J Equine Vet Sci 1991;11(4):232–4.
[52] Cruz AM, Barber SM, Grahn BH. Nasolacrimal duct injury following periorbital trauma with concurrent retinal choroidal detachment in a horse. Equine Pract 1997;19(8):20–3.
[53] McIlnay TR, Miller SM, Dugan ST. Use of canaliculorhinostomy for repair of nasolacrimal duct obstruction in a horse. J Am Vet Med Assoc 2001;218(8):1323–4.
[54] Valdez H, Rook JS. Use of fluorocarbon polymer and carbon fiber for restoration of facial contour in a horse. J Am Vet Med Assoc 1981;178(3):249–52.

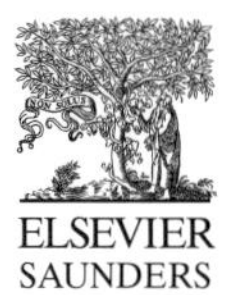
ELSEVIER
SAUNDERS

Vet Clin Equine 21 (2005) 217–230

VETERINARY
CLINICS
Equine Practice

Management of Complicated Wounds

Sam M. Hendrix, DVM*, Gary M. Baxter, VMD

Department of Clinical Sciences, College of Veterinary Medicine and Biomedical Sciences, Veterinary Medical Center, Colorado State University, 300 West Drake Road, Fort Collins, CO 80523, USA

The flight response is to blame for many injuries sustained by horses, and given the high energy involved in many incidents, the severity and extent of tissue involvement can be dramatic. These injuries can present the equine practitioner with a challenge; however, with appropriate therapy, many wounds have a surprisingly favorable outcome.

Degloving injuries

A limb that becomes entangled or trapped in fencing or other hazards can quickly sustain significant tissue damage. Degloving or avulsion injuries are not uncommon in equine practice, and their management can be challenging because of the prolonged treatment, cost, and sometimes unknown outcome [1]. Although degloving injuries can occur over other regions of the body, the most common sites for this type of trauma are the dorsal aspect of the metacarpus and/or metatarsus and the cranial aspect of the tarsus [1]. The longer a limb is entrapped and the harder the horse struggles to free itself, the more vascular, soft tissue, and bone damage is likely to occur. Some injuries that seem to be superficial and innocuous on the surface may involve vital structures surrounding the wound, however. Additionally, healing of wounds involving the distal limb is often delayed when compared with other areas of the body, further complicating the healing process.

Primary closure

The severity and duration of the degloving injury determine the best approach to treat the wound. Primary repair of the wound is always the best option if possible. In general, injuries that only involve loss of skin with maintenance of an intact blood supply respond favorably to primary repair.

* Corresponding author.
E-mail address: Samuel.hendrix@colostate.edu (S.M. Hendrix).

doi:10.1016/j.cveq.2004.11.011 ***vetequine.theclinics.com***

Although uncommon, recent injuries that are relatively uncontaminated and have minimal soft tissue swelling are also candidates for primary repair (Fig. 1). Many degloving injuries of the lower limb result in exposed bone or concurrent tendon injuries. Covering exposed bone or tendon with soft tissue is thought to decrease the chance of sequestrum formation and to improve healing. Also, closing as much of the wound as possible improves the cosmetic and functional outcome and lessens the amount of healing having to occur by second intention.

Delayed closure

Many degloving injuries are not identified for several hours or days, such that primary closure is often not an option. If there is significant swelling

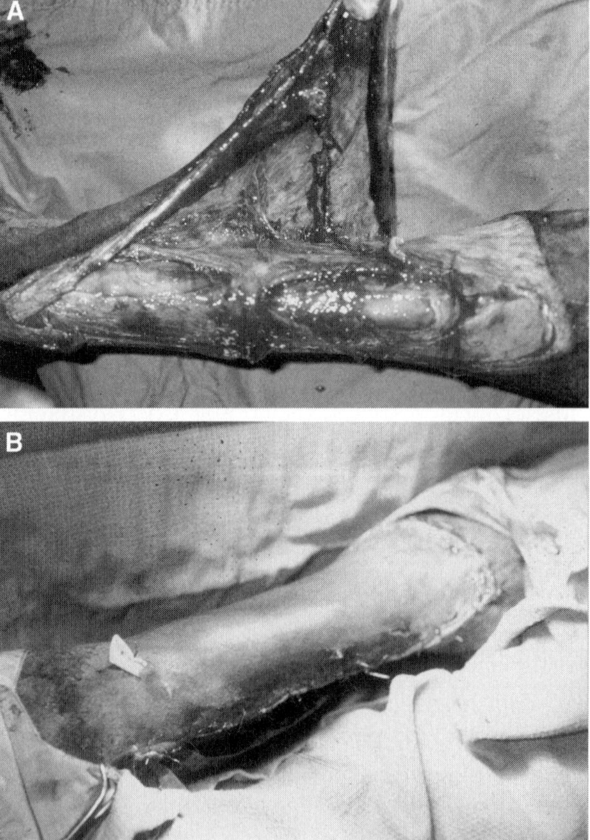

Fig. 1. (*A*) A degloving injury over the metatarsus with minimal secondary trauma or contamination. The long digital extensor tendon was transected (proximal is to the right). (*B*) Primary repair of the degloving injury shown in *A*. The extensor tendon could not be repaired, but the wound was closed and immobilized in a half-limb cast.

and contamination of the wound without loss of skin, delayed closure of the wound may be possible. Delayed closure of degloving injuries is performed infrequently by the authors, however. Aggressive management with direct debridement and lavage, followed by pressure bandaging to remove perilesional edema and contamination, is necessary in these cases. Wet-to-dry bandaging principles may be used to debride and remove much of the surrounding edema and debris. Initial treatment of the wound may require 2 to 3 days of debridement and bandaging before the wound is ready for closure. The wound edges can then be debrided and repaired in the absence of excessive swelling and contamination and with a reduced risk of infection. Use of tension sutures is often necessary to close the wound at this time, because wound retraction often occurs within a few days of injury.

Second-intention healing

Most degloving injuries result in a defect that involves the loss of a significant amount of skin directly at the time of injury or subsequently because of loss of blood supply. There is usually no choice in these injuries but to rely on second-intention healing. The goal in managing these severe injuries is to debride the wound of all necrotic tissue, followed by healing with healthy granulation tissue [1]. Debridement is usually performed by physical removal via sharp dissection of necrotic tissue combined with wound dressings and bandaging. During the initial healing phase, the wound should be covered with pressure bandages to minimize contamination of the tissues and to decrease motion at the wound site. External coaptation with splints or casts is usually unnecessary unless there is secondary extensor tendon involvement. In wounds with exposed bone, granulation tissue fails to cover nonviable bone, suggesting the formation of a sequestrum. The sequestrum needs to be removed to facilitate continued wound granulation. In many instances, the size of the wound may dictate subsequent skin grafting to allow complete healing. This procedure should be delayed for at least 6 to 8 weeks after injury to permit maximum wound contraction to occur before grafting.

Concurrent injury

Many degloving injuries of the metacarpus and/or metatarsus involve disruption of the underlying tendons and bone. Initial evaluation of most wounds should include radiographic evaluation to rule out secondary bone injury. Concurrent extensor tendon injury is usually identified by examination of the wound and is by far the most common secondary injury. Partial disruption of the flexor tendons may not be as readily apparent and may require ultrasonographic confirmation. Horses with concomitant extensor tendon injuries have a better prognosis for return to function than those with disruption of the flexor tendons. Approximately

50% to 75% of horses with extensor tendon injuries are likely to return to full use, whereas another 30% can be used for light riding [2–4]. In contrast, only 18% of those with flexor tendon injuries return to full use, with another 44% used for light riding [2].

Loss of the extensor tendon of the distal limb usually causes dorsal knuckling of the fetlock and an inability to extend the phalanges [3]. Management of extensor tendon disruption is based on supporting the dorsal aspect of the limb to counteract the pull of the flexor tendons on the palmar and/or plantar aspect of the limb. This is usually accomplished by splinting or casting the distal limb in extension [1,4]. Casting is usually used after primary repair of the tendon and wound or with small wounds that require minimal debridement. In most cases, the wound is managed by second-intention healing, and a rigid polyvinyl chloride (PVC) splint is applied to the dorsal or palmar and/or plantar aspect of the distal limb after wound bandaging. The bandage and splint, which maintain the limb in extension and prevent dorsal knuckling of the fetlock, are retained until normal limb function returns, which may vary from 3 to 6 weeks.

Nerve damage

There are probably many traumatic wounds in horses that damage nerves but that we fail to recognize as a result of our inability to diagnose these types of injuries. For instance, many heel bulb and pastern lacerations with significant bleeding probably have concurrent transection of the palmar or plantar digital nerve. This may or may not be recognized during examination of the horse or wound debridement; even if it were recognized, it would most likely not alter the treatment plan or prognosis. Unilateral transection of the palmar and/or plantar digital or palmar and/or plantar nerves associated with traumatic lacerations seems to cause minimal morbidity in horses. The palmar digital nerves regrow after transection in an attempt to reinnervate the affected area. Neuroma formation after nerve transection, although rare, can occur and may cause lameness, together with focal pain directly over the wound and nerve site. The lameness improves after local anesthetic is placed at the site of the neuroma. Surgical removal of the neuroma and associated nerve is the treatment of choice (Fig. 2), to which most horses respond favorably.

Nerve transection associated with wounds at other locations in the limb or trunk is uncommon or at least poorly recognized. Potential sites for concurrent nerve injury include the lateral aspect of the proximal radius and elbow, where the radial nerve lies fairly superficial, and the shoulder region, where lacerations and blunt trauma may contribute to suprascapular nerve injuries. Nerve injury in either location is uncommon, however. Injuries to smaller nerve branches most likely occur with all types of traumatic wounds but seem to have a minimal impact on wound healing. Occasionally, focal areas of wounds may be “hypersensitive” to touch, which may indicate

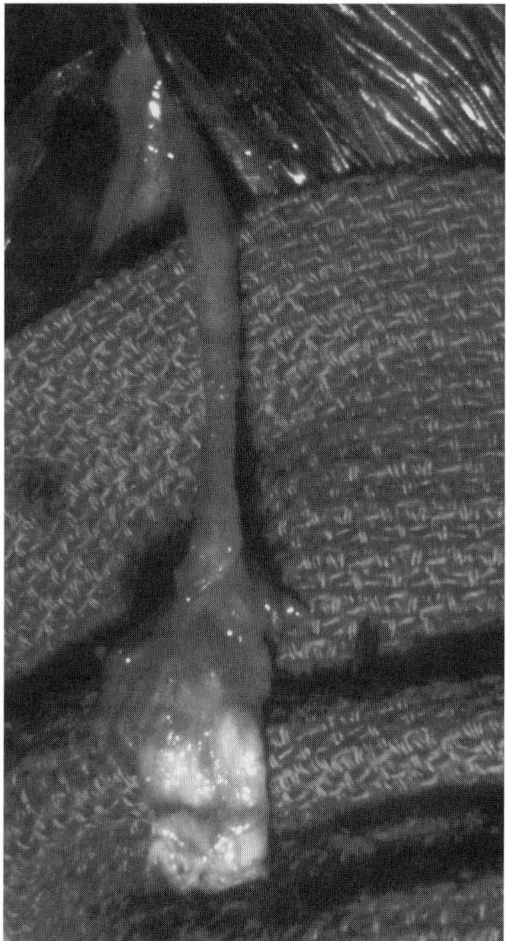

Fig. 2. Surgical removal of a painful neuroma that occurred secondary to a laceration over the pastern region.

previous damage to nerve branches with potential small neuroma formation. This hypersensitivity tends to resolve as the wound is covered with healthy granulation tissue.

Osseous sequestration and foreign bodies

The clinical presentation of horses with osseous sequestration and penetrating foreign bodies is similar in many ways. Medical management is usually unrewarding, and the clinical signs resolve only after removal of the offending foreign or necrotic material. The amount of secondary soft tissue scarring and bone remodeling is largely proportional to the time elapsed before surgical removal of the offending entity. Therefore, addressing these cases in a timely manner helps to return horses to full function without secondary complications.

Because of the lack of soft tissue protection, the distal limbs of horses are extremely susceptible to damage of the periosteum and underlying bone. With periosteal disruption, the underlying outer cortical bone is prone to develop ischemia, because the periosteum supplies blood to this zone. For a sequestrum to develop, secondary bacterial colonization around the site is also considered necessary. Cortical bone death occurs secondary to the alteration in blood flow. As the bone becomes necrotic, the dead section of bone becomes surrounded by inflammatory debris. This ischemic focus is highly susceptible to bacterial colonization and proliferation originating from the inciting trauma. This said, blunt trauma producing no external entry wound may result in sequestrum formation, indicating that bacterial inoculation may also occur via the bloodstream. This is most commonly seen with injuries to the metacarpal and/or metatarsal bones. These types of injuries nearly always develop a fistulous tract that eventually ruptures to the external environment through the skin.

Depending on the size of the devitalized bone fragment, the body may be able to resorb the sequestrum or expel it from the draining tract. Larger fragments usually persist and lead to more extensive clinical disease, however. The basis of persistence of the inflammatory focus is twofold. Because of the lack of vascularization, the immune response at the site is inadequate, leading to a chronic infection that persists in the face of a normal immune system [5,6]. Second, the relative lack of blood flow also thwarts the migration of osteoclasts to the site, hindering the natural resorption of bone. These events collectively result in a chronic inflammatory focus that the body cannot or only slowly resolves. Therefore, any wound with delayed healing should be closely evaluated for the possibility of a sequestrum.

The most common sites for sequestrum formation are those with a relative lack of soft tissue covering, such as the metacarpal and/or metatarsal bones, skull, calcaneus, distal radius, tibia, and phalanges (Fig. 3). The affected site most commonly involves some degree of soft tissue swelling and usually has a coexisting draining fistulous tract. There is usually not a significant lameness, but deep palpation over the sequestered bone generally produces a painful response [4,7].

Definitive diagnosis of osseous sequestration is made by radiographic evaluation of the involved site. Sequestra formation may not be readily noticeable on survey radiographs until 2 to 3 weeks after the inciting injury has occurred, however [8,9]. Correct radiographic orientation is necessary to identify most sequestra properly, and the use of oblique views of the region of interest is often essential. Contrast radiography may be useful to define the extent and location of a sequestrum.

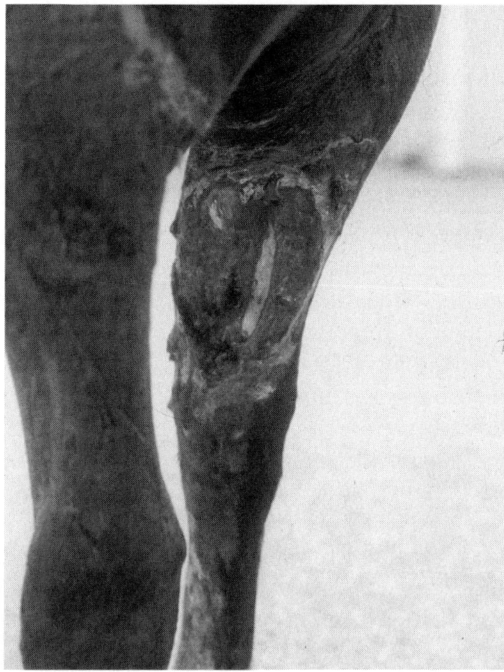

Fig. 3. A chronic nonhealing wound over the distal radius secondary to sequestrum formation.

The classic radiographic appearance of the chronic sequestrum is that of an isolated fragment of bone separated from the parent bone by a radiolucent sheath that represents the necrotic debris around the sequestrum. The surrounding healthy bone often has varying degrees of periosteal new bone, which forms the involucrum, or an envelope of viable bone surrounding the necrotic bone. The opening in the involucrum, known as the cloaca, represents the drainage site from the bone margin to the soft tissues. The early radiographic appearance of one or two radiolucent lines that lie beneath and run parallel to the outer cortex may help to predict potential osseous sequestration. Progressive separation of the bone results in a more distinct radiolucent line between the parent bone and the devitalized sequestered segment [7]. Ultrasound evaluation may also be of benefit in further localizing a fistulous tract and the bone fragment, but it is often underused [10]. The former is identified as an anechoic fluid- or gas-filled tract surrounded by echogenic fibrous scar tissue, especially in the chronic lesion. The highly echogenic bone fragment is usually surrounded by a pocket of fluid.

Many sequestra are diagnosed only after lengthy medical treatment without resolution of the chronic wound. A common history is that of a wound or draining tract that seems to resolve while on antibiotics but returns on discontinuing therapy. Medical management of this condition rarely results in complete resolution; however, it has been reported. The inflammatory debris and lack of vascular penetrance preclude the ability of the antibiotics to reach the bacteria imbedded within the sequestrum [11]. Surgical removal of the osseous sequestrum is the preferred method of treatment [5,6,8,12,13].

Preoperative bacterial culture and sensitivity testing of the tract and any associated abscessation may be useful in planning antibiotic therapy but is not considered essential. Environmental contamination during sampling can interfere with accurate identification of causative bacteria; however, needle aspiration or the use of a teat cannula may limit potential error. Culture of the deep tissue surrounding the sequestrum or the sequestrum itself is thought to provide the most accurate results. Until culture and sensitivity data are known, broad-spectrum antimicrobials should be used, because a variety of different bacteria may contribute to the infection. *Streptococcus* spp, *Staphylococcus* spp, *Pseudomonas* spp, *Enterobacteriaceae* spp, and anaerobes have all been identified in sequestra in horses [5].

Proper localization of the lesion is essential to plan the surgical approach for sequestrectomy. Along with the temperament of the horse and the financial constraints of the owners, the anatomic location of the lesion and the proximity and involvement of surrounding vital structures determine whether or not general anesthesia is necessary. The potential for complications is increased in the standing horse, particularly when the lesion is located adjacent to vital structures, such as joints or tendon sheaths. Complete resection and removal of the fistulous tract and sequestrum is best performed with the horse under general anesthesia. The tract should be dissected carefully from the adjacent soft tissue until the sequestrum is reached. If a clean and complete resection of the tract is achieved, primary closure of the skin defect is preferred. Therefore, it is important to be conservative in the amount of tissue removed, especially in wounds of the distal limbs. If complete resection of the contaminated tract is not possible, open drainage and second-intention healing represent the best choice.

All nonviable debris and bone should be removed. The surrounding bone should be curetted until the underlying healthy bone bleeds. Excessive bony proliferation may be removed with an osteotome or chisel to contour the bone. Healthy adjacent periosteum should be preserved if possible to minimize excessive bone remodeling.

Wounds left to heal by second intention should be covered with a nonadherent permeable or semiocclusive dressing to keep the bone moist and allow for granulation tissue formation. This is then covered with a protective bandage that is changed as often as needed based on the quantity of wound exudate. Once the defect has filled in with granulation tissue, skin grafts may be used to speed healing in large wounds, such as those on the dorsal aspect of the third metacarpal and/or metatarsal bone.

Most horses that develop sequestra have a good prognosis once the local infection has resolved. Return to full function after complete resolution of clinical signs is possible in most cases. In those horses that do not return to full function, secondary soft tissue, tendon, or bone damage sustained during the initial injury is the most likely factor leading to permanent problems.

Penetrating foreign bodies may present a similar clinical picture as that described for osseous sequestration. Many foreign bodies are only discovered after prolonged medical treatment that has been unsuccessful in resolving a local infection [1]. Many horses with foreign bodies present with a nonhealing persistent draining tract. Although some superficial foreign bodies can be expelled, most require surgical removal (Fig. 4).

The approach to the diagnosis and management of penetrating foreign bodies is similar to that for sequestra. Some foreign bodies may not be evident with survey radiographs, however, unless a gas line is evident secondary to bacterial infection. Objects like wood or plastic have the same radiodensity as soft tissue and are not visible on routine radiographs. Therefore, contrast radiography (fistulography), ultrasound, or probing the wound with a sterile metallic object may aid in the identification of a radiolucent foreign body [1,10].

Wounds involving a body cavity

Wounds over the trunk of the horse are fairly common, given the flight response of the horse, but few of these injuries penetrate the thorax or abdomen. Penetrating injuries to the chest or abdomen are often sustained as a result of the horse running into or jumping over a fixed object, such as a fence post, gate, fence, or tree (Fig. 5). Emergency management may be necessary in some cases of thoracic or abdominal penetration, because pneumothorax or bowel eventration may occur as a result of disruption to

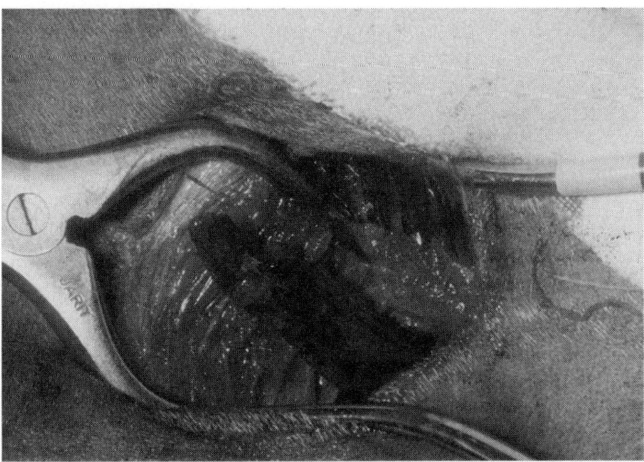

Fig. 4. A piece of wood identified in a wound tract that coursed over the right lateral aspect of the thoracic wall (cranial is to the right).

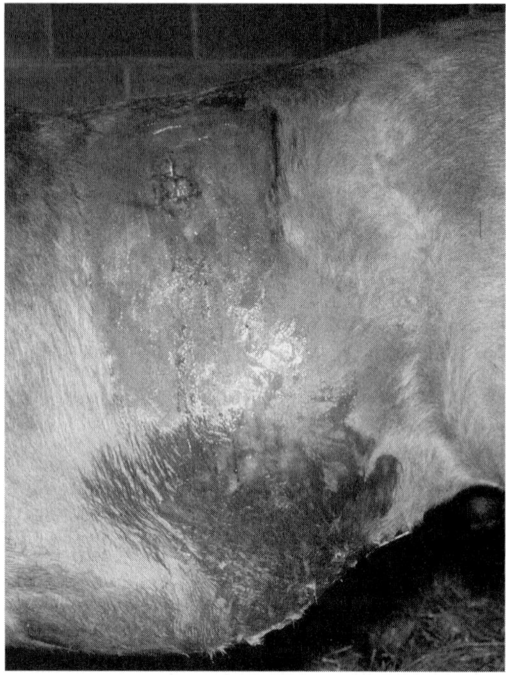

Fig. 5. Puncture wound over the dorsolateral aspect of the thorax and/or abdomen that resulted in pleuritis. Puncture wounds over this region may involve the thoracic or abdominal cavity or both if disruption of the diaphragm occurs.

the body wall [1,14]. Additionally, broad-spectrum antimicrobial therapy is essential with these injuries to prevent secondary infection within the thorax or abdomen.

Thoracic injuries

Clinical evaluation of a horse with a thoracic wound should initially focus on patient homeostasis. The horse should be closely evaluated for any evidence of respiratory distress, including flaring of the nostrils or short rapid breaths indicating a possible pneumothorax or pneumomediastinum. If suspected, the wound should be covered with a sterile airtight dressing to prevent further influx of air into the thorax [14]. Methods to document the presence of a pneumothorax are radiography (which is impractical in the field), ultrasound, and thoracocentesis. Diagnostic thoracocentesis may be performed by placing a catheter or 3.5-inch needle into the thoracic cavity and attaching a fluid extension line with sterile fluid (2–3 mL). If the fluid bubbles out of the extension, pneumothorax is confirmed; if the fluid is sucked into the thoracic cavity, it is unlikely that pneumothorax is present. Air within the thoracic cavity can also be easily confirmed with radiography, which may reveal secondary rib fractures, the presence of foreign bodies, or an atelectatic lung.

Emergency thoracocentesis and suctioning of air may be necessary as a life-saving procedure if the normally complete mediastinum is disrupted or if there is bilateral pleural cavity involvement. Tension pneumothorax (caused by a sucking wound) requires suctioning of air and treatment of the cause of the pneumothorax to prevent severe respiratory compromise [14]. Emergency evacuation of pleural air is achieved by active suction via a teat cannula or 14-gauge catheter placed high in the 13th intercostal space adjacent to the caudal margin of the rib. The teat cannula or catheter is attached to an extension line with a three-way stopcock and then to a 60-mL syringe or suction pump. The air is removed by active suction. As stated previously, the wound causing the condition must be covered to prevent continual entry of air. If available, intranasal oxygen may be beneficial in horses experiencing severe respiratory distress.

Once the horse is stabilized, further exploration of the wound is performed, preferably with the horse standing to avert further respiratory and cardiovascular compromise. General anesthesia may be used provided that the pneumothorax has been resolved. Because of the nature of these injuries, the wound should be thoroughly explored for the presence of foreign bodies or secondary rib fractures. Intercostal perineural local anesthesia facilitates a more thorough exploration as well as helping to control the pain that often accompanies these injuries [14]. Routine wound debridement and lavage should be performed, followed by removal of rib fragments, foreign bodies, and other debris that may be present within the depths of the wound. If possible, the wound should be closed primarily or covered with an airtight dressing and left to heal by second intention. Alternatively, the defect can be repaired with a primary muscle flap, diaphragmatic advancement flap, or prosthetic mesh [14]. In a horse with a wound over the lateral thorax, muscle pedicle flaps of the longissimus and external abdominal oblique muscles have also been used to close the defect [15].

Pleuritis secondary to thoracic trauma is uncommon if penetrating wounds are appropriately treated. Penetration of the thorax may not be readily apparent, however, thus delaying treatment. In one recent retrospective study, horses that developed pleuritis from chest wounds had a 50% mortality rate [16]. This further emphasizes the importance of identifying thoracic involvement accompanying these injuries and using broad-spectrum antimicrobials to prevent secondary pleuritis. Horses with acute, and especially chronic, chest wounds should be closely evaluated for secondary pleuritis by means of radiography, ultrasound, and fluid analysis obtained by thoracocentesis. In addition, depending on the location of the injury, concurrent involvement of the diaphragm may be present, leading to thoracic and abdominal cavity involvement. Thoracoscopy may be useful to help identify these attendant injuries as well as foreign bodies, such as wood, within accessible areas of the thoracic cavity [14].

Axillary wounds, although not penetrating chest wounds, may cause secondary pneumomediastinum and pneumothorax potentially leading to respiratory distress. These wounds often extend deep into the axilla along the thoracic wall and tend to suck in air. This initially leads to subcutaneous emphysema, which may progress to pneumomediastinum or pneumothorax [14]. Packing these wounds with sterile gauze and temporarily closing the skin over the defects or using stent bandages over the wounds helps to prevent air from moving into the tissues. The packing should be removed every 24 to 48 hours and the defect repacked until the defect has granulated. The horse should also be confined to a stall or cross-tied to minimize movement of the limb, which further minimizes the potential for subcutaneous emphysema. Horses with large axillary wounds should be closely monitored for the development of subcutaneous emphysema and impending pneumothorax.

Abdominal wounds

Wounds that enter the abdominal cavity are at risk for septic peritonitis and bowel eventration [1]. Large defects that involve an open abdominal cavity are emergency situations. Emergency first-aid treatment usually involves quickly closing the wound to prevent the bowel from exiting the wound. This may involve temporarily clamping or suturing skin over the defect or bandaging until exploration and repair of the wound can be performed [1]. If the bowel has spilled through the wound, it should be lavaged and returned to the abdomen as quickly as possible. With less obvious injuries, wound exploration, abdominocentesis, ultrasound, and rectal examination may all be used in various combinations to document whether a wound penetrates the peritoneal cavity. Most injuries involving the abdominal cavity are best treated with the horse under general anesthesia to permit thorough wound exploration, debridement, and primary closure. General anesthesia also facilitates complete abdominal lavage, thus minimizing secondary peritonitis. Abdominal drainage using large-bore catheters exiting the ventral abdomen may be necessary in horses with severe abdominal contamination. These drains may also be used for repeated lavage of the abdomen for several days after surgery. Large abdominal wall defects that cannot be closed primarily are usually bandaged and left to heal by second intention. Many of these defects need to be repaired at a later time (2–3 months) using a synthetic mesh implant [17].

Wounds involving major blood vessels

The most common location for wounds to involve a major blood vessel is the pastern region. Heel bulb or pastern lacerations occasionally transect the palmar digital vein or artery and can cause significant blood loss if not found soon after injury. In most cases, the bleeding can be controlled by applying pressure over the wound with a bandage. Alternatively, the severed ends of the vessels can be clamped for a short time before applying a bandage. This should be performed in the standing horse, because anesthesia to facilitate hemorrhage control is usually unnecessary and risky to the patient. Suturing of palmar digital vessels during repair of heel bulb or pastern lacerations is usually impossible, because the severed ends often retract into the wound. Even if the ends of the vessel could be identified, anastomosis is usually unnecessary because of the development of collateral circulation. Other locations in which wounds may involve a major blood vessel include the medial aspect of the tarsus (saphenous vein), the medial aspect of the distal radius (cephalic vein), and the lateral aspect of the metatarsus (great metatarsal artery). Because of the size of these vessels, ligation of the severed ends, if they can be identified, is considered the ideal approach. Anastomosis of a lacerated great metatarsal artery has been performed by one of the authors (GMB) but is probably unnecessary in most cases.

Summary

Most injuries, including those with significant tissue loss, can be successfully managed with proper therapy. With delayed healing, potential causes for the delay, such as sequestra, foreign bodies, and excessive motion, should be determined and treated to permit complete wound resolution. Horses have the innate ability to heal rapidly; however, minor injuries can quickly turn into complicated wounds, given the severity of the inciting trauma and the less than ideal environment in which the horses are housed. Wound management must focus on a combination of timely surgical and medical intervention to ensure the best potential outcome.

References

[1] Baxter GM. Wound management. In: White NA, Moore JN, editors. Current techniques in equine surgery and lameness. 2nd edition. Philadelphia: WB Saunders; 1998. p. 72–80.
[2] Foland JW, Trotter GW, Stashak TS, et al. Traumatic injuries involving tendons of the distal limbs in horses: a retrospective study of 55 cases. Equine Vet J 1991;23(6):422–5.
[3] Belknap JK, Baxter GM, Nickels FA. Extensor tendon laceration in horses: 50 cases (1982–1988). J Am Vet Med Assoc 1993;203(3):428–31.
[4] Bertone AL. Tendon lacerations. Vet Clin N Am Equine Pract 1995;11(2):293–314.
[5] Clem MF, Debowes RM, Yovich JV, et al. Osseous sequestration in horses, a review of 68 cases. Vet Surg 1988;11:2–5.
[6] Clem MF, Debowes RM, Yovich JV, et al. Osseous sequestration in horses. Compend Contin Educ Pract Vet 1987;9:1219–24.
[7] Moens Y, Verschooten F, DeMoor A, et al. Bone sequestration as a consequence of limb wounds in the horse. Vet Radiol 1980;21:40–4.
[8] Gift LJ, Debowes RM. Wounds associated with osseous sequestration and penetrating foreign bodies. Vet Clin N Am Equine Pract 1989;5(3):659–708.

[9] Booth LC, Feeney DA. Superficial osteitis and sequestrum formation as a result of skin avulsion in the horse. Vet Surg 1982;11:2–8.
[10] Cartee RE, Rumph PF. Ultrasonographic detection of fistulous tracts and foreign objects in muscles of horses. J Am Vet Med Assoc 1984;184:1127–32.
[11] Kahn DS, Pritzker KPH. The pathophysiology of bone infection. Clin Orthop 1973;96:12–9.
[12] Firth EC. Bone sequestration in horses and cattle. Aust Vet J 1987;64:65–9.
[13] Lewis RE, Heinze CD. Bone sequestration in the horse: diagnosis, radiography, and treatment. Proc Am Assoc Equine Pract 1970;16:161–70.
[14] Holcombe SJ, Laverty S. Thoracic trauma. In: Auer JA, Stick JA, editors. Equine surgery. 2nd edition. Philadelphia: WB Saunders; 1999. p. 382–5.
[15] Stone WC, Trostle SS, Gerros TC. Use of a primary muscle pedicle flap to repair a caudal thoracic wound in a horse. J Am Vet Med Assoc 1994;205(6):828–30.
[16] Lavoie JP, Pascoe JP, Ducharme N, et al. Penetrating wounds of the thorax in 15 horses. Equine Vet J 1996;28:220–4.
[17] Kawcak CE, Stashak TS. Predisposing factors, diagnosis and management of large abdominal wall defects in horses and cattle. J Am Vet Med Assoc 1995;206(5):607–11.

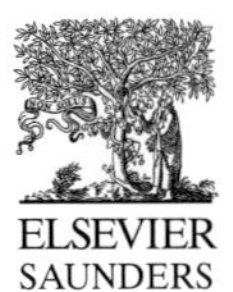

ELSEVIER
SAUNDERS

Vet Clin Equine 21 (2005) 231–239

VETERINARY
CLINICS
Equine Practice

Index

Note: Page numbers of article titles are in **boldface** type.

doi:10.1016/S0749-0739(05)00015-5

K

L

M

N

O

P

Changing Your Address?

Make sure your subscription changes too! When you notify us of your new address, you can help make our job easier by including an exact copy of your Clinics label number with your old address (see illustration below.) This number identifies you to our computer system and will speed the processing of your address change. Please be sure this label number accompanies your old address and your corrected address—you can send an old Clinics label with your number on it or just copy it exactly and send it to the address listed below.

We appreciate your help in our attempt to give you continuous coverage. Thank you.

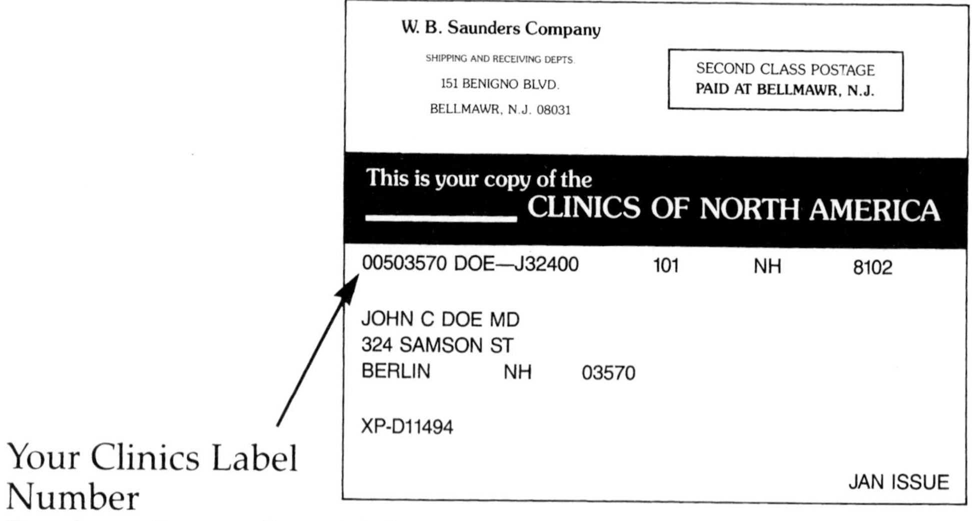

Copy it exactly or send your label along with your address to:
W.B. Saunders Company, Customer Service
Orlando, FL 32887-4800
Call Toll Free 1-800-654-2452

Please allow four to six weeks for delivery of new subscriptions and for processing address changes.